Facial Plastic Surgery Procedures in the Non-Caucasian Population

Editor

YONG JU JANG

FACIAL PLASTIC SURGERY CLINICS OF NORTH AMERICA

www.facialplastic.theclinics.com

Consulting Editor
J. REGAN THOMAS

November 2021 • Volume 29 • Number 4

ELSEVIER

1600 John F. Kennedy Boulevard • Suite 1800 • Philadelphia, Pennsylvania, 19103-2899

http://www.theclinics.com

FACIAL PLASTIC SURGERY CLINICS OF NORTH AMERICA Volume 29, Number 4
November 2021 ISSN 1064-7406, ISBN-13: 978-0-323-79888-4

Editor: Stacy Eastman
Developmental Editor: Ann Gielou M. Posedio

Facial Plastic Surgery Clinics of North America (ISSN 1064-7406) is published quarterly by Elsevier Inc., 360 Park Avenue South, New York, NY 10010-1710. Months of issue are February, May, August, and November. Business and Editorial Offices: 1600 John F. Kennedy Blvd., Suite 1800, Philadelphia, PA 19103-2899. Periodicals postage paid at New York, NY, and additional mailing offices. Subscription prices are $412.00 per year (US individuals), $895.00 per year (US institutions), $459.00 per year (Canadian individuals), $944.00 per year (Canadian institutions), $546.00 per year (foreign individuals), $944.00 per year (foreign institutions), $100.00 per year (US students), $100.00 per year (Canadian students), and $255.00 per year (foreign students). Foreign air speed delivery is included in all *Clinics* subscription prices. All prices are subject to change without notice. POSTMASTER: Send address changes to *Facial Plastic Surgery Clinics*, Elsevier Health Sciences Division, Subscription Customer Service, 3251 Riverport Lane, Maryland Heights, MO 63043. **Customer service: 1-800-654-2452 (US and Canada); 1-314-447-8871 (outside US and Canada); Fax: 314-447-8029; E-mail: journalscustomerservice-usa@elsevier.com (for print support); journalsonlinesupport-usa@elsevier.com (for online support).**

Reprints. For copies of 100 or more of articles in this publication, please contact the Commercial Reprints Department, Elsevier Inc., 360 Park Avenue South, New York, NY 10010-1710. Tel.: 212-633-3874; Fax: 212-633-3820; E-mail: reprints@elsevier.com.

Facial Plastic Surgery Clinics of North America is covered in *MEDLINE/PubMed* (*Index Medicus*).

Contributors

CONSULTING EDITOR

J. REGAN THOMAS, MD
Professor, Facial Plastic and Reconstructive Surgery, Department of Otolaryngology–Head and Neck Surgery, Northwestern University Feinberg School of Medicine, Chicago, Illinois, USA

EDITOR

YONG JU JANG, MD, PhD
Professor and Department Chair, Department of Otolaryngology, Asan Medical Center, University of Ulsan College of Medicine, Seoul, Korea

AUTHORS

KYOUNG HWA BAE, MD
Department of Oculoplasty, Kim's Eye Hospital, Seoul, Korea, Seoul, Republic of Korea

JI SUN BAEK, MD
Department of Oculoplasty, Kim's Eye Hospital, Seoul, Korea, Seoul, Republic of Korea

YUN HEE CHOI, MD
Co-director of Aone Plastic Surgery, Board Certified Anesthesiologist, Yongin-si, Gyeonggi-do, Republic of Korea

JAE WOO JANG, MD, PhD
Department of Oculoplasty, Kim's Eye Hospital, Seoul, Korea, Seoul, Republic of Korea

YONG JU JANG, MD, PhD
Professor, Department of Otolaryngology, Asan Medical Center, University of Ulsan College of Medicine, Seoul, Korea

HAK-SOO KIM, MD
Labom Plastic Surgery Clinic, Seoul, Korea

IN-SANG KIM, MD
Labom Plastic Surgery Clinic, Seoul, Korea

YOON-JI KIM, DDS, MS, PhD
Assistant Professor, Department of Orthodontics, Asan Medical Center, College of Medicine, University of Ulsan, Seoul, Republic of Korea.

TAEK KEUN KWON, MD, PhD
Director of Aone Plastic Surgery, Board Certified Plastic Surgeon, Yongin-si, Gyeonggi-do, Republic of Korea

BU-KYU LEE, DDS, MS, PhD
Professor, Department of Oral and Maxillofacial Surgery, Asan Medical Center, College of Medicine, University of Ulsan, Seoul, Republic of Korea

HAN-TSUNG LIAO, MD, PhD
Professor, Division of Trauma Plastic Surgery, Department of Plastic and Reconstructive Surgery, Craniofacial Research Center, Chang Gung Memorial Hospital, College of Medicine, Chang Gung University, Taoyuan, Taiwan

HYUN MOON, MD
Department of Otolaryngology, Asan Medical Center, University of Ulsan College of Medicine, Seoul, Korea

SANGHOON PARK, MD, PhD
Chief, Department of Facial Bone Surgery, ID Hospital, Seoul, South Korea

STEPHEN S. PARK, MD
Department of Otolaryngology–Head and Neck Surgery, University of Virginia, Charlottesville, Virginia, USA

JOSE A. PATROCINIO, MD, PhD
Professor Emeritus, Department of Otolaryngology, Medical School, Federal University of Uberlandia, Uberlandia, Minas Gerais, Brazil

LUCAS G. PATROCINIO, MD, PhD
Chair, Department of Otolaryngology, Medical School, Federal University of Uberlandia, Uberlandia, Minas Gerais, Brazil

TOMAS G. PATROCINIO, MD, PhD
Private Practice, OTOFACE, Uberlandia Medical Center, Uberlandia, Minas Gerais, Brazil

HYUNG MIN SONG, MD, MS
Drsong4u Aesthetic Plastic Surgery Clinic, Gangnam-gu, Seoul, Korea

JENICA SU-ERN YONG, MBBS
Department of Otolaryngology–Head and Neck Surgery, KK Women's and Children's Hospital, Singapore

MAN-KOON SUH, MD
JW Plastic Surgery Center, Seoul, Korea

KHANH NGOC TRAN, MBBS, FRACS
Drsong4u Aesthetic Plastic Surgery Clinic, Gangnam-gu, Seoul, Korea

Contents

Foreword: Facial Plastic Surgery Procedures in the Non-Caucasian Population ix

J. Regan Thomas

Preface: Facial Plastic Surgery for the Non-Caucasian Population xi

Yong Ju Jang

Asian Facelift 471

Taek Keun Kwon and Yun Hee Choi

The Asian facelift requires an adaptation of current techniques to achieve a desired aesthetic outcome. Cultural differences and differences in anthropomorphologic features alter a patient's vision of beauty and youthfulness. Rejuvenation of the aging Asian face mandates a set of strategies, including understanding cultural aspects of Asian patients, anatomy of Asian patients, and appropriate techniques based on these cultural and anatomic considerations. For stable application and results, the surgeon must understand surgical facial anatomy. If performed properly, facelifts can improve facial balance and can yield aesthetically more appealing results. The deep plane facelift technique presented is well suited for Asian patients.

Forehead Lift for Asians 487

In-Sang Kim and Hak-Soo Kim

Asians have anatomic and clinical characteristics to be considered before forehead lift. Because of the anatomic characteristics of Asians, for the better outcomes of blepharoplasty or augmentation rhinoplasty, forehead lift as a combined surgery must be considered beforehand. Forehead lift is frequently indicated in young Asian patients. Endoscopic browlift without visible scar is favored for patients, and it can be done in a modified multiplane fashion for better outcomes in patients with thick and redundant skin. There are rare but severe complications of endoscopic forehead lift, such as motor nerve paresis and diplopia, although they are temporary in most cases.

Lower Eyelid and Midface Rejuvenation: Suborbicularis Oculi Fat Lift 497

Han-Tsung Liao

The lower eyelids and midface are considered to be a contiguous aesthetic unit although they are different anatomic structures. Through in-depth understanding of complex anatomy and aging theory and appropriate surgical strategies according to the type of aging, surgical outcome of aging lower eyelid/midface can be more and more predictable. This article discusses the characteristics and theories of aging and 5 types of lower eyelid/middle face aging based on 4 key factors, namely, protruding fat in the orbital, excess skin on the lower eyelid, sagging midface and soft tissue deflation. Various combinations of surgical strategies are adopted accordingly.

Incisional Blepharoplasty for the Asian Eye 511

Hyung Min Song and Khanh Ngoc Tran

The goal of Asian blepharoplasty is to create a lid crease configuration that resembles the natural-appearing crease found in other Asians. Because the Asian upper eyelid contains more prominent preseptal fat resulting in greater lid fullness, soft tissue work in blepharoplasty of the Asian eye is even more diverse and essential than that of whites in order for there to be the sustainability of the eyelid crease. Hence, Asian blepharoplasty should be performed specifically following the orbital anatomy of Asians. This article details the incisional method of blepharoplasty to create natural-appearing creases for Asians with single eyelids.

Nonincisional Blepharoplasty for Asians 523

Kyoung Hwa Bae, Ji Sun Baek, and Jae Woo Jang

Various nonincisional techniques for double eyelid surgery have been introduced in the past. They are simple, noninvasive, and efficient techniques to create a double eyelid. The authors prefer the full-thickness single continuous method using the 7-0 nylon, round long needle. Appropriate choice of the patients and surgical method results in a natural, esthetically pleasing eyelid and decreases the loss of eyelid crease.

Cosmetic Bone-Contouring Surgery for Asians 533

Sanghoon Park

The major needs for cosmetic facial bone surgery come from anatomic differences in facial shape and in personal preference. Especially when consulting patients with different national or ethnic backgrounds, careful attention should be paid during consultation for the ideal or desirable facial shape that they have in mind. Patients generally seek a slim and smooth-contoured face. Surgery of the cosmetic facial bone has developed from surgical experiences in facial bone trauma and congenital anomalies. A limited approach is recommended for satisfactory aesthetic outcome. Surgeons should understand the basic procedures of L-shaped osteotomy of the zygoma and intraoral mandible reduction.

Recent Trends in Orthognathic Surgery in Asia 549

Yoon-Ji Kim and Bu-Kyu Lee

Anatomy and standards of beauty are different between Asians and Westerners. Unlike Westerners, Asians have a wide and prominent jaw shape but prefer a slim and soft face shape. To achieve this goal, maxillary setback and/or posterior impaction surgeries are popular among upper jaw surgery, and various adjuvant surgeries are performed simultaneously on the mandible to obtain the so-called oval shape or V-line face. In addition, according to the development of virtual surgery software and orthodontic treatment techniques, the surgery-first approach is now accepted as a reliable option for orthognathic surgery if it is indicated.

Special Considerations in Facial Reconstruction in the Non-White Patient 567

Jenica Su-ern Yong and Stephen S. Park

The principles of facial reconstruction are well established and some unique modifications apply to the non-White population. Anatomic and physiologic distinctions to this group give rise to alterations in design and surgical planning. Different ethnic groups have different skin anatomy and physiology and that should be taken into consideration. Healing differs among the different ethnic groups, affecting the final result regardless of method chosen. Variations in aesthetic units can lead to different flap selection and design. These should be considered for this population to maximize aesthetic outcomes and patient satisfaction.

Approach for Rhinoplasty in African Descendants **575**

Lucas G. Patrocinio, Tomas G. Patrocinio, and Jose A. Patrocinio

The main objectives of rhinoplasty in African descendants are to improve the definition and projection of the nasal tip, augment the dorsum, and reduce the alar base. Open rhinoplasty using costal cartilage graft, with lateral crural tensioning and septal extension graft associated with en bloc dorsal augmentation is the workhorse. Cartilage resections should be minimal. Oral isotretinoin and triamcinolone injection may improve tip definition. Surgical success ultimately depends on the ability of the surgeon to accurately identify the anatomic variables and reconcile these anatomic realities with the patient's aesthetic expectations and his or her sense of ethnic identity.

Cosmetic Augmentation Rhinoplasty for East Asians **589**

Man-Koon SUH

Symmetric pocket formation and meticulous implant carving are the most critical parts of nasal dorsal augmentation using implants. Innovative three-dimensional printed nasal implants can exactly fit the nasal dorsal contour, decreasing the chance of deviation and malpositioning. Vertically oriented folded dermal graft technique can avoid the high resorption rate of conventional dermofat grafts. Multilayered costal cartilage graft technique for dorsal augmentation can minimize warping and difficulty in the graft carving. Derotation graft allows supple and movable nasal tip while enabling enough tip lengthening, even if the septal extension graft is the most commonly performed procedure for short nose correction.

Special Consideration in Rhinoplasty for Deformed Nose of East Asians **611**

Yong Ju Jang and Hyun Moon

Typical Asian deformed nose has many different types: concave nasal dorsum, low nasal dorsum, wide nasal dorsum, deviated nose, convex nasal dorsum, saddle nose, short-nose deformity, and deformities involving irreversible damage of skin/soft tissue envelope are the most representative ones. The key concept in Asian rhinoplasty is augmentation in all different forms of nasal deformities. Augmentation of the nose consists of framework, tip, and dorsal augmentation. Septal extension grafting and tip grafting are 2 maneuvers with profound importance in augmentation of lower two-thirds of the Asian nose. Dorsal augmentation is central concept in beautifying all different types of deformed noses, even the hump nose.

FACIAL PLASTIC SURGERY CLINICS OF NORTH AMERICA

FORTHCOMING ISSUES

February 2022
Modern Approaches to Facial and Athletic Injuries
J. David Kriet and Clinton D. Humphrey, *Editors*

May 2022
Facial and Nasal Anatomy
Sebastian Cotofana, *Editor*

August 2022
Injectables and Nonsurgical Rejuvenation
Jessyka G. Lighthall, *Editor*

RECENT ISSUES

August 2021
Facial Paralysis
Travis T. Tollefson and Jon-Paul Pepper, *Editors*

May 2021
Oculoplastic Surgery
John B. Holds and Guy G. Massry, *Editors*

February 2021
Preservation Rhinoplasty
Sam P. Most, *Editor*

Foreword

Facial Plastic Surgery Procedures in the Non-Caucasian Population

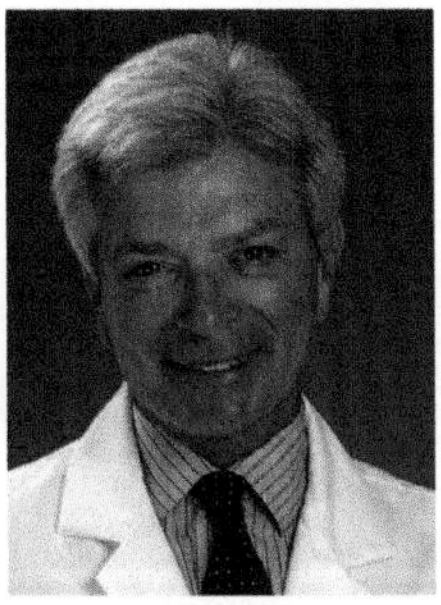

J. Regan Thomas, MD
Consulting Editor

Most of the literature and the instructional information publications regarding facial plastic surgery procedures has historically been from North American or European sources. Because of that history, much of the focus and development of clinical surgical information and facial plastic procedures has been described utilizing a Caucasian patient base. However, there has been tremendous growth and expansion internationally in the interest in facial plastic procedures, and accordingly, the ethnic patient population base has greatly expanded. This broadening of interest of the patient populations has stimulated the appropriate growth of attention and clinical expertise to successfully treating a wide and inclusive group of patient candidates.

All races and ethnicities share a desire for facial attractiveness and aesthetic appearance. There are certain ethnic differences in facial anatomy, and the surgical and treatment goals must recognize and accommodate those desired outcomes. This *Facial Plastic Surgery Clinics of North America* issue has incorporated the insights and guidance of guest editor, Yong Ju Jang, MD, PhD, to develop a clinically insightful discussion and technically applicable issue covering non-Caucasian patient requirements and useful procedures.

Dr Yong Ju Jang has assembled a group of expert authors to discuss their successful techniques of a variety of facial plastic surgery procedures. This key group of procedures is discussed by the contributing authors and accordingly will be a useful reference for expertly treating an ethnically wide range of patients. All the contributing authors are well-recognized experts in the procedures that they are discussing. Their expertise and experience provides through this issue a clinically useful resource for our readership to use in their own clinical environments.

Facial Plastic Surgery Clinics of North America continues to provide genuine insight into the various aspects of the multiple components included in the realm of facial plastic surgery. Our readership will continue to be able to assemble the practical clinical reference materials to benefit their practices and their patient populations through our ongoing coverage and descriptions such as found in this issue.

J. Regan Thomas, MD
Facial Plastic and Reconstructive Surgery
Department of Otolaryngology–
Head and Neck Surgery
Northwestern University School of Medicine
60 East Delaware Place
Chicago, IL 60611, USA

E-mail address:
regan.thomas@nm.org

Facial Plast Surg Clin N Am 29 (2021) ix
https://doi.org/10.1016/j.fsc.2021.08.012
1064-7406/21/© 2021 Published by Elsevier Inc.

Preface
Facial Plastic Surgery for the Non-Caucasian Population

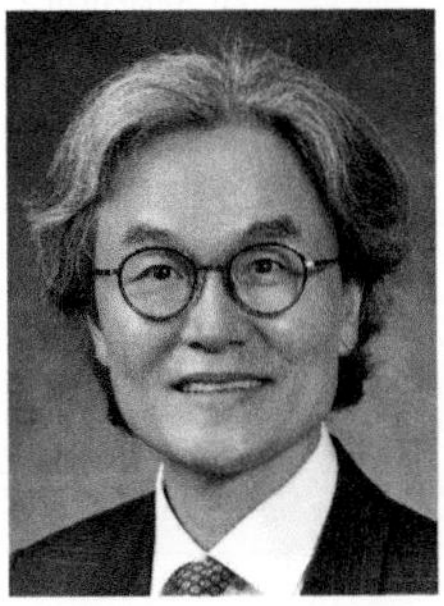

Yong Ju Jang, MD, PhD
Editor

Unlike other surgery aimed at removing tumor or inflammation, facial plastic surgery is unique in that the anatomic characteristics of the patients largely determine the very success of the surgical outcome. The ultimate goal of facial plastic surgery is changing the anatomic structure of the face in ways favored by the subjects or general population. General anatomic differences between ethnicities have tremendous importance in planning and executing various facial plastic surgery procedures.

Undeniably, most contemporary plastic surgery procedures have been pioneered, developed, and refined by numerous giants in the field, mostly North American or European. Furthermore, ethnic Caucasians from North America and Europe have been the most represented in terms of patient volume. Hence, the basic surgical techniques and nuances, and scientific knowledge pertaining to facial plastic surgery have been developed predominantly for Caucasian populations.

Seeking facial beauty and normalcy is a universal human desire. In this era of globalization, increased demand for facial plastic surgery is a phenomenon sweeping all ethnicities of all countries.

Certainly, people from different ethnic backgrounds have different facial anatomies. Accounting for these differences requires particular attention and study of each. Unfortunately, there is a relative lack of available literature specific to the non-Caucasian population. In that regard, publishing a special issue dedicated to the non-Caucasian population is a truly timely and necessary undertaking.

It was an honor to edit this special issue. As editor, I followed these principles: the content should be comprehensive; the authors should be experts who are keen to teach and have unique areas of interest; and the content should be most up-to-date. With those considerations in mind, I invited 11 facial plastic surgeons from Korea, Taiwan, Brazil, and the United States. Thankfully, all the invited authors willingly agreed to contribute and put in phenomenal effort for their articles. The issue covers facial rejuvenation, blepharoplasty, facial reconstruction, facial bone contouring surgery, and rhinoplasty. All articles provide explicit features that can only be created by masters of their fields. I believe that this special issue will serve as a useful reference not only for non-Caucasian patients but also for Caucasian patients who have similar anatomic features with other ethnicities.

Facial Plast Surg Clin N Am 29 (2021) xi–xii
https://doi.org/10.1016/j.fsc.2021.06.011

I am happy to highlight that this issue features cosmetic bone contouring surgery, a popular and important method of facial cosmetic surgery particularly in East Asia, which is a rare a practice in the other part of the world. One possible shortcoming I wish to remedy in the future is the heavy focus on facial plastic surgery procedures for East Asians, which can be justified to some degree considering a significant anatomic and cultural difference between the East Asians and other ethnicities. I hope this collective endeavor of the contributing authors can help the readers get a better understanding of the facial plastic surgery for non-Caucasians, leading to better surgical outcomes and better patient care.

Yong Ju Jang, MD, PhD
Department of Otolaryngology
Asan Medical Center, University of Ulsan College of Medicine
88, Olympic-ro 43-gil
Songpa-gu, Seoul 05505
South Korea

E-mail address:
3712yjang@gmail.com

Asian Facelift

Taek Keun Kwon, MD, PhD*, Yun Hee Choi, MD

KEYWORDS

- Asian facelift • Deep plane • Facial anatomy • Retaining ligaments

KEY POINTS

- Specific cultural and anthropomorphologic differences require a different approach to restore facial youthfulness and attractiveness.
- Knowledge of anatomic structures of the face and neck is essential to understanding surgical procedures and to achieving better results.
- The deep plane facelift technique presented in this article is well suited for face and neck rejuvenation of Asian patients.

Aging signs appear on the face and neck due to the natural aging process, facial expressions in daily life, effects of gravity, and exposure to the sun. As people get older, the appearance and shape of the face are altered, leading to a sagging appearance of the cheeks, excess skin along the jawline and prominent jowls, sagging skin and excess fat in the neck, and decreased skin elasticity and texture. Therefore, a proper rejuvenation procedure can be chosen based on the causes.

Facelift surgery rejuvenates the middle and lower thirds of the face and upper neck. The procedure is individualized to a patient's needs, and the plastic surgeon tailors techniques accordingly. Various techniques have been introduced for facelifts and neck lifts, and they are differentiated and compared by their different dissection planes. Modern facelift surgery was initiated by Skoog,[1] who elevated a cervicofacial flap deep to the platysma and the superficial fascia of the face. Anatomic descriptions of the superficial musculoaponeurotic system (SMAS),[2] retaining ligaments, and danger zones further enhanced understanding of the intricacies of facial anatomy. The current classification of facelift categories includes the subcutaneous lift, SMAS manipulation, deep plane and composite lift,[3,4] short scar and minimal invasive technique, and any combination of these. The 2 most common current facelift techniques are the deep plane rhytidectomy and SMAS manipulation. There are a limited number of studies objectively comparing the 2 techniques.

The deep plane facelift utilizes a plane of dissection below the SMAS and platysma of the face and neck, allowing for the direct lysis of key facial retaining ligaments and the mobilization of superficial soft tissue.[3,4] This is important to support the thicker and heavier tissues of the Asian face to create a more rejuvenated appearance and one that will last longer. The deep plane approach also allows access to the buccal fat pads (BFPs) of the cheeks, which are larger in the Asian face, so that they can be reduced.

The Asian face can be quite different from the white face in many respects. Some of the unique characteristics of the Asian face, versus those of white individuals, to consider during an Asian facelift include a wider and flatter face; more prominent malar bone and mandibular angle[5,6]; weaker bone structure, especially in the lower region of the face; thicker and heavier soft tissues that cause more sagging in the lower face; and more prominent, droopy BFPs. Therefore, the chief problem is tissue drooping while having fewer wrinkles on their face. Due to their relatively thick skin, the weight of their tissue is considerably more than in other groups, and performing facelift surgery is more difficult.

Many Western plastic surgeons emphasize the importance of midcheek lifts. Vertical vector

18-6, Ihyeon-RO 29BEON-GIL, Giheung-gu, Yongin-si, Gyeonggi-do, Republic of Korea
* Corresponding author.
E-mail address: aone8101@naver.com

Facial Plast Surg Clin N Am 29 (2021) 471–486
https://doi.org/10.1016/j.fsc.2021.06.001

deep plane rhytidectomy provides significant long-term augmentation of volume in the midface. For several reasons, the midcheek lift in Asians is less important than for whites. Lifted midcheek tissue tends to come back down because it is difficult to support the thicker and heavier skin of Asians using only suture suspensions. During recovery, patients complain that their cheekbones appear more prominent and swelling lasts longer because of the elevated thick tissue. Lambros[7] described that changes in the volume of cheek fat, either loss or gain, rather than ptosis account for an aged appearance. The craniofacial skeleton undergoes many changes as individuals mature. Retrusion of the lower maxilla has been observed in older patients compared with younger cohorts. Therefore, in Asians, the midcheek region should be approached in a different way from that in whites. If a midcheek lift is required, volume augmentation in this region should be considered rather than a vertical lift. Many surgeons started adopting fat injection as part of their strategy to replace lost volume. Fat grafting can be used successfully to offset the apparent width of the Asian face by placing fat along the anterior jawline and upper cheek to make the lower cheek and outer jawline appear less heavy.

ANATOMY

Knowledge of anatomic structures of the face and neck is essential to understanding surgical procedures, achieving better results, and avoiding injury to important structures, including sensory and motor nerves. The soft tissues of the face are arranged concentrically into 5 basic layers that are bound together by a system of facial retaining ligaments[8]: (1) the skin; (2) subcutaneous fat; (3) SMAS; (4) loose areolar tissue that includes retaining ligaments, space, and deep facial fat; and (5) periosteum and deep fascia. The subcutaneous layer has different thicknesses based on the location and patient. The third layer is the SMAS layer, and all of the facial muscle motor nerves are deep to this plane. Layer 4 is the layer that undergoes the most change, consisting of alternating spaces and ligaments.

Superficial Musculoaponeurotic System

The SMAS is a well-defined portion of the superficial facial fascia that divides the deep and superficial adipose tissue of the face and forms a continuous sheath through the face and neck, and its thickness varies by patient and region of the face.[2] The fibromuscular layer of the SMAS integrates with the superficial temporal fascia and frontalis muscle superiorly and with the platysma muscle inferiorly (**Fig. 1**A). The SMAS acts as a central tendon for the coordinated muscular contraction of the face and provides the functional role of movement for expression. The SMAS plays a vital role in the facelift procedure, and surgical maneuvering and tightening of the SMAS allow for facial rejuvenation (see **Fig. 1**B).

Retaining Ligament

The retaining ligaments of the face are important in understanding concepts of facial aging and rejuvenation. These are fibrous attachments that fix the superficial layers of the face to the underlying deeper tissues to support the facial soft tissue in their normal anatomic position, thereby resisting gravitational change. Retaining ligaments of the face serve a dual purpose as they relate to facelift surgery. The ligaments act as the entryway to the midface and also serve a sentinel role with regard to peripheral facial nerve branches.[9]

Furnas was the first to describe the anatomy of the retaining ligaments of the face. Their superficial extensions form subcutaneous septa that separate facial fat compartments. Their main significance relates to their surgical release in order to achieve the desired aesthetic outcome. When performing facial aesthetic surgery, plastic surgeons should choose a plane of dissection, release the appropriate ligaments depending on the desired aesthetic goals, and avoid nerve injury by using the ligaments as anatomic landmarks.

Descriptions of the retaining ligaments are variable in the literature, and different interpretations of anatomy, several classifications, locations, and nomenclature systems have been proposed.[10] Despite the variation in published descriptions, the zygomatic retaining ligament (ZRL) occupies a predictable anatomic location given its relationship to the body and arch of the zygoma (**Fig. 3**A). Furnas described the zygomatic ligaments as stout fibers that originate at or near the inferior border of the anterior zygomatic arch, behind the insertion of the zygomaticus minor muscle, and insert in the skin serving as an anchoring point. In Mendelson and colleagues'[8] description, zygomatic ligaments start just lateral to the zygomaticus major muscle, where they identified the location of the strongest ligament, and continue medially across the origins of the zygomaticus major and minor and levator labii superioris. Alghoul and colleagues[9] showed the ZRLs originating along the entire length of the zygomatic arch extending onto the malar body. During the release of the major zygomatic ligaments, the zygomatic and buccal rami of the facial nerve are found caudal to the zygomatic

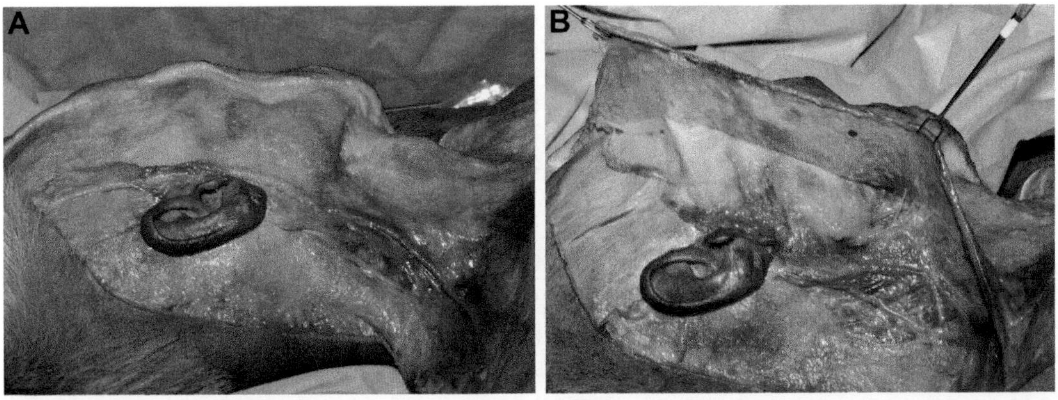

Fig. 1. The SMAS integrates with the superficial temporal fascia and frontalis muscle superiorly and with the platysma muscle inferiorly (*A, B*).

ligaments, because it is here that these nerve branches pass from deep fascia to an immediate sub-SMAS plane.

The masseteric retaining ligament (MRL), on the other hand, is less predictable and varied in location given that they are condensations of the deep fascia.[10] The mean vertical distance between the main ZRL and upper MRL was 11 mm[9] (**Fig. 2**). The MRL arises from the masseteric fascia over the masseter muscle. Their relationship to the muscle is controversial. Although some anatomic studies have shown the ligaments arising along the anterior border of the masseter, others have shown them to arise 1 cm to 2 cm posterior to the anterior border and even from the middle portion of the muscle.[10] The MRL is an important landmark for the zygomatic and buccal facial branches (see **Fig. 3**B).

The mandibular osteocutaneous ligaments usually is a very stout band or bands that originate from the periosteum of the mandible inferior to the mental foramen at approximately the lateral border of the origin of the depressor anguli oris muscle (**Fig. 4**).[11] These ligaments fix this muscle and its investing fascia and continue to the dermis by a condensation of fibrous septae in the superficial fat layer. The terminal branch always is cranial to this ligament, with a distance of approximately 10 mm.

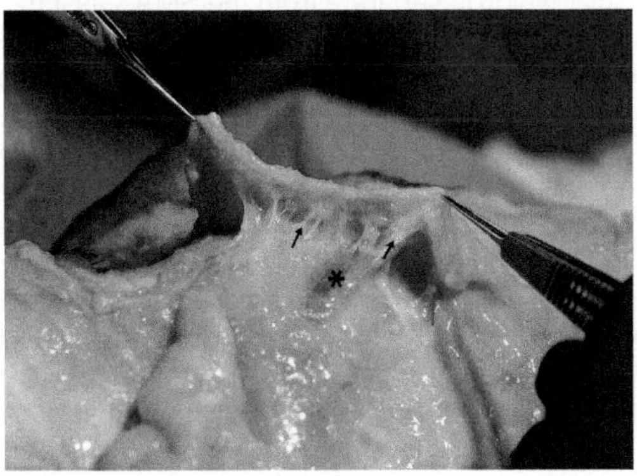

Fig. 2. Cadaver dissection of the right malar area. The zygomatic cutaneous retaining ligament is marked with the black arrow. Zygomaticus major (*) and upper masseteric ligament (*red arrow*).

Buccal Fat Pad

The BFP that Bichat described in 1802 is an important structure that contributes to cheek and facial contour. The BFP consists of a main body and 4 extensions: buccal, pterygoid, superficial, and deep temporal. The buccal extension is the most superficial segment of the fat pad and imparts fullness to the cheek (**Fig. 5**). More than half of the BFP mass is the body and the buccal extension together. The ptotic lower portion of the buccal extension may contribute to jowl formation. The BFP is an important anatomic structure in relation to the masticatory muscle, facial nerve, and parotid duct. The zygomatic and buccal branches of the facial nerve lie superficial to the buccal extension. The parotid duct passes through the entire lateral surface of the BFP or penetrates it.

Jowls

The jowls and labiomandibular folds are classic signs of aging. These generally are areas of concern for the appearance of many men and women as they age. Correction of the jowls and labiomental folds are 2 of the most essential elements for a successful facelift. The jowl is the combination of the fat compartment in the lower face sliding downwards and weakening of the facial ligaments, including mandibular ligament and septum, causing a loss of definition in the jawline, chin, and neck area (**Fig. 6**).

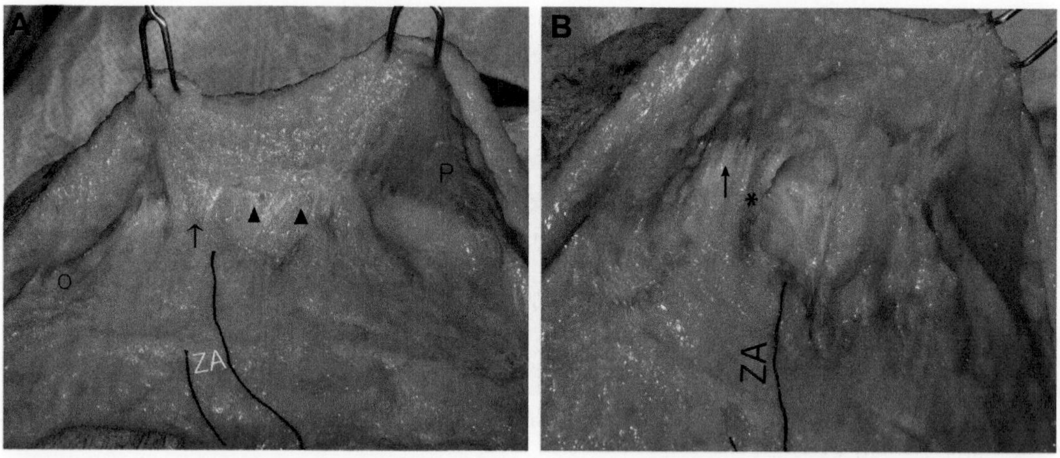

Fig. 3. Cadaver dissection of the right cheek. (*A*) Arrows point to the location of the zygomatic ligament and arrowheads point to the masseteric ligament. (*B*) After release of the zygomatic and masseteric ligaments, the zygomatic and buccal rami of the facial nerve are found. Platysma (P), orbicularis oculi (O), and zygomatic arch (ZA).

Facial Nerve

The facial nerve has a complex pattern, and there is considerable variability among patients. The incidence of injury to the facial nerve during a standard rhytidectomy has been reported in 2% of patients. All terminal branches of the facial nerve run below the SMAS. The protection provided by the SMAS is variable, and the temporal branches are the least protected. The course of the temporal branch has been described in detail in the literature. One of the most widely used clinical estimates for the course of frontotemporal branch of the facial nerve is the Pitanguy line, defined as a line drawn from a point 0.5 cm inferior to the tragus to a point 1.5 cm superior and lateral to the eyebrow. The Pitanguy line is not accurate to estimate the course and depth of the frontal branch, but it is simple to understand the course of the frontal branch and is close to the anterior limit of the danger zone.

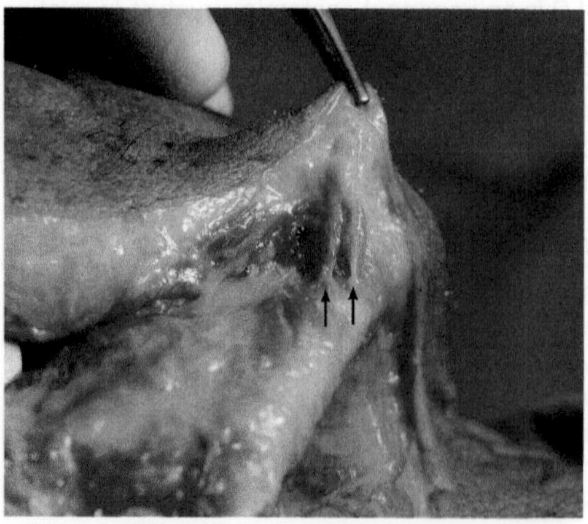

Fig. 4. The arrows indicate the mandibular ligament. The mandibular ligament is an osteocutaneous ligament that arises from the anterior third of the mandible and inserts directly into the dermis.

Two plastic surgeons' facial dissections demonstrated that the frontal branch travels within the innominate fascia, a fibrofatty layer deep to the SMAS, as it crosses the zygomatic arch into the temporal region. Agarwal and colleagues[12] showed that the frontal branches are located consistently within the innominate fascia, a fibrofatty layer deep to the SMAS and superficial temporal fascia (**Fig. 7**). Trussler and colleagues[13] showed that the frontal branch is protected by a deep layer of the parotid temporal fascia, which is separate from the SMAS as it traverses the zygomatic arch. Division of the SMAS above the arch in a high-SMAS facelift is safe when using the technique described in that study.

The zygomatic and buccal branches emerge from the parotid gland and run over the masseter muscle under the parotid-masseteric fascia (**Fig. 8**.). The exact point where they pierce the deep fascia is variable but is in the vicinity of the anterior border of the masseter. The ZRL and MRL can aid in identification of these nerve branches. The upper zygomatic subbranch passes between the major zygomatic cutaneous ligament and upper masseteric cutaneous ligament, deep to the deep fascia and under the upper third of the zygomaticus major muscle. The area 1 cm below the zygomaticus major muscle,

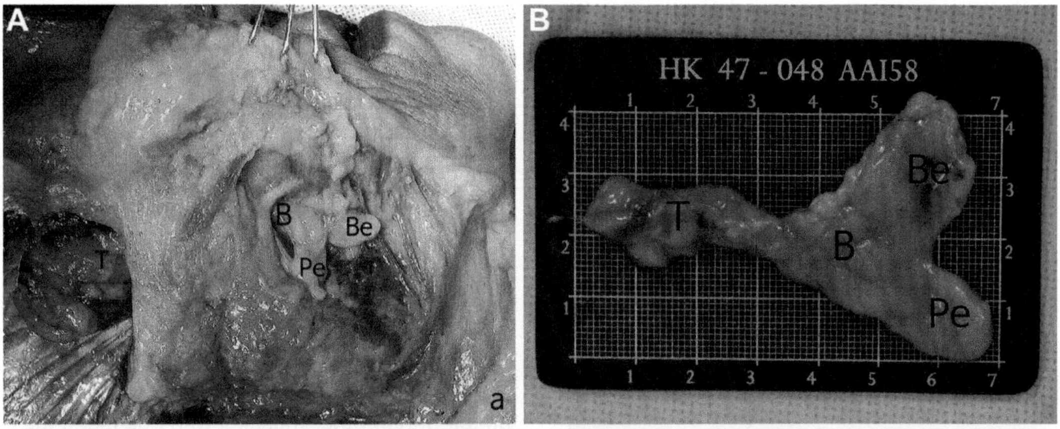

Fig. 5. Cadaver dissection of the buccal fat. (*A*) The body and 3 extensions of the buccal fat. (*B*) Removed buccal fat from the masticatory space. Body (B), buccal extension (Be), pterygoid extension (Pe), and temporal extension (T).

therefore, has been labeled a "sub-SMAS danger zone."[9] The lower zygomatic subbranch runs immediately inferior to the upper MRL in a more superficial plane than the upper branch.[8,10,11] The buccal branch crosses through the lower masseteric ligament. The buccal ramus is thought to be the most commonly injured facial nerve branch during facelift surgery, but the clinical effect seldom is noted owing to rich arborizations and abundant interconnections.

The cervical branch exits the parotid gland and passes behind the angle of the mandible anteroinferiorly from its emergence at the caudal end of the parotid, coursing under the platysma as it innervates the muscle (**Fig. 9**). Disruption of this nerve can lead to lip depressor dysfunction, which often is confused with injury to the marginal mandibular nerve with pseudoparalysis.

The marginal mandibular branch (MMB) runs toward the mandibular angle in a subplatysmal plane before turning across the body of the mandible. The nerve runs deep to the platysma and superficial to the facial vessels throughout its course to supply the muscles (see **Fig. 9**). The relation of the MMB with the inferior border of the mandible is extremely important surgically. The position of this branch is variable when posterior to the facial artery but always above the inferior border of the mandible when anterior to the facial artery.[14] Thus, the facial artery can be used as an important landmark in the course of the nerve (see **Fig. 9**B).

Neck Anatomy

The aging process exerts an impact on each anatomic element of the cervical region to varying

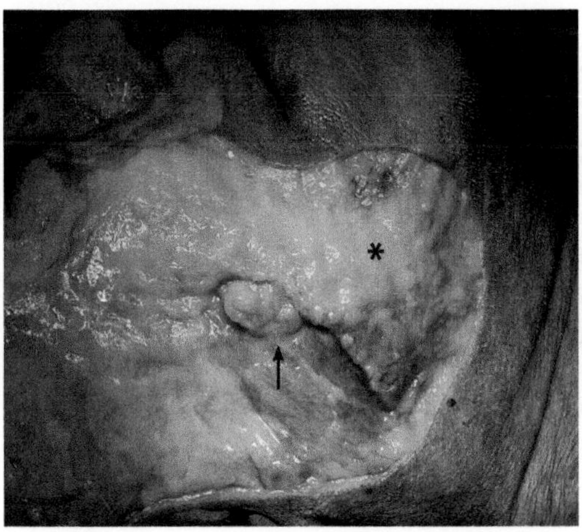

Fig. 6. Fat compartments forming the jowl. Subcutaneous fat (*) and prolapsed buccal fat (*arrow*).

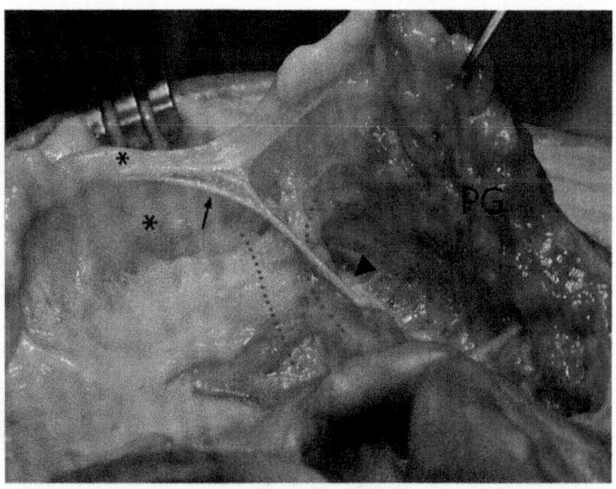

Fig. 7. Cadaver dissection of the right face. The parotid gland (PG) is reflected inferiorly. The outline of the zygomatic arch is denoted with red dots. The frontal branch (*arrow*) travels within the innominate fascia (*). The arrowhead marks the zygomatic branch.

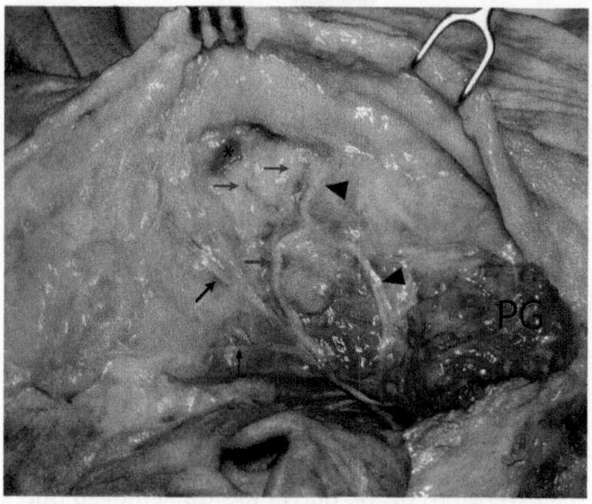

Fig. 8. The zygomatic (*red arrows*) and buccal (*arrowheads*) branches emerge from the parotid gland and run over the masseter muscle under the parotid-masseteric fascia. The parotid gland (PG) is reflected laterally. The star indicates the zygomaticus major. The frontal branches (*black arrows*) run within the fibrofatty layer.

degrees in each patient. Each element of the contributing anatomy should be identified preoperatively. The platysma is a broad muscle and covers most of the anterior and lateral aspect of the neck. On the lateral side of the neck, just underneath the platysma, is the external jugular vein, which can be seen descending from the angle of the mandible. The great auricular nerve (GAN) and other cervical cutaneous nerves run superficial to the sternocleidomastoid muscle (SCM) and deep to the platysma. Understanding the anatomic relationships of 3 structures, the GAN, external jugular vein (EJV), and platysma, is important for a safe neck dissection (**Fig. 10**).

The cervical fascia consists of concentric layers of fascia that compartmentalize structures in the neck. These fascial layers are defined as the superficial fascia and deep fascia with sublayers within the deep fascia. The superficial cervical fascia encloses the platysma muscle and is associated closely with the subcutaneous adipose tissue. The superficial layer of deep cervical fascia (investing layer) is what plastic surgeons commonly refer to simply as the "deep cervical fascia."

The platysma is a superficial thin and flat muscle that covers a broad area and has minimal direct attachment to the bone and is indirectly stabilized with the skeleton by ligaments, so it is more affected than other muscles with age (see **Fig. 1**). The platysma can vary in thickness depending on gender, age, and size. The primary innervation of the platysma is by the cervical branch and occasionally aberrant innervation by the MMB. The platysma has variable decussation with fibers from the other side 1 cm to 2 cm below the mandible. Depending on their mode of decussation, they display 3 anatomic variants. As a part of aging, its medial fibers attenuate or thicken to create platysmal bands.

The EJV and its tributaries drain the majority of the external face. It is formed by the union of the posterior auricular vein and posterior division of the retromandibular vein. These 2 veins combine immediately posterior to the angle of mandible, forming the EJV. The EJV has a relatively superficial course down the neck. It descends down the neck within the superficial fascia, runs obliquely and inferiorly superficial to the SCM, crosses the transverse cervical nerve, and lies parallel with the GAN posterior to its upper half (see **Fig. 10**). The EJV varies considerably in its size, course, and formation.

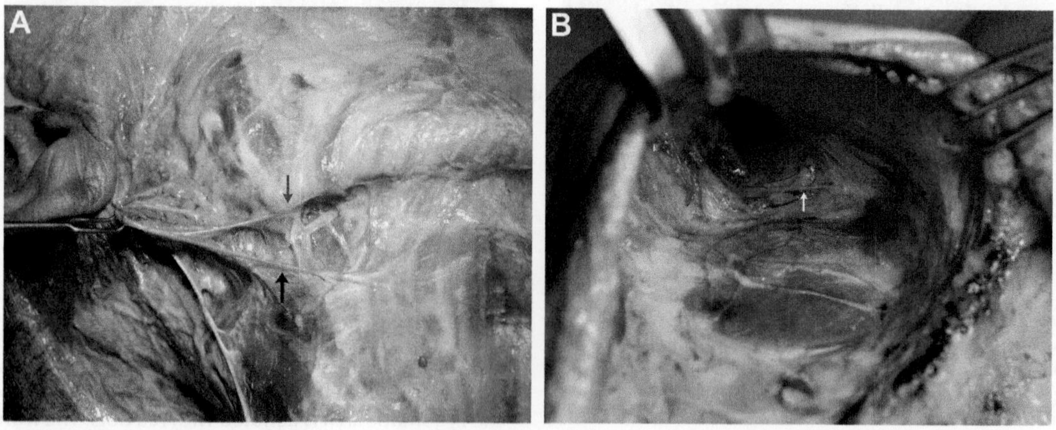

Fig. 9. (*A*) The cervical (*black arrow*) and MMB (*red arrow*). (*B*) The marginal mandibular nerve (*white arrow*) can be seen crossing the facial vessels.

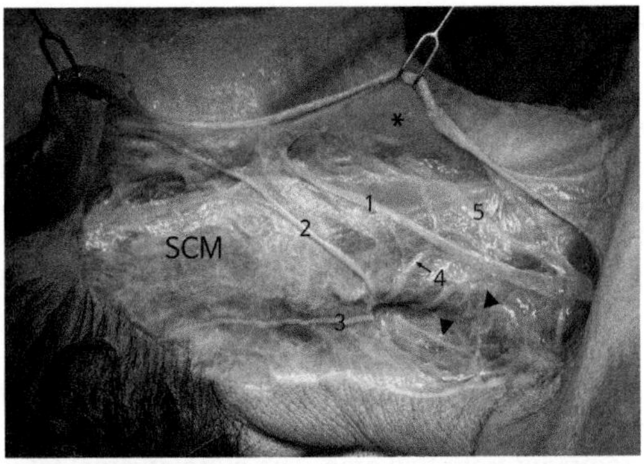

Fig. 10. Cadaver dissection of the right neck. The spatial relationship of 3 structures—the GAN, EJV, and platysma—is important for a safe neck dissection. EJV (1), GAN (2), LON (3), transverse cervical nerve (4), common facial vein (5), platysma (*), supraclavicular nerve (*arrowheads*), and SCM.

The anterior rami of the C1-4 vertebrae constitute the cervical plexus and provide sensory innervation to the neck, clavicle, and skin surrounding the ear. The GAN is the largest ascending branch of the cervical plexus. The GAN originates from the cervical plexus at levels of C2 and C3 spinal roots, encircles the posterior border of the sternocleidomastoid, runs beneath the investing fascia on the sternocleidomastoid, or occasionally perforates the deep fascia and ascends on the deep fascia. Therefore, when elevating a skin flap in the lateral neck, keeping the SCM fascia intact often, but not always, prevents injury to the GAN. On reaching the parotid gland, it lies approximately 1 cm posterior to the EJV and divides into multiple branches in the proximity of the inferior pole of the parotid gland, coursing anterior and posterior to the earlobe, supplying sensation to the skin overlying the posteroinferior aspect of the auricle and the skin overlying the parotid gland and anteroinferior aspect of the auricle[15] (see **Fig. 10**). Overall, the most common nerve injury caused by facelift surgery is the GAN, which occurs in up to 7% of procedures, most likely a product of its anatomic location and superficial course. The classic external landmark for locating the nerve is at the midbelly of the SCM muscle, 6.5 cm inferior to the bony external auditory canal.

The lesser occipital nerve (LON) is derived mainly from the C2 and sometimes C3 nerve root and usually is smaller in diameter compared with the GAN. It ascends along the posterior margin of the sternocleidomastoid (see **Fig. 10**). Near the cranium, it perforates the deep fascia and divides into branches. It supplies the superior ear and the mastoid area with considerable anatomic variation. It is not uncommon for the LON to run superficially in the subcutaneous layer after penetration of the investing layer. The LON has been described as less important than the greater auricular nerve.

The cervical retaining ligaments anchor the platysma and soft tissues of the neck to the deep cervical fascia and deeper skeletal structures. Feldman[16] described the retaining ligaments and filaments of the neck. The platysma-mandibular ligament attaches the platysma-SMAS layer to the mandibular periosteum. The platysma-auricular ligament is a fascial condensation that extends from the posterior border of the platysma to the dermis of the inferior auricular region (**Fig. 11**). During surgery, these fibrous attachments serve as a landmark for the proximity of the GAN and the posterior border of the platysma.

PREOPERATIVE PREPARATION

As with any other facial plastic procedure, patient evaluation and selection are important in the entire treatment plan. The surgeon should keep in mind that failing to plan is planning to fail. During the patient interview and history taking, evaluation of the psychological aspects of the patient must be done carefully.

The surgeon must know the patient's desire and progression of aging and explain the procedure required, including risks and benefits. Preoperative preparation entails the control of concurrent illnesses. Blood pressure, diabetes, and other chronic systemic illnesses should be well managed. Certain medical conditions or lifestyle habits also can increase the risk of complications. The following factors may present a significant risk or result in unfavorable results after facelift. Blood-thinning medications or supplements increase the risk of hematomas after surgery. Medical

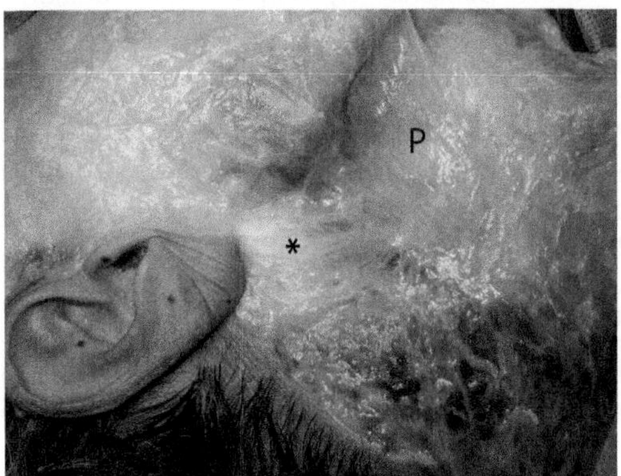

Fig. 11. The platysma auricular ligament (*) arises from the parotid fascia and anchors the posterior border of the platysma (P) and SCM fascia.

conditions, such as poorly controlled diabetes or high blood pressure, increase the risk of poor wound healing, hematomas, and heart complications. Smoking significantly increases the risk of poor wound healing, hematomas, and skin loss.

With the patient sitting upright, several important anatomic landmarks are outlined preoperatively, including the path of the temporal branch of the facial nerve and the deep plane entry point. The Pitanguy line is the approximate location of the seventh nerve and should be drawn routinely out when doing any surgery in this area. Areas, such as the jowls, prominent bands in the platysma, and collection of submental fat, are the most improved areas after a facelift procedure. Thorough examination of these regions gives valuable clues about the treatment plan. Careful evaluation of the neck and its relationship to the lower third of the face leads to selection of the appropriate procedure to meet a patient's goals.

ANESTHESIA

Facelifting procedures can be performed under intravenous monitored anesthesia or general anesthesia. Regardless of the type of anesthesia used, the key to successful surgery is effective local anesthesia. Adequate local infiltration into the subdermal plexus and subcutaneous tissue provides the necessary vasoconstriction for optimal surgery. A local anesthetic solution that has both rapid onset and prolonged duration of analgesia is optimal. A combination of lidocaine and bupivacaine with epinephrine fulfills these criteria.

OPERATIVE PROCEDURE

The surgical procedure described in this article introduces a method based on the deep plane dissection published by Hamra.[3] The traditional deep plane technique lifts the SMAS, platysma, and skin as a compound unit with a thicker, well-vascularized flap. The flap is elevated in a sub-SMAS dissection in the inferior cheek, transitioning to a supra-SMAS plane immediately superficial to the zygomaticus muscles in the superior medial cheek (**Fig. 12**).

Submental Approach

The submental approach is performed at the beginning of the rhytidectomy procedure in the presence of submental fat accumulation and severe submental skin laxity, including platysmal bands. The procedure begins with a submental crease incision along the submental crease with a length of about 4 cm. When submental liposuction is performed, it removes supraplatysmal fat from the submental and submandibular region. Liposuction creates numerous tunnels in the subcutaneous plane that facilitates subcutaneous flap elevation. Platysmaplasty for the central correction of platysma bands may be followed by elevation of the submental skin flap. After identification of the anterior border of the platysma and its laxity, platysmaplasty is performed using medial edge plication or by the excision of redundant medial platysma (**Fig. 13**). If subplatysmal fat causes fullness in the submental region, excess fat is removed from this area. The subplatysmal fat is more vascular and fibrous and is difficult to remove with a suction cannula. If it is removed sharply, the surgeon encounters bleeding.

For digastric muscle hypertrophy and/or lower position of the hyoid bone, partial resection of the anterior belly of digastric muscle should be considered. In microgenia, the obtuse cervicomental angle and short neck are produced, and this can be solved by chin augmentation using fat or an implant via a submental approach. Because Asians tends to have less severe neck skin laxity than whites, if they simply have supraplatysmal fat accumulation, mild platysmal bands, good skin elasticity, a submental approach is not required, and posterosuperior platysma tension alone produces satisfactory results.

Incision and Skin Flap Elevation

All incisions on the scalp or along the scalp-skin interfaces must be made precisely parallel to the hair follicles to avoid injury to them. The anterior temporal hairline incised perpendicular to the hair

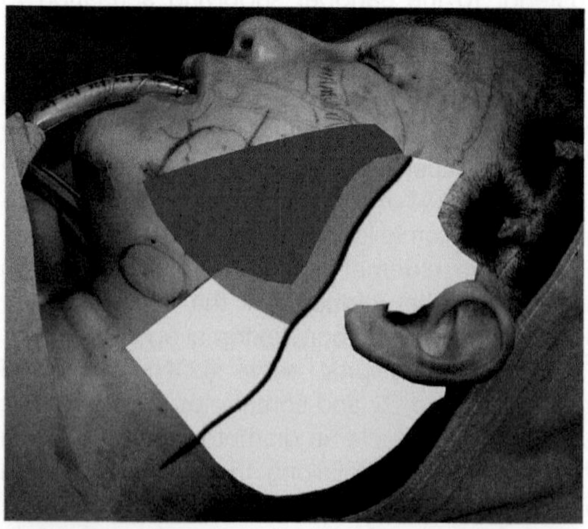

Fig. 12. The area of the subcutaneous (yellow and orange) and sub-SMAS (orange and red) dissection is illustrated. The black line indicates an incision for deep plane entry.

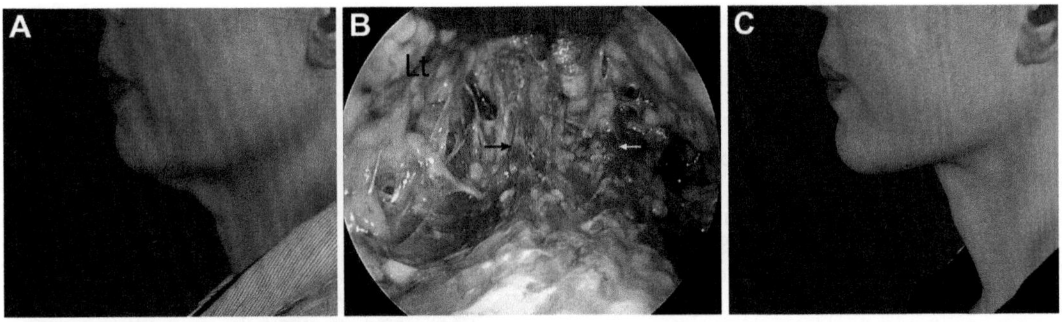

Fig. 13. Correction of the platysmal bands. (*A*) Preoperative photograph, (*B*) the platysmal bands, and (*C*) postoperative photograph.

shafts beginning slightly above the level of the lateral canthus. The incision is tracked along the inferior hairline of the sideburn, into the hairless recess between sideburn and auricle, turning downward into the preauricular crease, continuing retrotragally, and then following the crease of the lobule-facial junction (**Fig. 14**A). The incision is continued posteriorly along the auriculomastoid sulcus, and the direction is change slightly at the level of the superior crus, following the anterior occipital hairline for about 1 cm and extending into the occipital hair 5 cm to 7 cm in length, depending on neck aging (see **Fig. 14**B). Posteriorly along the auriculomastoid sulcus, the incision should continue a few millimeters into the posterior conchal cartilage rather than directly in the sulcus. This method helps minimize the inferior descent of the posterior auricular scar to a more visible location with age.

Once the incision has been performed, the subcutaneous flap initially is dissected with a no. 10 scalpel and countertraction is applied manually by an assistant to maintain uniform thickness of the flap (**Fig. 15**). The surgeon should consistently palpate the thickness of the flap for any irregularities with his nondominant hand. The anterior extent of the skin flap dissection of the face is from the lateral canthus to the line connecting the mandible angle.

The skin and sternocleidomastoid fascia are tightly adhered in the mastoid area, making tissue elevation difficult. Beginning the dissection in the postauricular area posteriorly or inferiorly helps the surgeon identify the proper plane more superiorly and anteriorly. There is a risk of injury to GAN, the LON and the EJV during a lateral neck dissection; thus, the proper dissection plane is important. Once the posterior margin of the platysma has been approached, the plane can be developed rapidly with broad spreading movements of the dissecting scissors. After completion of the subcutaneous elevation (see **Fig. 15**), additional direct

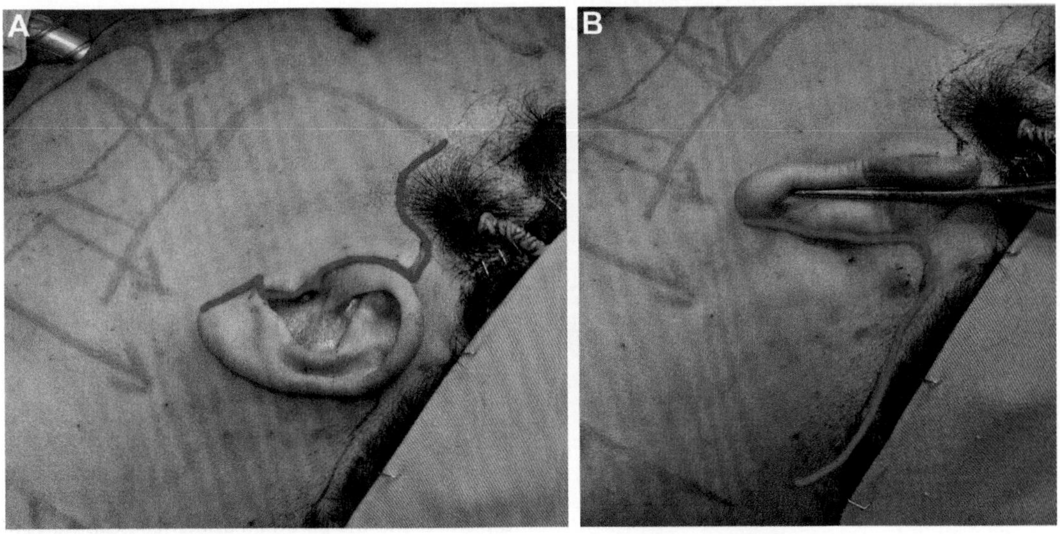

Fig. 14. Surgical marking for (*A*) facial and (*B*) neck incisions has been completed.

excision of the fat and liposuction can be performed around the entire neck.

Deep Plane Dissection

After completely elevating the subcutaneous flap, the dissection plane is changed from superficial to deep to the SMAS and platysma (see **Fig. 12**). Careful manipulation of the SMAS layer is key in determining stability for satisfactory results. The upper and lower margin of the zygomatic arch and the Pitanguy line are marked (**Fig. 16**). An incision for deep plane entry is then made through the SMAS with a no. 10 scalpel, located 2 cm anterior to the Pitanguy line to avoid injury to the frontal branch of the facial nerve. Many doctors have recommended a deep plane entry point from the angle of the mandible to the lateral canthus, but, in Asians, the extent of the skin dissection should be performed more anteriorly than in whites, and the SMAS incision should be located slightly posteriorly rather than at the recommended line to prevent skin dimpling when the SMAS is tightened.

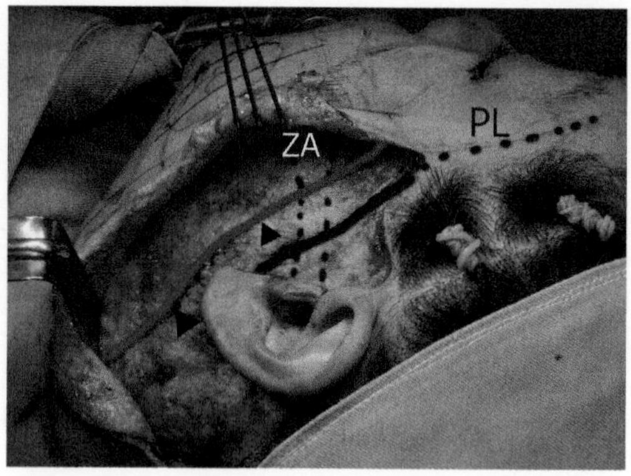

Fig. 16. The incision for deep plane entry is marked (*red line*). The Pitanguy line (PL) and the zygomatic arch (ZA).

First, the deep plane dissection begins from the lower region of the face over the masseter muscle. The SMAS is elevated from the parotid fascia and the dissection advances anteriorly. There is a natural glide plane (premasseteric space) between the SMAS and the parotid-masseteric fascia. This area is relatively avascular and separates easily. The muscle fibers of the platysma usually are visible on the undersurface of the flap and used as guide for the dissection (**Fig. 17**). From the anterior border of the parotid gland, translucent masseteric muscle fascia can be seen, and in patients who have abundant deep facial fat on the muscle fascia, the risk of injury to underlying structures, such as the MMB, is reduced. Blunt dissection is advanced anteriorly to the area beneath the subcutaneous jowl fat. The inferior limit of the sub-SMAS dissection in a deep plane facelift is the inferior border of the mandible; this protects the MMB. Another dissection end point is the facial artery, which can be visualized in the subplatysmal plane.

After dissection of the inferior cheek, attention then is directed to the malar and midportion of the cheek. Compared with the inferior cheek, the plane of dissection is not clear; discerning the correct plane of dissection can be difficult in this region and important structures, such as the facial nerve, the transverse facial artery, and the parotid duct ,run closely together; therefore, tissue elevation in this area is more risky than that of the inferior third of the face.

The dissection remains subcutaneous above the level of the zygomatic arch to the orbicularis

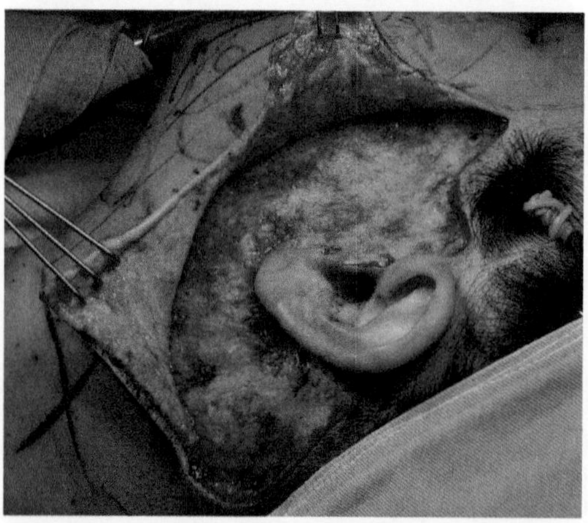

Fig. 15. The skin flap dissection of the face and neck.

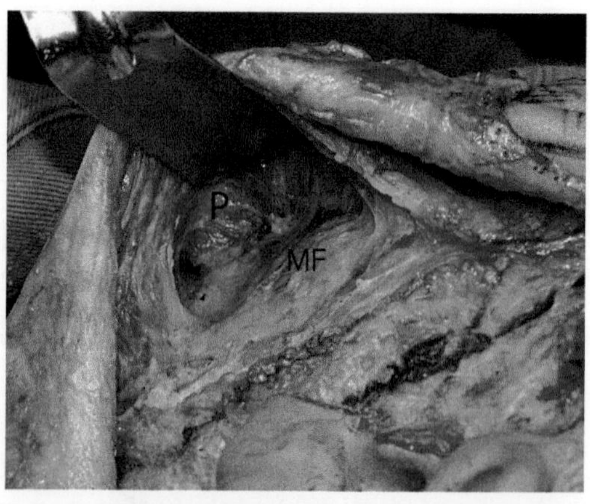

Fig. 17. The composite skin and SMAS flap are elevated off the parotid-masseteric fascia. There is a natural glide plane (premasseteric space) between the SMAS and the parotid-masseteric fascia. Platysma (P) and masseteric fascia (MF).

oculi. As the dissection proceeds anteriorly, a small perforating branch of the transverse facial artery is encountered before zygomatic and MRL is identified completely (see **Fig. 3**B). This is addressed carefully with bipolar cauterization. Further dissection forward exposes a strong zygomatic cutaneous ligament and masseteric cutaneous ligament (**Fig. 18**). Complete ligamentous release requires elevation of the composite flap to the anterior border of the masseter. After cutting these retaining ligaments, the zygomaticus major surrounded by fat is identified. At this point, the dissection should be transitioned from sub-SMAS to the subcutaneous layer to avoid injuring the zygomatic nerve branches. The zygomatic branch travels beneath the zygomaticus major muscle but may give off a fine branch superficial to the muscle, which innervates the orbicularis oculi laterally. The extent of the dissection is determined by the amount of midface laxity. After the upper masseteric ligaments have been lysed completely, the surgeon should stop the SMAS dissection because maximum soft tissue release has been obtained, and there is no advantage to continuing to dissect anteriorly, where the zygomatic and buccal branches are more superficial and prone to injury.

The jowls are among the most common complaints of patients and among the most difficult for which to attain long-lasting results. Ptotic jowls may be corrected with release of the platysma-mandibular insertion and the mandibular ligament tightening the platysma and the SMAS. The platysma is inserted tightly into the mandible around the facial artery. It consistently is found that platysma fibers attach to the mandible at the anterosuperior border of the facial artery (**Fig.19A**). After releasing it, the mandibular retaining ligament is encountered in the anteromedial position of the platysma insertion (see **Fig. 19**B). Occasionally, the marginal mandibular nerve traveling superficial to the facial artery is encountered. The jowls affected by hypertrophy of the superficial and deep fat should be corrected by direct fat removal and liposuction. If excessive jowls exist due to buccal fat pseudoherniation, this may be addressed at this time. A conservative excision of buccal fat is indicated. Only a small amount of fat should be removed initially to prevent over-resection.

Finally, the posterior border of the platysma is released from the fascial attachments of the SCM. Dissection starts from the mandibular angle area where the SMAS, platysma and SCM interface with each other. The dissection extends inferiorly along the posterior border of the platysma 5 cm to 6 cm below the angle of the mandible. This procedure releases the dense fascial attachments of the platysma from the SCM, which allows for lateral mobilization of the platysma in the neck. The posterior border of the platysma is reliably located just anterior to the greater auricular nerve, which always is identified and serves as a useful landmark (see **Fig. 10**). Before fixation of the SMAS, fat injection is performed in areas requiring volume augmentation, including the midcheek area.

Superficial Musculoaponeurotic System Fixation and Closure

Once the SMAS flap has been elevated and adequately released, the SMAS flap then is suspended, working inferiorly to superiorly, with several half-mattress sutures using 2-0 polydioxanone (PDS) placed along the cuff of the platysma and SMAS at the deep plane entry point (**Fig. 20**). Three key point sutures are performed followed by additional fixations between them for resuspension. The flap is placed under a moderate amount of tension and then rotated through a medially based arc. At first, the platysma is anchored to the mastoid fascia in a vertically oblique vector of approximately 30° to improve neck contour, and the lower cheek platysma is attached to the tympanomastoid fascia (Lore fascia) in a superolateral vector of approximately 45° to define the jaw line and improve the jowls. The upper midface SMAS is anchored to the deep temporal fascia in a vertically oblique vector of approximately 60°, parallel to the long axis of the zygomaticus major or perpendicular to the nasolabial fold, but this vector should be individualized to the patient. Additional multiple fixation sutures between the key sutures helps ensure that tension is distributed evenly along the flap.

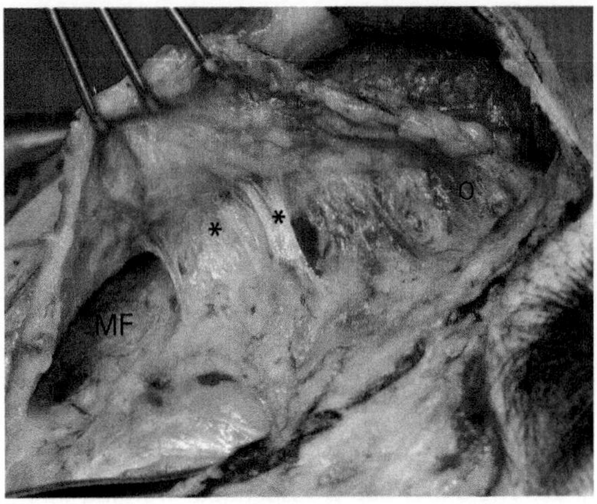

Fig. 18. The zygomatic (right *) and MRL (left *). Orbicularis oculi (O) and masseteric fascia (MF).

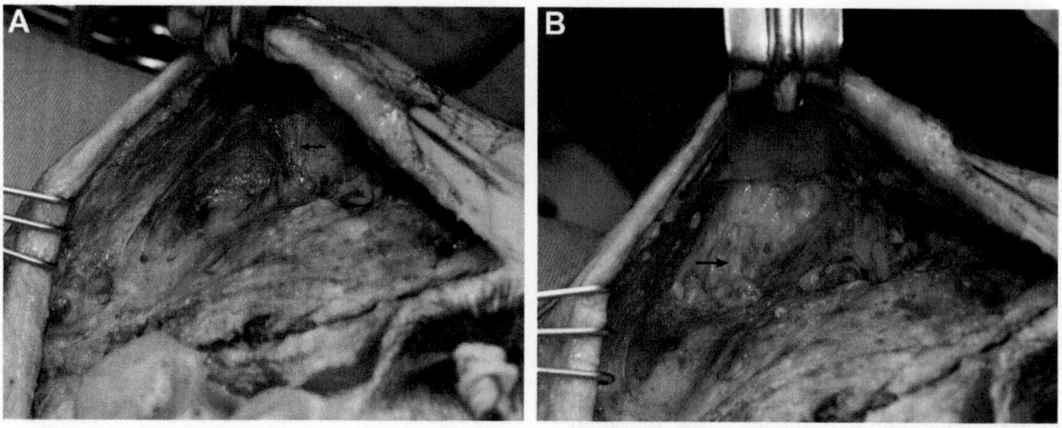

Fig. 19. The platysma insertion and mandibular retaining ligament. (*A*) Arrow indicates the platysma insertion around the facial artery. (*B*) After cutting the platysma insertion, the mandibular retaining ligament is encountered anteromedial to the platysma insertion (*arrow*).

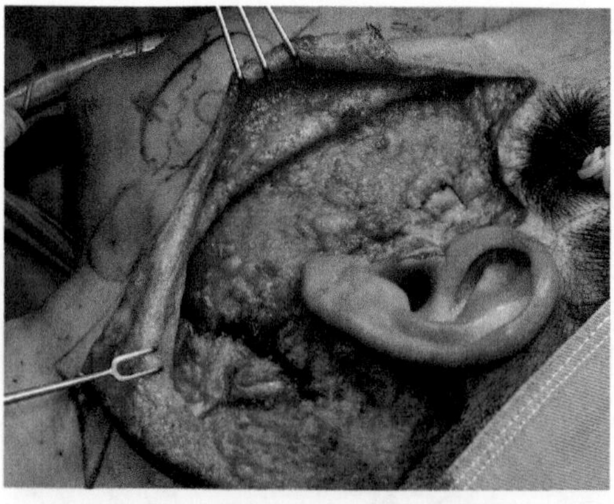

Fig. 20. The SMAS flap is suspended, working inferiorly to superiorly, with several half-mattress sutures using 2-0 PDS.

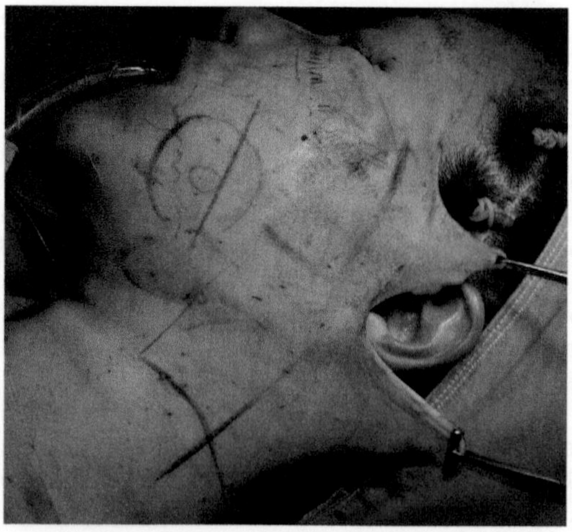

Fig. 21. The redundant skin is excised a meticulously and suspended in a similar vector as the deep plane flap to allow for tension-free skin closure.

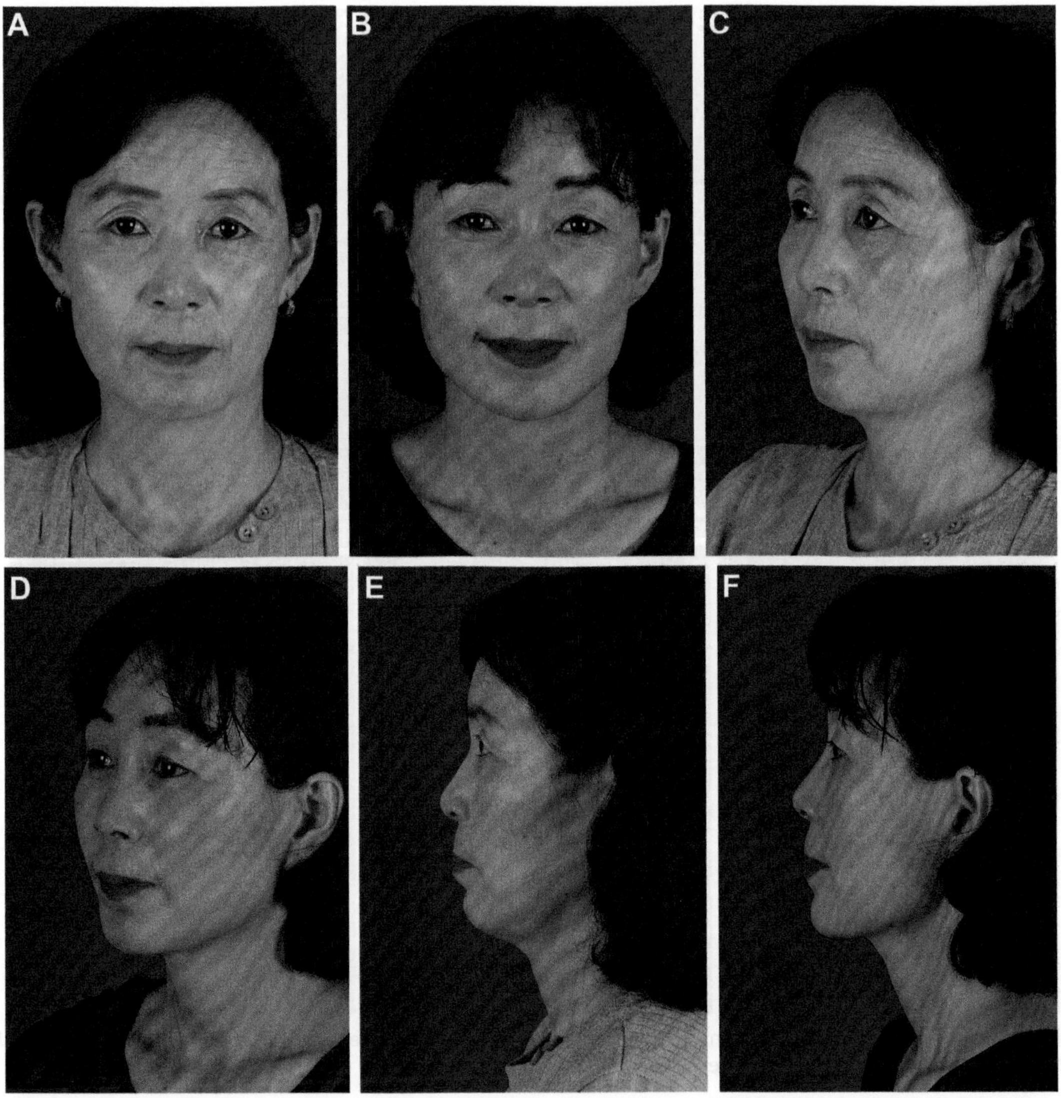

Fig. 22. Postoperative views at 10 months of a 55-year-old woman after a deep plane face lift, endobrow lift, and lower lid blepharoplasty. Preoperative views (*A*, *C*, and *E*). Postoperative views (*B*, *D*, and *F*).

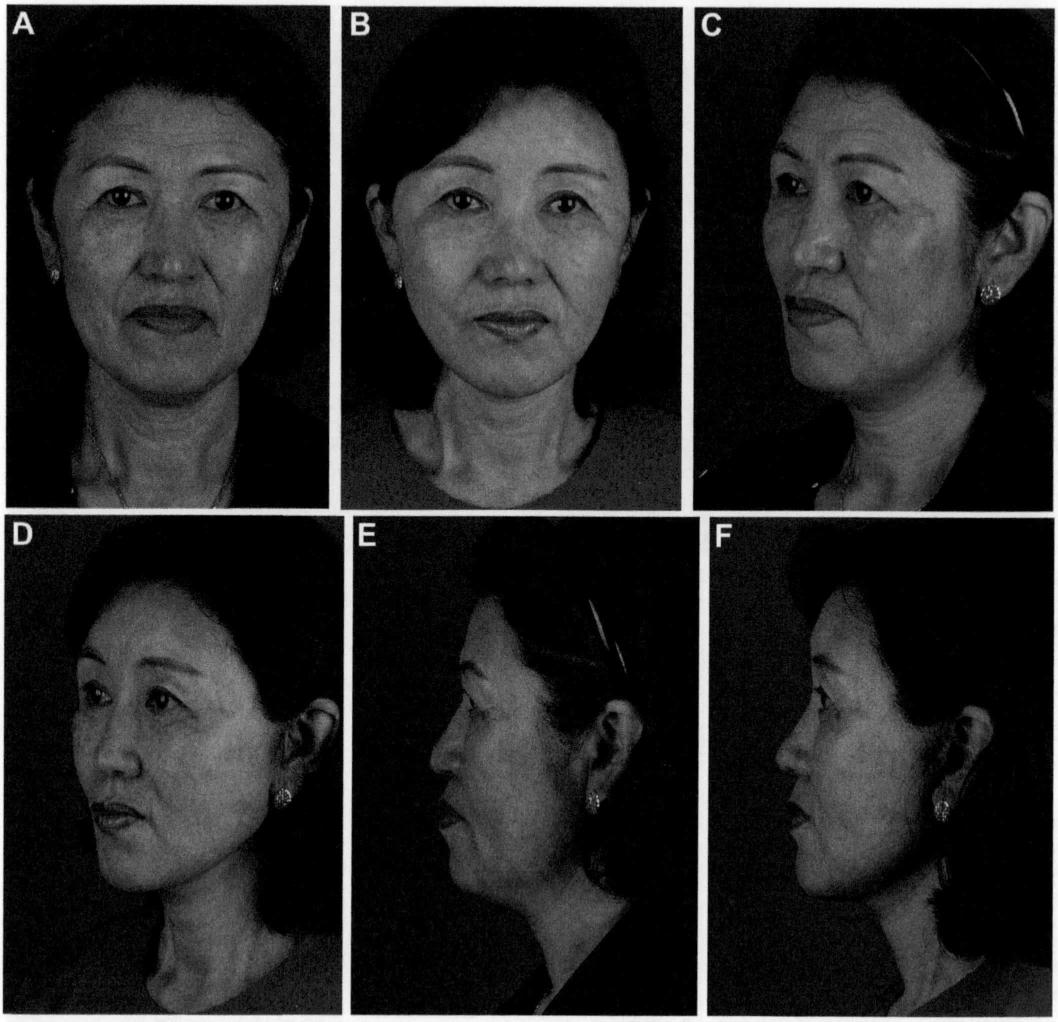

Fig. 23. Postoperative views at 22 months of a 61-year-old woman after a deep plane face lift, endobrow lift, and lower lid blepharoplasty. Preoperative views (*A*, *C*, *E*). Postoperative views (*B*, *D*, *F*).

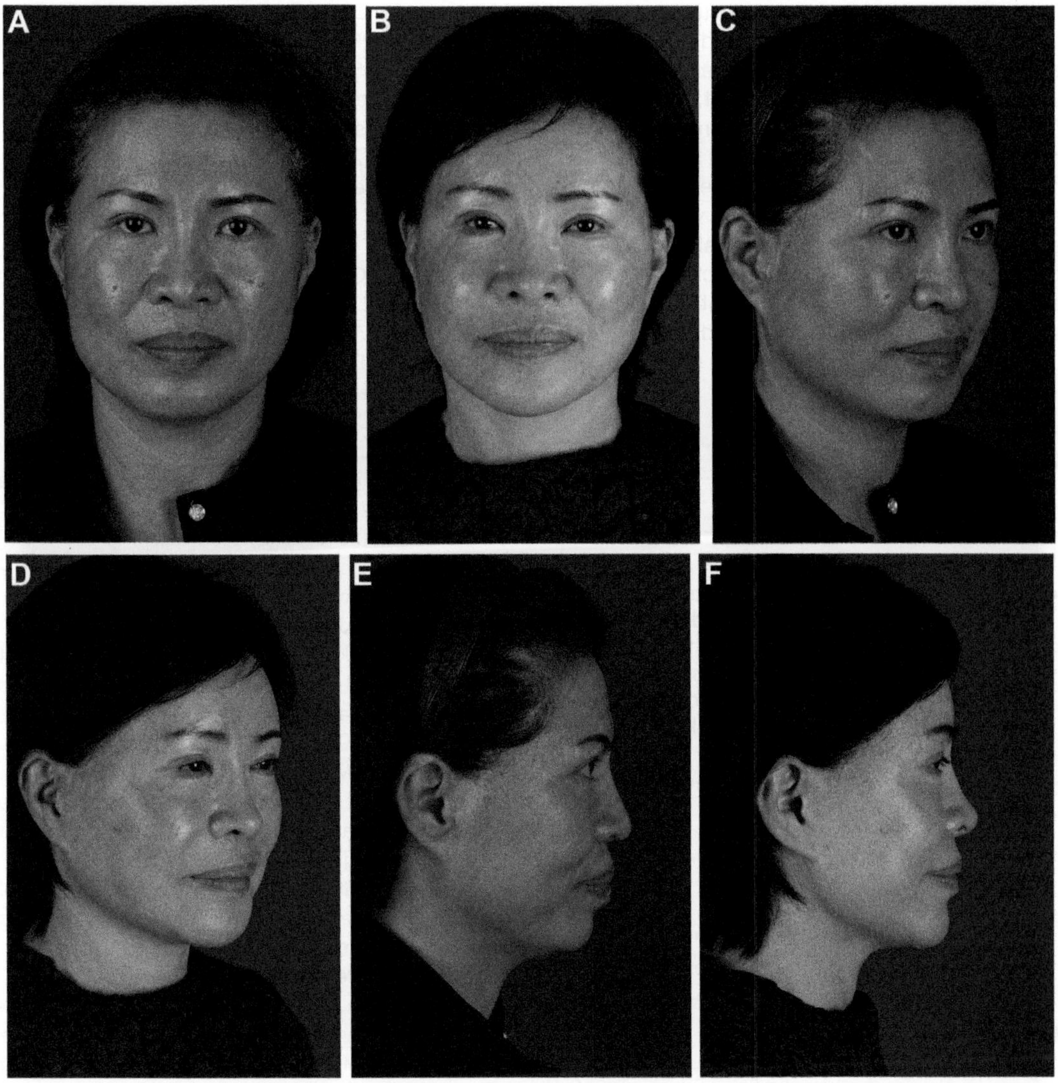

Fig. 24. Postoperative views at 7 years of a 64-year-old woman after a secondary facelift, canthoplasty, endobrow lift, and revisional rhinoplasty. Preoperative views (*A, C, E*). Postoperative views (*B, D, F*).

After resuspension of the SMAS, the redundant skin is meticulously excised and suspended in a similar vector as the deep plane flap to allow for tension-free skin closure (**Fig. 21**). Before final skin closure, a small drain is inserted through a stab incision posterior to the occipital hairline which is removed the following day. Placement of a bulky, noncompressive facelift dressing completes the process.

COMPLICATIONS

The complex flap created by the deep plane dissection is well vascularized, and this makes it resistant to many rhytidectomy complications. Hematoma is the most common early complication following facelift surgery. The most common cause of hematoma is related to uncontrolled blood pressure. The rate of hematoma formation is reported to be as low as 1.8%. Infections are rare, reported in only 0.3% to 0.6% of cases. Skin slough rates also are low, reported in 2.7% of cases, and the incidence of injury to the facial nerve during a standard rhytidectomy has been reported in 2% of the patients.

SUMMARY

The deep plane technique begins in the subcutaneous plane in the preauricular area, moves to the sub-SMAS layer distally, and the ligaments attached to the SMAS within the midface are cut and vertically or superolaterally sutured. Rejuvenation of the aging Asian face mandates a unique set of strategies that include understanding the cultural aspects of the Asian patient, the anatomy of the Asian patient, and the techniques that re appropriate based on these cultural and anatomic considerations. If properly performed, the facelift can improve facial balance and yield a more aesthetically appealing result. In Asians, the goal of the facial and neck lift is to create a well-defined jaw line, deep cervicomental angle, and depressed submandibular area; and midcheek lift is less important than lower face lift (**Figs. 22–24**).

CLINICS CARE POINTS

- In Asians, the deep plane facelifts are effective particularly in obtaining a defined jaw line; and the blood supply to the flap is enough, so the risk of flap necrosis is minimal. Because wide dissection of the face and neck is required, however, there is risk of hematoma and nerve injury.

DISCLOSURE

The authors have nothing to disclose.

REFERENCES

1. Skoog T. New methods and refinements. In: Tord S, editor. Plastic surgery. 1st edition. Stockholm: Almgrist and Wicksell International; 1974. p. 300–30.
2. Mitz V, Peyronie M. The superficial musculo-aponeurotic system (SMAS) in the parotid and cheek area. Plast Reconstr Surg 1976;58(1):80–8.
3. Hamra ST. The deep-plane rhytidectomy. Plast Reconstr Surg 1990;86:53–61.
4. Hamra ST. Composite rhytidectomy. Plast Reconstr Surg 1992;90:1-13. Plast Reconstr Surg 1998; 102(3):843–55.
5. Guo MK. Cephalometric standards of Steiner analysis established on Chinese children. Taiwan Yi Xue Hui Za Zhi 1971;70(2):97–102.
6. Lam SM. Aesthetic strategies for the aging Asian face. Facial Plast Surg Clin North Am 2007;15(3): 283–91.
7. Lambros V. Observations on periorbital and midface aging. Plast Reconstr Surg 2007;120:1367–76 [discussion: 1377].
8. Mendelson BC, Jacobson SR. Surgical anatomy of the midcheek: facial layers, spaces, and mid cheek segments. Clin Plast Surg 2008;35(3):395–404.
9. Alghoul MB, O McBride J, Zins JE. Relationship of the zygomatic facial nerve to the retaining ligaments of the face: the subSMAS danger zone. Plast Reconstr Surg 2013;131(2):245e–52e.
10. Alghoul M, Codner MA. Retaining ligaments of the face: review of anatomy and clinical applications. Aesthet Surg J 2013;33(6):769–82.
11. Stuzin JM, Baker TJ, Gordon HL. The relationship of the superficial and deep facial fascias: relevance to rhytidectomy and aging. Plast Reconstr Surg 1992; 89:441–51.
12. Agarwal CA, Mendenhall SD III, Foreman KB, et al. The course of the frontal branch of the facial nerve in relation to fascial planes: an anatomic study. Plast Reconstr Surg 2010;125:532–7.
13. Trussler AP, Stephan P, Hatef D, et al. The frontal branch of the facial nerve across the zygomatic arch: anatomical relevance of the high-SMAS technique. Plast Reconstr Surg 2010;125:1221–9.
14. Dingman RO, Grabb WC. Surgical anatomy of the mandibular ramus of the facial nerve based on the dissection of 100 facial halves. Plast Reconstr Surg Transplant Bull 1962;29:266–72.
15. Biglioli F, D'Orto O, Bozzetti A, et al. Function of the great auricular nerve following surgery for benign parotid disorders. J Craniomaxillofac Surg 2002; 30(5):308–17.
16. Feldman JJ. Surgical anatomy of the neck. In: Feldman JJ, editor. Necklift.. 1st edition. Stuttgart (Germany): Thieme; 2006. p. 106–13.

Forehead Lift for Asians

In-Sang Kim, MD*, Hak-Soo Kim, MD

KEYWORDS

• Forehead lift • Asian • Endoscopic • Complication • Diplopia

KEY POINTS

- For Asians, there are special anatomic and clinical considerations in performing forehead lift.
- Forehead lift has powerful clinical effects when it is combined with augmentation rhinoplasty and blepharoplasty.
- For the best outcome of the forehead lift in Asians, the dissection planes, incisions, and skin resections can be diversified.
- There are rare complications related to the endoscopic forehead lift, such as temporal facial nerve injury and diplopia.

INTRODUCTION

The rejuvenation of the upper third of the face is the key to the restoration of the patient's youthful appearance, because the aging changes are often most pronounced in the upper one-third of the face. The aging changes of the upper face include forehead rhytides, sagging eyebrows, hooding of the upper eyelids, and periorbital wrinkles. Continuous muscle contractions lead to horizontal rhytides by the frontalis muscle, vertical glabellar rhytides by the corrugator supercilii muscle, and crow's-feet by the orbicularis oculi muscle. In addition to repeated muscle contraction, tissue sagging also contributes to the aging changes.

Besides gravitational pull, deflation of skin and subcutaneous tissue, gradual volume loss of bone and muscle in the frontal, temporal, and orbital regions are related to the tissue sagging. The eyebrows begin to descend with infrabrow tissue, which is sagging and bulging over the eyelids. Ptotic brows and combined dermatochalasis of eyelid skin leads to the hooding of the upper eyelids. Horizontal rhytides in the nasal root also develop with sagging soft tissue in the region accentuated by the action of the procerus muscle. Combined effects of these changes clinically result in the appearance of aging face with a sense of fatigue, anger, or sadness.

With the emergence of endoscopic facial surgery in the 1990s, endoscopic forehead lift has evolved to an alternative to the classic forehead lifts with decreased numbness, smaller invisible scars, and shorter recovery period. Now the endoscopic brow lift is regarded as a standard procedure with long-term favorable outcomes.[1]

Despite its numerous advantages, the endoscopic browlift is often criticized for a high recurrence rate, ranging up to 9% in some studies, and still there is no consensus on which forehead lift technique is the most reliable and safe.[2] Endoscopic browlift has some clear disadvantages in patients with thick furrowed skin, and high arched foreheads. In these patients, still there is a role for the classic coronal or subcutaneous forehead lifts and they can be done as solitary or combined procedures with endoscopic browlift.

DISCUSSION

There are anatomic and clinical differences for Asians that should be considered carefully before the forehead lift operation. Asians tend to have thicker skin and ligamentous attachments in forehead. Relieving the heavy soft tissue load in glabella, subbrow, upper eyelids, and radix area by forehead lift has a great clinical significance when it is performed in combination with other facial plastic surgeries, such as rhinoplasty and blepharoplasty.

Labom plastic surgery clinic, Gangnam-daero 600, Dongshin B/D 3F, Seoul, Korea
* Corresponding author.
E-mail address: drbe0911@gmail.com

Facial Plast Surg Clin N Am 29 (2021) 487–495
https://doi.org/10.1016/j.fsc.2021.06.002

Special Considerations for Asians

Double-eyelid surgery

The double-eyelid surgery is the most common aesthetic procedure in East Asian countries. When evaluating a patient seeking the double-eyelid surgery, the upper eyelids should be evaluated in contiguity with the eyebrows and forehead.[3]

Roughly 50% of East Asians have some form of supratarsal folds (ie, double-eyelid creases[4]) and others do not. Asians without double-eyelid creases have characteristics of puffy eyelids and heavy infrabrow soft tissue. Because of abundant orbital fat that is overlying the tarsal plate, insertion of the levator aponeurosis to the dermis is hindered.

Heavy infrabrow tissue is related to thick skin and bulky subcutaneous fibrofatty layer and orbicularis oculi muscle. The retro-orbicularis fat, preaponeurotic fat, and pretarsal fat contribute to the thick eyelid skin. For these patients, when the supratarsal fold is surgically created along the thick eyelid skin, an unnaturally deep fold under the overhanging plump eyelid skin is created giving the unnatural operated look.[5]

In case of elderly patients who exhibit redundant eyelid skin with dermatochalasis and concurrent brow ptosis, browlift must be considered to relieve the skin excess before or in combination with blepharoplasty.

Likewise, for a more satisfying outcome of the double-eyelid surgery in younger patients with heavy eyelids, the heavy soft tissue load in the infrabrow-eyelid area must be relieved first by the browlift before or in combination with the double-eyelid surgery (**Fig. 1**). In the same regard, for a patient who wants to increase the height of preexisting supratarsal creases, the surgeon must consider the browlift first if there is fullness of soft tissue over the upper eyelids.

Ideally, endoscopic browlift proceeds first, and at least a month and ideally 6 or more months later, double-eyelid surgery is performed. If double-eyelid surgery and the endoscopic browlift are done concurrently as combined surgeries, supratarsal creases are created first in a modestly lower position before the browlift. When the brow with infrabrow soft tissue is elevated and eyelid skin is stretched thin by the browlift, supratarsal creases on a thinned skin are more natural and shallower in shape.

Considering that the patients seeking the double-eyelid surgery are commonly young-aged, endoscopic browlift is the most suitable browlift procedure because of completely hidden scars.

Augmentation rhinoplasty

Augmentation rhinoplasty is one of the most popular aesthetic procedures in Asian countries. Although rhinoplasty and brow modification is a powerful combination, there has been little attempt to integrate analysis of the nose and brows, even though modification of the nasal-glabellar relationship maximizes the results for patients seeking rhinoplasty.[6] Brow elevation with modifications of the glabellar muscles deepens the nasion, creates concavity, elongates the overall nasal length, and also makes the brow-tip aesthetic line narrower and more defined (**Fig. 2**).

One of the most common mistakes by surgeons doing augmentation rhinoplasty for Asian patients is overaugmentation of the radix. Asians have flat foreheads, and the nasofrontal angle is shallow and it is rather a gentle smooth curvature than an

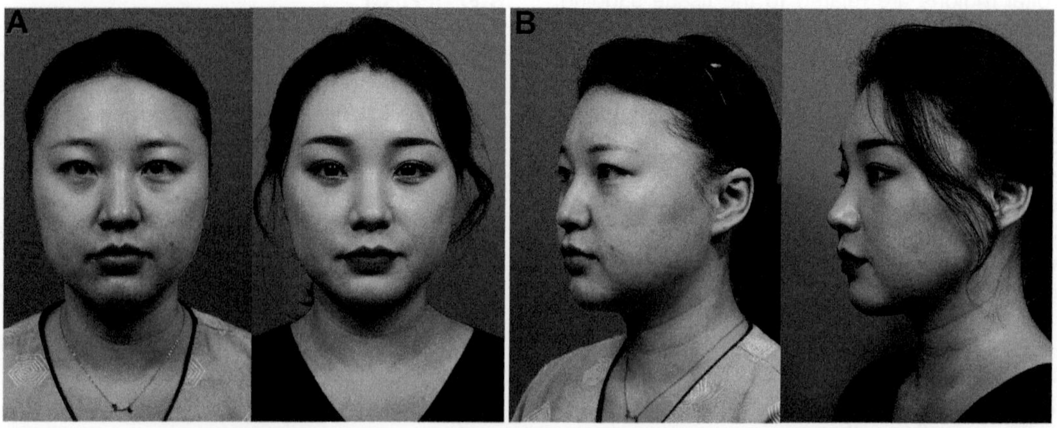

Fig. 1. A 31-year-old female patient who wanted to improve heavy and puffy appearance of her eyes, and to increase the height of supratarsal creases. After relief of heavy soft tissue load in the eyelids by endoscopic browlift, brighter open appearance of eyes is noticed and supratarsal creases are exposed wider.

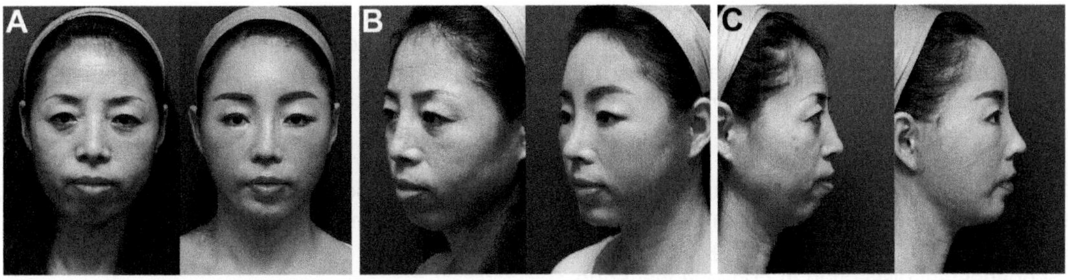

Fig. 2. A 46-year-old female patient who had a flat forehead and full nasal root. Augmentation rhinoplasty was done, which was combined with endoscopic browlift and forehead augmentation with fat injections. Enhanced brow-tip aesthetic lines and elongation of the nose by browlift are noticed. Other procedures include facelift, chin augmentation, and lower blepharoplasty.

angle, especially in females. This is the reason why forehead augmentation surgery with fat injections or alloplastic implants is common in Asian countries.

In elderly Asians, brow ptosis aggravates the ill-defined nasion with the flat nasofrontal angle and fullness of radix, where overaugmentation of radix results in an unnatural operated look that is aesthetically detrimental especially for female patients. Some younger Asian patients may also exhibit soft tissue crowding in the glabellar area, which is usually combined with heavy infrabrow soft tissue and puffy eyelids with variable degree of brow ptosis.

Browlift is remarkably beneficial in these patients as a combined surgery with augmentation rhinoplasty. Browlift relieves the fullness of the radix opening the nasofrontal angle and increases the glabella-to-nasion distance to make room for an amount of augmentation. Also the brow-tip aesthetic line is more enhanced with elevation of brows. The general length of the nose is elongated also, because browlift moves the nasal starting point higher by removing the bulging soft tissue in the nasal root, which sets the soft tissue nasion in a lower position.

As in the case of double-eyelid operation, endoscopic browlift is always preferred as a combined procedure with augmentation rhinoplasty for younger patients, because of hidden scars.

Browlift should be considered before augmentation rhinoplasty for the patient as follows:

- Patients with full radix, ill-defined nasion.
- Patients with flat forehead and low-set brows.
- Patients with flat nasofrontal angle, who nevertheless want significant amounts of radix augmentation.
- Secondary patients who complain that their nose still looks "heavy" following a primary rhinoplasty.[6]
- Patients who have a history of foreign body injections in the glabella and nasal root.

Brow shape

Numerous attempts have been made to define the ideal shape and position of the eyebrows. However, although there are certain basic principles, the aesthetic ideal cannot be generalized and must be assessed in relation to sex, ethnicity, orbital shape, eye prominence, and overall facial proportions. Preferred eyebrow for any individual is influenced by culture, fashion, and the era in which one lives.[7]

Culturally, Korean women in the present time may prefer flatter shape of the brows, compared with White women who prefer a more arched and laterally upward shape of the brows. This cultural difference is well witnessed in the brow make-up by Korean and Korean-American women. It is noticeable that the flatter and fuller brow shape is preferred by Korean women living in Korea and the more arched and slimmer brow shape preferred by Korean-American women raised in America.

Some Western surgeons try to keep the medial brow at a lower level while elevating the lateral brow, minimizing modifications of brow depressor muscles. However, for Korean women, moderate amount of medial brow elevation is well accepted and even desired by many. It is reported that the head-up type and the horizontal type of the brow were preferred for the young-looking brows by Korean women,[8,9] and this preference is more evident in young Korean women. Therefore, modification for brow depressor muscles should be sufficient enough to mobilize the medial brow in most Asian patients, if it is not contraindicated in such cases who have downturned or droopy eyebrows.

Thick skin and dense ligamentous attachments

Asians generally have thicker skin than Whites. Asian male patients often have thicker forehead skin with deep transverse folds, and ligamentous attachments of the skin to the underlying bone are also dense and stout making surgical dissection more difficult. Heavy and firm forehead skin may predispose to incomplete correction or relapse of forehead rhytides with the standard endoscopic forehead lift, which may fall short in providing an adequate rejuvenation of the thick skin with deep folds.

Endoscopic browlift without skin excision does not address the problem of skin laxity or redundancy in the forehead effectively in patients who has the skin as a main problem (**Fig. 3**).

Subperiosteal dissection in conventional endoscopic browlift is not effective to detach the fibrous septae between the muscle and the dermis to soften severe forehead creases.[10] In this regard, for Asian patients with heavy thick forehead skin, coronal/subgaleal/subcutaneous forehead lifts or variations of endoscope-assisted multiplane forehead lifts may be considered. Elderly patients with redundant skin and severe wrinkles also benefit from the multiplane approach with some skin excisions.[10]

Various endoscope-assisted multiplane forehead lifts have been suggested, such as biplanar endoscopic forehead lift,[11] subcutaneous endoscopic forehead lift,[12] and endoscopic temporal brow lift.[2] Endoscopic browlift with skin excision in the central forehead through minicoronal or trichophytic incision is another option (**Fig. 4**).

Skin excision through the trichophytic incision does not elevate the hairline in contrast to the coronal browlift. In this procedure, approximately 1.5 to 2.0 cm of skin is removed to elevate the brow and forehead. This approach can also provide restoration of an elevated hairline to a more youthful lower position while still elevating the brow, forehead, and nasal radix (**Figs. 5** and **6**).[13]

Canthal tilt

Another consideration is the positive canthal tilt or the Mongolian slant of Asians. Restoration or accentuation of the positive canthal tilt by browlift is beneficial for most Asian patients. However, there are patients who are concerned with their subjectively or objectively excessive canthal tilt, and they do not want to aggravate the sharp or temperamental appearance. This disfavor is more noticeable in younger patients with naturally pronounced positive canthal tilt. For those patients, dissection is minimized at the lateral orbit, where resistant fibrous attachment, that is, the thickened lateral orbicularis retaining ligament, also called the "lateral orbital thickening" or "precanthal tendon," is present. Temporal suspension is also minimized during the temporal fixation.

In contrast, dissection and myotomies in the medial brow area are more emphasized to ensure

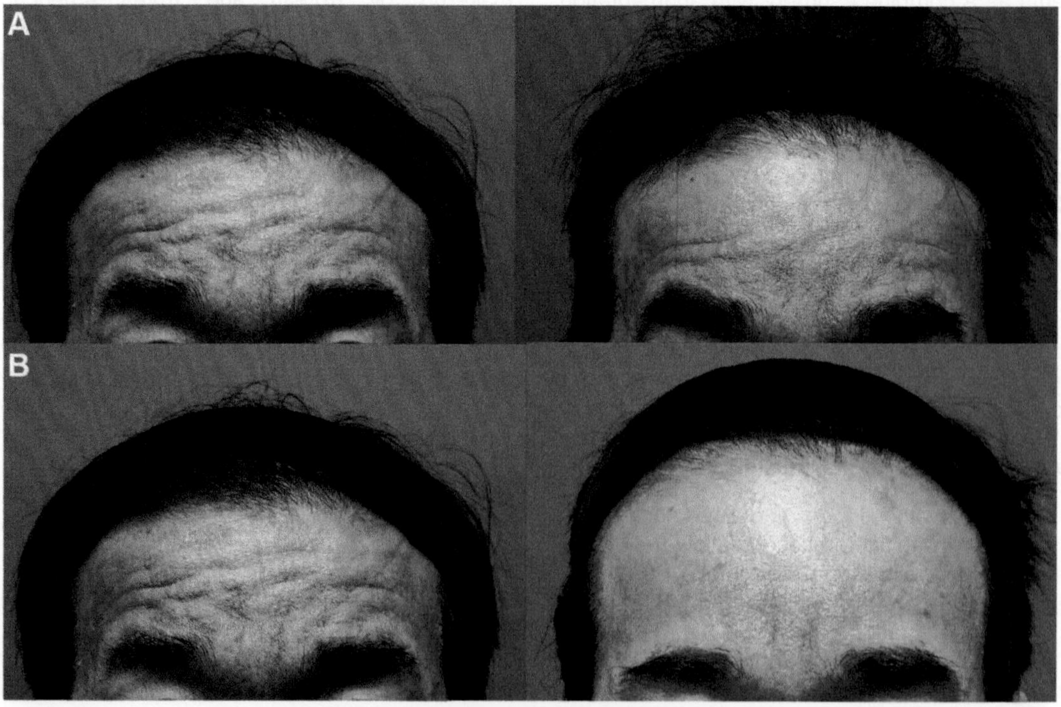

Fig. 3. A 61-year-old male patient with thin hairs. (*A*) Left, preoperative. Right, 4 months after endoscopic browlift. Mild but insufficient improvement requiring a revision surgery. (*B*) Left, preoperative. Right, 2 months after revision forehead lift by coronal lift.

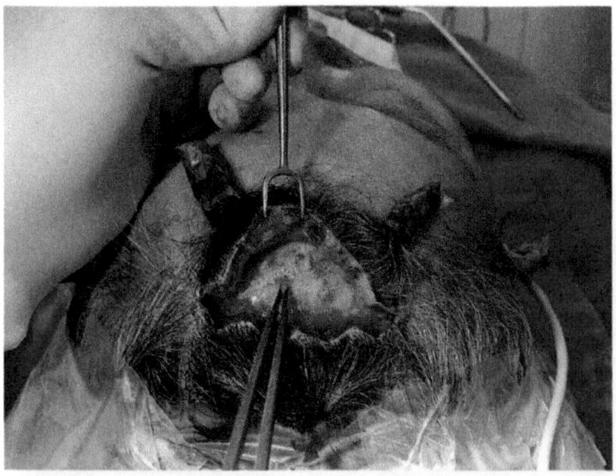

Fig. 4. Minicoronal browlift incision for skin excision and subgaleal dissection in the central forehead combined with typical endoscopic browlift through slit incisions for subperiosteal dissection.

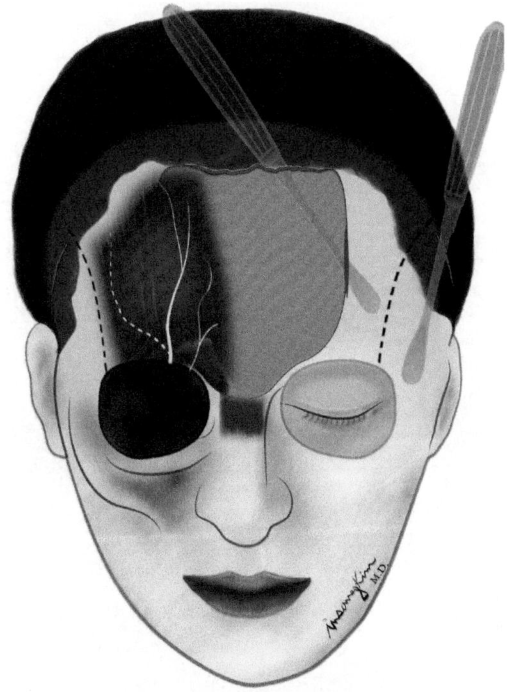

Fig. 5. A multiplane method of skin excision through trichophytic incision and central subgaleal dissection (*pink area*), and lateral endoscopic browlift (*blue area*). The central subgaleal pocket is connected to the lateral subperiosteal and temporal pockets through the slit incisions (*blue line*) from medial to lateral.

a softer or brighter appearance. The "surprised look" by overdissection of the medial brow is usually less of a problem in Asian patients.

SURGICAL TECHNIQUES

Detailed descriptions on operative techniques of endoscopic browlift are available in other articles. The authors' techniques are summarized next.

For most patients, five incisions are made within the hair-bearing scalp as follows:

- A single 15-mm midline incision.
- Bilateral 15-mm incisions at the level of the lateral canthus, which is variable medially or laterally according to the desired brow shape.
- Bilateral 25-mm incisions in the temporal area.

Through the midline and paramedian incisions, a periosteal elevator is inserted and the periosteum is raised in a blind fashion inferiorly to a level approximately 2 cm above the supraorbital rim. Temporal pocket is created right on the deep temporal fascia under direct vision and illuminated by a headlight.

Then a periosteal elevator is placed through the temple incision and the two dissection pockets, central and temporal, are connected from lateral to medial. Under endoscopic control, the temporal pocket is further dissected preserving the sentinel vein and other zygomaticotemporal veins and nerves as much as possible. The lateral orbital rim is dissected in the supraperiosteal or subperiosteal plane. It is important to release soft tissue attachments including the lateral orbital thickening down the lateral orbital rim, and inferiorly to the zygomatic body and medial zygomatic arch. The orbicularis oculi is the only muscle depressing the lateral brow, which is weakened with scissors.

Dissection proceeds further in the central pocket to the supraorbital rim. At the inferior end of the temporal ridge, release of the thickened temporal adhesion, which is the orbital ligament, is essential.

The periosteal and galeal attachments along the supraorbital rim are divided from lateral to medial before the supraorbital nerve is identified. If the dissection is sufficient, the yellow retro-orbicularis oculi fat is visualized.

Next the central portion of the brow between the two supraorbital nerves is addressed. The periosteum is divided, and the glabellar muscles are visualized within the overlying galeal fat pad. The first and largest muscle encountered is the corrugator supercilii. Medially the corrugator takes its origin at the superior orbital rim and superolaterally it interdigitates with the frontalis muscle. Transverse portion of the corrugator travels more inferiorly and horizontally, and oblique portion of the corrugator travels more superiorly. In the midline, the procerus fibers runs vertically, and the

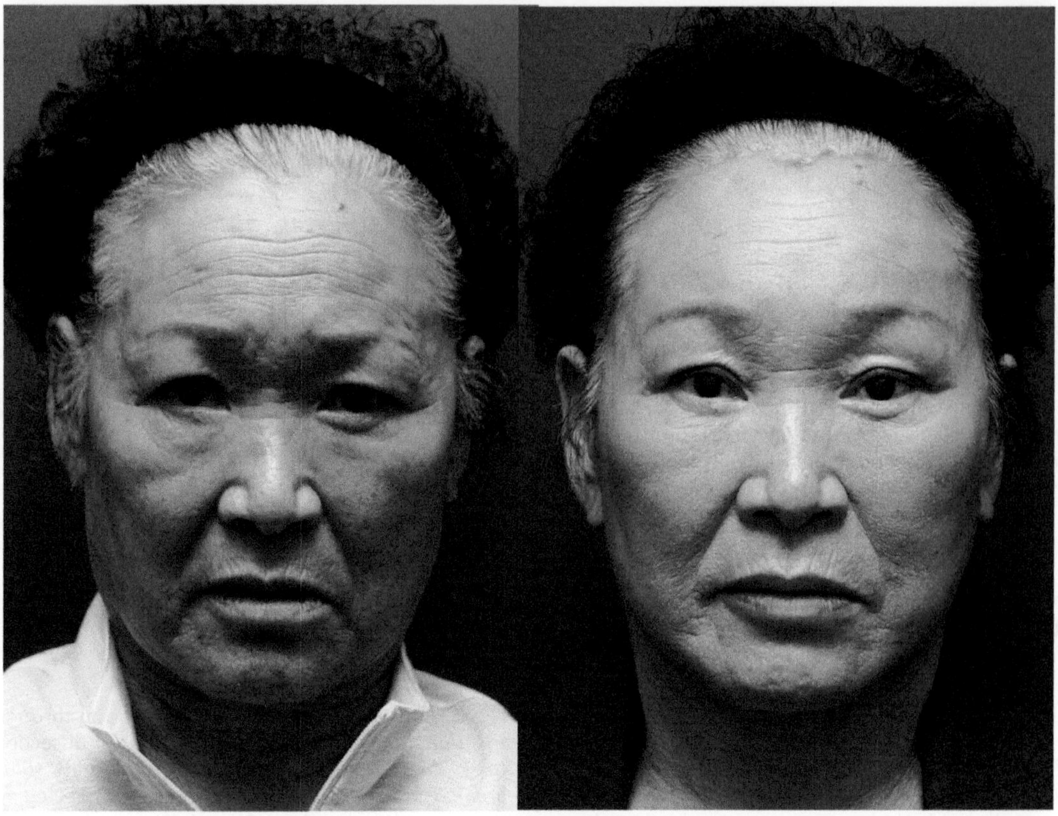

Fig. 6. A 73-year-old female patient who had endoscopic browlift combined with trichophytic skin incision and subgaleal dissection in the central forehead. Reduction of forehead height, improvement of forehead wrinkles, and brow elevation are noticed.

depressor supercilii rises vertically behind the origin of the corrugator.

Biting forceps or bipolar electrocautery are used to strip away the muscles. Bipolar cautery has advantages over endoscopic forceps to minimize bleeding, to reduce readhesion of muscles, and to reduce traction injuries of nerves. However, it should be used cautiously in the vicinity of superomedial orbital rim, because of the potential thermal conduction and subsequent indirect injury to the structures inside the orbit, such as trochlea and extraocular muscles.

While doing myotomies, small branches of the supratrochlear nerve are encountered along with small artery and veins. Injury to some of the supratrochlear nerve branches is inevitable, although related problems are usually clinically insignificant.

When the depressor supercilii and procerus muscles are stripped away, subcutaneous fat comes into view, and the surgeon should be cautious not to tear the thin skin. Lateral to these muscles, the light-colored medial orbicularis oculi muscle is seen behind the supratrochlear nerve fibers.

For the fixation, cortical bone tunneling with suture fixation method is used. In our experience, this method is strong and stable enough for most patients if the soft tissue release is adequate.

Absorbable 3–0 PDS (Ethicon, Inc, Somerville, NJ) suture was used for the fixation in the past; however, suture granulomas and inflammation during hydrolysis were observed frequently. Therefore now the authors use the 3–0 Vicryl (Ethicon, Inc) instead, although the soft nature of the suture material makes it difficult to insert it into the bone tunnel, requiring a guide nylon suture.

The Vicryl suture holds its tensile strength for approximately 2 to 3 weeks in tissue and is completely absorbed by hydrolysis within 56 to 70 days.[14] In our experience, the shorter duration of support by the Vicryl suture compared with the PDS did not correlate with the increased relapse or premature loosening of the fixation. It may be attributable to the readhesion of soft tissue to the bone, which is sufficiently firm to hold the tissue in place stabilizing the forehead skin flap before loosening of the Vicryl suture.

The Endotine device (Coapt Systems, Palo Alto, CA) is useful in cases with severe brow ptosis or with heavily folded skin where maximum fixation is required. However, dislocation of the device, palpability, sharp shooting pain on palpation, variable degree of discomfort, and a lack of lateral compared with central lift are reported as related problems.[15] The high cost of the device is the main disadvantage.

In Asians, combined forehead augmentation during forehead lift with fat injections is frequently required. However, possible dislodging of the engaged skin on the device during the forehead fat injection is another related problem with the Endotine device.

COMPLICATIONS OF ENDOSCOPIC BROWLIFT

Relapse

Revision rates of endoscopic browlift are known to be less than 1%.[1] Relapse in the early postoperative period is usually caused by a lack of soft tissue release. Ligamentous attachments along the supraorbital and lateral orbital rim must be released completely. Periosteum and galea must be released completely along the orbital rims identifying the retro-orbicularis oculi fat.

Even with inadequate soft tissue release, skin traction may simulate an elevation of the brow without substantial movement of deeper tissues at the glide plane level. If a browlift fails months after surgery, possible causes are loss of fixation or unfavorable anatomy of the patient.[16]

Some patients may have a stronger orbicularis oculi muscle activity, which depresses the brow laterally. The lateral orbicularis should be resected or denervated during browlift to weaken its action. Some patients may have absence of galeal reflection adhering the lateral brow to the lateral supraorbital rim, which causes absence of the galeal fat pad as a gliding plane over the lateral brow and congenitally downturned brows.

Some patients have loose and heavy skin. By endoscopic browlift with subperiosteal dissection, the heavy skin of these patients is not addressed effectively. Techniques incorporating some skin excision in the central or temporal incision sites may be considered instead or in combination with endoscopic browlift.

Nerve Injury

The most dreaded complication is injury to the temporal branch of the facial nerve. Temporary neuropraxia of the temporal branch of the facial nerve is the potential problem, which typically resolves completely in 6 months to 1 year. Permanent injury is extremely rare and its reported incidence is less than 0.1%.[16]

The most common complication after endoscopic browlift is postoperative paresthesia. Temporary neuropraxia from traction is a common side effect in the supraorbital and supratrochlear nerves. Inadvertent injury to supratrochlear nerve branches during corrugator resection is common. Patients are counseled preoperatively about the slow but steady recovery over 6 months to 1 year.

Some patients may experience severe forms of dysesthesias, such as shooting, burning pain, or intractable pruritus,[1] which can prolong for more than 1 year. However, typically the symptoms eventually subside, and to relieve the symptoms, prescription of neuromodulators, such as gabapentin, may be helpful.

Patients may experience headaches and significant nausea and vomiting immediately after surgery and for a few postoperative days in some patients, which arise from muscle tension, nerve traction, and stimulation of pressure points by surgical maneuvers or by the drain insertion. Antiemetic drug is routinely administered after surgery to mitigate the symptoms.

Alopecia

Hair follicle injury may be caused by incision, electrocautery, and tight sutures causing ischemia of hair follicles. Telogen effluvium may occur around the incision lines or distantly from the incision lines. Incisions should be made parallel to hair shafts and electrocautery should be judiciously used. Deep subcutaneous sutures and use of staples for closure of incisional wounds decrease the skin tension and decrease the chance of ischemia of hair follicles. Scar alopecia around an incision may be observed for 6 to 12 months, and in most cases hair regrows. Permanent alopecia may be managed with simple excision and/or hair transplantation.[1]

Hematoma

Hematoma may occur most frequently around the glabellar area, because of the supraorbital and supratrochlear vessels and resection of depressor muscles in the area. The sentinel vein in the temple also is a cause of hematoma.

Hematoma formation or significant bruising around the eyes and face with or without chemosis delays the early social recovery and decreases the patient's overall satisfaction with the surgery. Saline irrigation at the conclusion of surgery and routine postoperative Jackson-Pratt drain placement along the superior orbital rim are helpful to decrease hematoma and bruise.

Contour Irregularity

Uneven return of frown muscle action appears if the corrugator muscle resection has not been symmetric or incomplete. Balanced myectomy of corrugator rather than myotomy is recommended. Muscle resection using a bipolar cautery to prevent readherence of muscle fibers is helpful besides bleeding control.

When a large volume of corrugator is resected, a surface contour deformity may result. Contour irregularity is treated by fat grafting at the time of the surgery or later after surgery when it is revealed.

Lagophthalmos

Considering the typical age group of browlift patients, medical history should be carefully taken for the upper and lower eyelid procedures. Patients with a history of upper blepharoplasty or browpexy are at a higher risk of developing lagophthalmos from skin shortage. If lower lid laxity from prior lower lid surgeries is present, lagophthalmos adding to the preexisting lid laxity induces or aggravates the epiphora and exposure keratitis, requiring canthoplasty/canthopexy in some patients.

Brow Asymmetry

For brow asymmetry, bony configuration of forehead, temple and orbit, eyebrow shape, depressor and elevator muscle tone, and activity are involved. Excessive asymmetric activity of the frontalis, which can be a result of compensation for unilateral ptosis, can cause persistent postoperative brow asymmetry. Therefore thorough preoperative examination is required.

For the correction of brow asymmetry, stronger traction and fixation for the lower side is necessary. In contrast, periosteal release is limited for the higher side. Orbicularis oculi myotomy on the depressed brow side is helpful to elevate the brow to a more symmetric position.

If brow asymmetry exceeds 6 mm, unilateral forehead lift is recommended.[12] To symmetrize the asymmetrical brow shape, the fixation points may be placed asymmetrically.

Diplopia

Diplopia is a rare complication but it is severely distressing to the patient and the surgeon. Recently, Shim and colleagues[17] reported six cases of diplopia after endoscopic browlift. All the patients exhibited superior oblique palsy in the report.

In our institute, we have experienced five cases of postoperative diplopia over a 3-year period (2017–2020) for about 520 endoscopic browlift cases. Although diplopia was temporary and completely resolved for all patients, typically it persisted for a few months and it persisted for up to 4 months in one patient. Characteristically diplopia was aggravated on downward gaze during walking downstairs, reading books, and driving.

One of the most probable explanations is the indirect progression of thermal damage to the trochlea or extraocular muscles during myotomies or bleeding control using the electrocautery. Thermal injury to tissue is accompanied by inflammation, progressive thrombosis, or tissue damage of surrounding area. In this regard, electrocautery at the superomedial orbital rim should be done with extreme caution to avoid indirect thermal injury to the trochlea and/or to the superior oblique muscle or its fascia. However, direct structural damage, which can be permanent, is unlikely considering the range of surgical dissection and inaccessibility of the area.

In all of our cases with diplopia, bipolar electrocautery was used for myotomies of depressor muscles. Diplopia has not occurred in cases where only endoscopic forceps or scissors were used for myotomies.

There are other possible explanations for diplopia, such as hemorrhage or hematoma around the trochlea, which can arise from the excessive traction,[18] edema/swelling, or local anesthetic toxicity of extraocular muscles.

Reassurance to the patient and safety warning in driving and stair-walking is required.

SUMMARY

There are some anatomic and clinical differences for Asians, which should be considered carefully when doing forehead lift. The browlift is a powerful combination surgery for the double-eyelid surgery and the augmentation rhinoplasty, which are the most common aesthetic procedures in Asian countries. Endoscopic browlift is successful and beneficial in most Asian patients when it is indicated, and it can be done in a modified multiplane fashion for better outcomes in patients with thick and redundant skin.

CLINICS CARE POINTS

- Asians tend to have thicker skin and ligamentous attachments in forehead.
- For a better outcome of the double-eyelid surgery in Asians, if heavy soft tissue is

present in the infrabrow-eyelid area, it must be relieved by forehead lift beforehand.

- For a better outcome of augmentation rhinoplasty in Asians, forehead lift is considered beforehand to deepen the nasion, to define brow-tip aesthetic line more, and to relieve fullness of radix.
- Surgical dissection, skin excision, and fixation in forehead lift are individualized according to the desired brow shape, canthal tilt, and tissue laxity.
- There are rare but severe complications of endoscopic forehead lift, such as motor nerve paresis and diplopia, although they are temporary in most cases.

DISCLOSURE STATEMENT

The authors have nothing to disclose.

REFERENCES

1. Lee H, Quatela VC. Endoscopic browplasty. Facial Plast Surg 2018;34(2):139–44.
2. Rohrich RJ, Cho MJ. Endoscopic temporal brow lift: surgical indications, technique, and 10-year outcome analysis. Plast Reconstr Surg 2019; 144(6):1305–10.
3. Lam VB, Czyz CN, Wulc AE. The brow-eyelid continuum: an anatomic perspective. Clin Plast Surg 2013; 40(1):1–19.
4. Lu TY, Kadir K, Ngeow WC, et al. The prevalence of double eyelid and the 3D measurement of orbital soft tissue in Malays and Chinese. Sci Rep 2017; 7(1):14819.
5. Choi Y, Kang HG, Nam YS. Three skin zones in the Asian upper eyelid pertaining to the Asian blepharoplasty. J Craniofac Surg 2017;28(4):892–7.
6. Daniel RK, Kosins A, Sajjadian A, et al. Rhinoplasty and brow modification: a powerful combination. Aesthet Surg J 2013;33(7):983–94.
7. Gunter JP, Antrobus SD. Aesthetic analysis of the eyebrows. Plast Reconstr Surg 1997;99(7):1808–16.
8. Hwang SJ, Kim H, Hwang K, et al. Ideal or young-looking brow height and arch shape preferred by Koreans. J Craniofac Surg 2015;26(5):e412–6.
9. Jung GS, Chung KH, Lee JW, et al. Eyebrow position and shape favored by Korean women. J Craniofac Surg 2018;29(3):594–8.
10. De Cordier BC, de la Torre JI, Al-Hakeem MS, et al. Endoscopic forehead lift: review of technique, cases, and complications. Plast Reconstr Surg 2002;110(6):1558–68.
11. Ramirez OM. Endoscopically assisted biplanar forehead lift. Plast Reconstr Surg 1995;96(2):323–33.
12. Daniel RK. Endoscopic forehead lift. Aesthet Surg J 2001;21(2):169–78.
13. Niamtu J 3rd. The subcutaneous brow- and forehead-lift: a face-lift for the forehead and brow. Dermatol Surg 2008;34(10):1350–61.
14. Ethicon product catalog. Available at: https://www.jnjmedicaldevices.com/sites/default/files/user_uploaded_assets/pdf_assets/2020-12/ETHICON-Wound-Closure-Catalog-115681-190531.pdf. Accessed January 28. 2021.
15. Chowdhury S, Malhotra R, Smith R, et al. Patient and surgeon experience with the Endotine forehead device for brow and forehead lift. Ophthal Plast Reconstr Surg 2007;23(5):358–62.
16. Nahai F, Saltz R. Endoscopic plastic surgery. 2nd ed. St. Louis: Qualtiy Medical Publishing Inc.; 2008.
17. Shim JS, Chung JM, Kim TM. Diplopia following endoscopic brow lift. Eur J Plast Surg 2020. [Epub ahead of print].
18. Mavrikakis I, DeSousa JL, Malhotra R. Periosteal fixation during subperiosteal brow lift surgery. Dermatol Surg 2008;34(11):1500–6.

Lower Eyelid and Midface Rejuvenation
Suborbicularis Oculi Fat Lift

Han-Tsung Liao, MD, PhD[a,b,c,d,*]

KEYWORDS

• Lower eyelid surgery • Midface lift • SOOF lift • Fat grafting

KEY POINTS

- Knowing the anatomic structure of ligament, spaces, and superficial/deep fat compartment in lower eyelid/midface helps to ensure good outcomes.
- The theories of aging process and theirrelation to anatomic structure must be understood.
- Selection of surgical strategies is made according to the degree of the 4 aging factors: baggy lower eyelid, redundant of lower eyelid skin, fat deflation and malar descent.
- We provide a detailed description of the surgical method and effect of orbicularis oculi muscle and suborbicularis oculi fat lift in midface rejuvenation.

INTRODUCTION

The lower eyelid and midface are a central component of face. The degree of aging in these areas determines most of the "old" look of the patient. However, solving only lower baggy eyelid is no longer considered enough to achieve a "younger looking" visage and even results in a "tired looking" face if the patient has aging signs simultaneously coming from the midface or the lid–cheek junction, such as a tear trough deformity, nasojugal fold, malar fat ptosis, or midcheek groove. Although the lower eyelid and the midface are different anatomic structure, nowadays the current concepts consider they are aesthetic contiguous units, which should be managed simultaneously for optimal rejuvenation results[1].

FACIAL ANATOMY OF LIGAMENTOUS STRUCTURE, SPACE, AND FAT COMPARTMENT

The midcheek is defined from the upper limits of the lateral canthus level to the lower limits of the oral commissure level. It can be divided into a bony support part, on which soft tissue is supported by maxilla and zygoma (midface), and an unsupported part, which is include the orbital cavity (lower eyelid) and oral cavity (upper lip).[2] Although the anatomy of these areas is complex, recent cadaver studies and advanced tools have defined the anatomic structure of the middle cheek clearly, especially the ligamentous structures, spaces, and superficial/deep fat compartments. An understanding of the aging-related anatomic structure allows surgeons to adopt corresponding surgical strategies and also make the surgical outcome more predictable.

Ligament Structure

The ligamentous structure supports the soft tissues on top of the underlying bones or muscles.[3] The relaxation of the ligamentous structure causes these soft tissues to hang on the loosening ligament line. Furthermore, resorption of the bone to which the

[a] Division of Trauma Plastic Surgery, Department of Plastic and Reconstructive Surgery, Chang Gung Memorial Hospital, Linkou, Taiwan; [b] Craniofacial Research Center, Chang Gung Memorial Hospital, College of Medicine; [c] Chang Gung University, Taoyuan, Taiwan; [d] Department of Plastic Surgery, Xiamen Chang Gung Memorial Hospital, China
* Corresponding author. Division of Trauma Plastic Surgery, Department of Plastic and Reconstructive Surgery, Craniofacial Research Center, Chang Gung Memorial Hospital, College of Medicine, Chang Gung University, 5 Fuxing Street, Taoyuan 333, Taiwan
E-mail address: lia01211@gmail.com

Facial Plast Surg Clin N Am 29 (2021) 497–509
https://doi.org/10.1016/j.fsc.2021.06.003
1064-7406/21/

ligament is attached or soft tissue deflation or descent results in grooves or depressions in the related ligamentous structure, such as a tear trough deformity or groove (tear trough ligament), palpebral–malar deformity (orbital retaining ligament), midcheek deformity or groove (zygomaticocutaneous ligament), or nasolabial deformity (maxillary ligament). The ligamentous structure can divide the midcheek into the lid–cheek, malar, and nasolabial zones.[4]

Spaces

There are several spaces in the midcheek between the retaining ligament structures that provide gliding planes for movement of superficial over deep structures. Usually, no important structures pass within these spaces, which can be opened by blunt dissection easily in this avascular space. Three key spaces are identified and related for dissection in midface lift: the preseptal, prezygomatic, and premaxillary spaces.

Preseptal space

This inferior boundary of this space is palpebral origin of the orbicularis oculi muscle (OOM) medially and the orbicularis retaining ligament (ORL) laterally. The lateral boundary is the lateral orbital thickening. The floor and roof of the space is formed by the orbital septum and preseptal and pretarsal OOM, respectively. Hence, the space is located in the lower eyelid predominately. The space provides an ideal dissection plane for lower eyelid surgery.[2]

Prezygomatic space

The triangular prezygomatic space is bounded superiorly by the ORL, inferiorly by the zygomatic ligament, and posteriorly by the preperiosteal fat; the origins of zygomaticus major and minor and anteriorly by orbital part of OOM and suborbicularis oculi fat (SOOF). Around midpupil line, the upper ORL boundary merges with its lower boundary into the vertex of the triangular space. This space helps the surgeon to approach the malar area and to identify the SOOF structure for a midface lifting procedure.[5]

Premaxillary space

The premaxillary space is bounded superiorly by the tear trough ligament and the origin of the orbital part of OOM; inferiorly by maxillary ligament; medially by the nasal side wall, levator labii superioris alaeque nasi, and nasalis; and laterally by a 5-mm-wide loose areolar tissue. The floor is the levator labii superioris and the roof is the orbital part of the OOM. The release of the tear trough ligament and the origin of the palpebral and orbital OOM is considered to be adequate when the dissection is going into the premaxillary space and the levator labii superioris can be seen.[2]

Fat Compartment

The face can be layers of the following structures: skin, superficial subcutaneous fat, superficial musculoaponeurotic system, deep fat, and deep fascia or periosteum. The superficial subcutaneous fat and deep fat of the midcheek are highly compartmentalized. Rohrich and Pessa[6] performed a facial anatomic study by injecting methylene blue into facial soft tissue and tracked its diffusion by natural septa boundaries to further identify the different facial compartments. The midcheek superficial fat can be divided into orbital fat compartment, cheek fat compartment, and nasolabial fat (NLF) compartment. The inferior orbital fat of the orbital fat compartment is located in the lower eyelid with the lower boundary being the ORL. The NLF lies anteriorly to the deep medial cheek fat and medially to the SOOF; the superior border is the ORL. The superficial cheek fat compartment comprises the medial cheek fat, middle cheek fat, and lateral temporal cheek fat. The superficial medial cheek fat lies lateral to the NLF and the upper border is the ORL and the lateral orbital compartment. The inferior orbital fat, NLF, and superficial medial cheek fat are often referred to as malar fat. The deep fat, which lies below the superficial musculoaponeurotic system, is either anterior or posterior to the mimetic muscle. The deep fat includes the SOOF, which lies deep to the subcorbicularis oculi muscle with medial and lateral components and the deep medial cheek fat, which is located deep to the upper lip levators with a medial and a lateral part. The medial deep medial cheek fat lies deep and medial to NLF and the lateral deep medial cheek fat lies deep to the superficial medial cheek fat. The deflation and hypertrophy of different fat compartments with age causes the aged appearance in midface.[7,8]

AGING APPEARANCE OF LOWER EYELID AND MIDFACE

An aging lower eyelid/midface has characteristics of (1) wrinkles and redundant skin of lower eyelids (**Fig 1**A), (2) baggy lower eyelids (see **Fig 1**A), (3) vertical elongation of lid–cheek junction (see **Fig 1**C); (4) tear trough deformity/nasojugal fold (see **Fig 1**B); (5) a palpebral–malar groove (see **Fig 1**B); (6) a visible inferior orbital rim (see **Fig 1**A); (7) a V deformity or depression (see **Fig 1**B); (8) a midcheek groove with a Y deformity (see **Fig 1**D); (9) a midface descend; and (10) a prominent nasolabial fold (see **Fig 1**).[8]

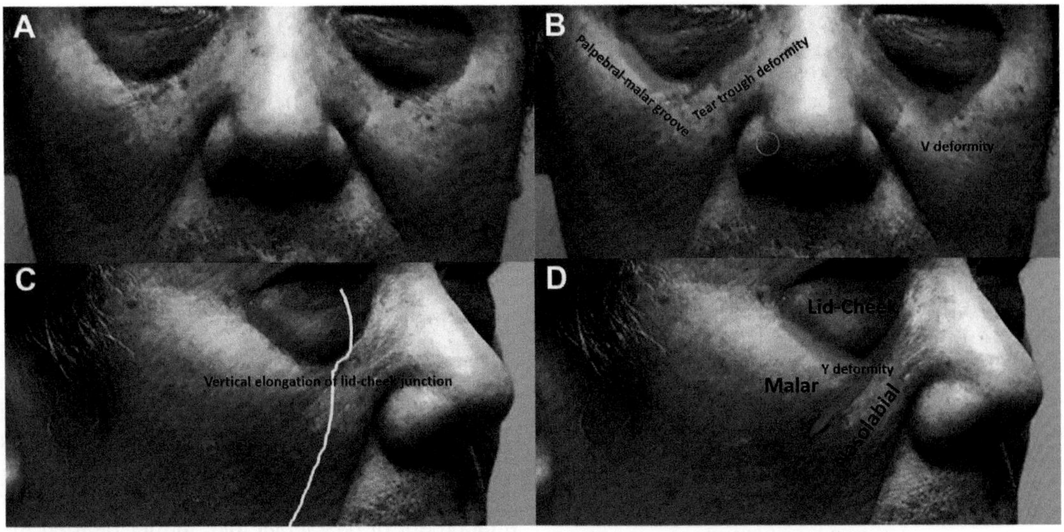

Fig. 1. Demonstration of the characteristics of aging.

Baggy Lower Eyelids

Protrusion of the orbital fat is caused by distension of the globe suspension system (capsulopalpebral fascia [CPF], Lockwood's suspensory ligament, lateral canthus tendon, and orbital septum), which results in the globe descend. The lowering globe further compresses the intraorbital fat with subsequent forward displacement.[9]

Tear Trough Deformity

The investigators found that a tear trough deformity is due to a lack of fat under the level of inferior arcus marginalis and the true osseocutaneous tear trough ligament between the palpebral and the orbital OOM.[10] The tear trough ligament is derived from maxillary bone and inserts into dermis through the intersection between the palpebral and the orbital OOM. The triangular gap formed by the junction of OOM, medial lip elevators, and levator alaeque nasi also contributes to tear trough formation.[11] The tear trough deformity may be congenital or be enhanced by aging process of maxillary bone resorption or the deep medial cheek fat deflation or malar fat decent.[10]

Palpebral Malar Groove

The origin of OOM is attached firmly medial to the inferior orbital rim to the level of the medial corneoscleral limbus. However, when it goes further laterally, the muscle is only attached to the rim indirectly by orbital retaining ligament.[12] The orbital retaining ligament is a bilamellar structure with a distance of 5 to 7 mm between the upper and the lower lamella. The distance narrows medially, lengthens centrally, and narrows again laterally until the ORL merges with the lateral orbital thickening. With the aging process, the tear trough deformity extends laterally along the laxity of the ORL and results in a palpebral malar groove. The deflation of inferior orbital fat and deep lateral cheek fat or descend malar fat causes the central V deformity with a hollowing of the central area under the deepening lid–cheek junction (tear trough and palpebral malar groove).[11] The Y deformity is formed if the V deformity connects from the tear trough depression medially to the midcheek groove laterally.[2] The Y deformity can separate the midcheek into the lid–cheek, malar, and nasolabial zones.

AGING THEORY OF THE MIDCHEEK

Before lower eyelid and midface surgery, surgeons should know the theory of aging. Five theories were postulated, including skin aging, ligament loosening, skeletal atrophy, gravitational soft tissue descent, and soft tissue volume loss.

Skin Aging

The process of aging skin is via both intrinsic and extrinsic factors.[8,13] The characteristics of intrinsic skin aging are the flattening between the interface of epidermis and dermis, the thinning of dermis and subcutaneous tissue, the loss of elasticity of skin owing to disorganization and reduction of elastic fiber, and the decreased number of fibroblast and its production of collagen types 1 and III.[13,14] The majority of external factors are owing to photoaging and tobacco consumption. Both factors can be independent or have a synergic negative effect on skin and causing premature wrinkles by production of intracellular reactive oxidative intermediates resulting in impairing the collagen synthesis, the production of abnormal elastin and proteoglycan, and thinning of the epidermis.[15] Furthermore, the repetitive dynamic expressive muscle contractions such as OOM cause fine and deep wrinkles around the periorbital region. Combining this pathophysiology, aging skin shows fine wrinkles or deep depressed rhytids with laxity and redundance of the skin. Because the skin of the lower eyelid is thinner than that of the midface, the appearance of aging lower eyelid skin is more obvious than aging midface skin.

Skeletal Aging

Several authors observe that the facial skeleton continues remodeling through life by comparing young and old facial bone morphology with 3-dimensional computed tomography scans. The outcome shows the posterior displacement of the maxillary, resorption of the superomedial and inferolateral orbital rim, and the pyriform aperture.[16–18] The resorption of this midfacial skeleton further pulls back the retaining ligament and results in greater depression or hollowing at the ligament area, such as the tear trough–nasojugal groove and its lateral extension palpebromalar groove by the tear trough–ORL or midcheek groove by the zygomaticocutaneous ligament. Furthermore, the midface soft tissue migrates inferiorly owing to the loss of support by the retruded maxillary. This process further enhances the aging appearance of nasal labial fold and V and Y deformities.

Ligament Loosening

The retaining ligament is considered to function as binding the soft tissue from the dermis to the underlining skeletal periosteum or the deep fascia of the parotid gland and masseter muscle. Mendelson and colleagues have described clearly the ligament structures (tear-trough–ORL, zygomaticocutaneous ligament) and spaces (preseptal, prezygoma, premaxillary) in between the structure and underlines 3 segments (lid–cheek, malar, and nasolabial) in the midface.[2,4] In youth, the ligament is firm, the space is tight, and it is able to hold and stabilize the soft tissue. However, the repeated facial expression and dynamic movement of the soft tissue in the midface with the intrinsic aging process loosens the ligament structure and makes the space expand. The weakness of the ligament structure and expansion space leads to soft tissue descent in the boundaries of these spaces. They also address that totally releasing the tear-trough–orbital retaining ligament is the key point to lift the ptotic midface structure.[19]

Gravitational Soft Tissue Descent

The concept of the midface lift surgery is based on the soft tissue descent owing to gravity at the midface region. In youth, the malar fat stabilizing the upper midface part can cover the inferior orbital rim and blend the lid–cheek junction. Owing to ligamentous attenuation and gravity effect, the malar fat loses support and descends inferiorly. This inferior migration leads to the unveiling of the inferior orbital rim and the obvious tear trough deformity, palpebral malar groove, a V-shaped deformity, and a Y deformity with the midcheek groove. The migrated malar fat, which is accumulated and hanging above the line of the muscular attachment of nasolabial fold, further deepen the aging appearance of nasolabial fold. However, the aging midface appearance can be reverted 10 to 15 years when the patient is in the supine position.[8] When the patient is lying down for the surgery, you can find the bulging baggy eyelid is decreased; the tear trough, palpebral malar depression, midcheek groove, and prominent nasolabial fold are diminished owing to the descended malar fat that drifts back to the original position and makes the hollowing groove appear full again. This phenomenon further supports the gravitational theory of midface aging.

Soft Tissue Volume Loss

The volumetric theory of facial aging is described by Lambros[20] and the concepts are gradually accepted and popularized recently through research by Rohrich and Passa.[20] The main concept is compartmentalization of the facial soft tissue. The aging of midface appearance results from the deflation or hypertrophy of different fat compartments. The fat tissue can generally be divided into superficial and deep compartments. The tear trough or nasojugal groove is resulted from the deflation of deep periorbital fat (medial SOOF) followed by the loss of smooth blend between the medial SOOF and the superior border of malar fat (the lid–cheek junction). The further deflation of deep medial cheek fat and deep medial cheek fat makes the ptosis of the superficial medial cheek fat and NLF and leads to elongation of the tear trough laterally, with a visible inferior orbital rim and V deformity of the central medial cheek hollowing and prominent of nasolabial fold. Hence, the volume augmentation over the deep compartment fat can greatly diminish the tear trough, V deformity, and nasolabial fold and create more fullness of the anterior cheek and smooth the lid–cheek junction.[6,21] These points further elucidate the importance of volumetric theory in midface aging. A trend of aging is found with the gradual deflation of the deep facial compartment and hypertrophy of some superficial compartments, especially the inferior part adjacent to the natural crease.

ALGORITHM FOR THE MANAGEMENT OF THE LOWER EYELID AND MIDFACE

The management of midface rejuvenation depends on the severity of aging in skin laxity, prominence of baggy eyelids, midface descent, and/or midface volume deficiency. The most important thing is to achieve a balance between surgeon's technique and the patient's expectation. Hence, there is no single surgical technique that can solve all kinds of lower eyelid and midface problem. The surgeon should examine the patient carefully, discuss the procedure and expectations in detail with the patient, and provide various techniques, listing their advantages and disadvantages. This author's choice of surgical technique is based the following 4 aging factors of the lower eyelid and midface, namely, lower baggy eyelids, Skin laxity or redundancy of the lower eyelid, superficial/deep fat compartment deflation, and midface decent.

Lower Baggy Eyelid

If the patient has the sign of bulging fat herniation over the lower eyelid, the appropriate surgical strategy is either fat transposition or fat excision with CPF/septum hernia repair, depending on the signs of aging.[22–24] Usually, for lower eyelid bulging fat without a tear trough deformity, visible inferior orbital rim, or V deformity, fat excision with a CPF hernia repair procedure is suffiecient.[9,24,25] However, if the tear trough deformity, V deformity/depression, or visible inferior orbital rim are noted, the bulging fat is transposed to cover and augment the depression area of these deformity. Be careful with patients who have psuedoherniation of the lower baggy eyelid, in which the fat is not herniated or excessive, and the appearance of psuedoherniation is due to the severe depression of tear trough deformity and V deformity and skeletonization of inferior orbital rim. In this situation, the fat cannot be excised or transposed to avoid a hollowed appearance of the lower eyelid postoperatively. Instead, CPF hernia repair to avoid herniation in the future with a midface lift and/or fat grafting over the depressed area to blend the lid–cheek junction results in better outcome. Transconjunctval or subciliary approach depends on the skin laxity of the lower eyelids. If the patient is young and the skin is tight, a transconjunctival is preferred. In contrast, if the patient is old and redundant skin of the lower eyelid is noted and a midface lift will be performed in the same time, a subciliary incision is preferred.

Skin Laxity or Redundant of Lower Eyelid

The thinnest skin is found over the lower eyelid; redundancy and laxity of skin at this region is more and more obvious as age advances. Hence, skin removal is inevitable for the recovery of the youthful lower eyelid. Although skin tightening by laser or chemical peeling can achieve a similar result, the effect is better in Caucasian than Asian patients. After laser resurfacing or peeling hyperpigmentation, which are commonly seen in Asian patients, dark circles and a sleepy appearance result. The skin removal should be both conservative to avoid postoperative ectropion and liberal enough to achieve the desired aesthetic outcome. There is no standard or scientific rule to judge how much skin should be removed to achieve the best aesthetic result and avoid complications. Fortunately, as surgeons perform more cases and gain more experience, they develop better judgment for the skin excision. In general, after midface lifting by medial and lateral SOOF anchoring to the inferior orbital and lateral orbital periosteum, respectively, the patient is instructed to open their eyes and mouth to their maximum degree, and the width of skin excision can be judged at this time. The cutting line of lower skin muscle flap is just above the upper margin of subciliary incision without forcefully pulling the lower skin–muscle flap upward. This is one reasonable method to judge skin removal. The other method is the pinch test, where the patient sits in front of surgeon and the surgeon uses the curved forceps to pinch the skin that needs to be removed from the incision line and see if it causes ectropion. The least width of pinched skin that does not cause ectropion is the skin you can remove.

Superficial and Deep Fat Compartment Deflation

Soft tissue volume loss and skeletal resorption over the midface lead to the pseudoptosis of malar fat. The inferior migration of malar fat owing to the loss of support by posterior displacement of the midface skeleton and deep medial cheek fat compartment deflation further elongate the tear trough depression from the medial to the lateral side of inferior orbital rim, which is named the palpebral malar groove. These structures make the inferior orbital rim skeletonized and visible, the V deformity or depression owing to central hollowing below the visible inferior orbital rim, and the Y deformity or depression if the depression along the zygomatico–cutaneous ligament is obvious.

Hence, the strategy to solve the volume loss is fat graft augmentation over the deep portion of midface fat compartment to give the support of the superficial fat compartment and fullness of the cheek and further fat graft contouring in the superficial fat compartment to blend the lid–cheek junction, depression, and any irregular area.

Midface Decent

A midface lift can correct the malar fat descent resulting from a gravitational effect and ligamentous laxity. The reposition of malar fat can diminish the visible of inferior orbital rim and V-deformity/depression and make the upper anterior cheek more fullness. The dissection planes are reported either via subperiosteal or preperiorsteal plane through the prezygomatic and premaxillary spaces. The subperiosteal approach has been often used previously owing to its simplicity and the concept of whole composite flap lift including the skin, OOM, SOOF, and the zygomatic major and minor muscle and lip levators.[26,27] Fixation can be either on the deep temporal fascia via a transtemporal approach or on lateral orbital thickening and inferior orbital rim via a subciliary approach. However, prolonged swelling, ecchymosis, and other possible complications are noted with this approach. The intact tight periosteum cannot be lifted until the distal inferior periosteum is released. Hence, an intraoral incision is sometimes needed, which in turn carries the risk of infection. Furthermore, because the ligament structure from the periosteum to the dermis remains intact, the deformity owing to the tear trough ligament and ORL complex cannot be resolved completely. During the animation and speech process, before the periosteum is firmly attached to the new position, the contraction of the levator lip, zygomatic major and minor muscles cause the midface descent to recur readily. With a clear understanding of the anatomic structure of the midface, preperiosteal dissection is now safer and more effective for the midface lift.[1,19,27–29] Preperiosteal dissection through the bloodless and predissected prezygomatic and premaxillary space can actually break the ligament connection from periosteum to dermis and separate the superficial component (skin, OOM, and SOOF) from the deep structure (lip levator muscle, zygomatic major and minor). Hence, the superficial components can easily slide upward on the deep structure. The superficial components will not be affected by contraction of the deep animated muscle. These advantages mean that it has less swelling and ecchymosis compared with subperiosteal dissection, and it can raise the malar fat more stably without being disturbed by deep muscle pulling.

Surgical Strategy According to the Four Aging Factors

Based on the 4 key aging factors, different surgical strategies can be adopted (**Table 1**). If the patient only has volume loss-predominant aging (type I aging) with tear trough groove and/or midcheek groove and nasolabial fold. The volume augmentation by autologous fat grafting or fillers is sufficient to solve patient's problem. In type II aging, some patients present with prominent and protruding baggy lower eyelids without skin aging, volume deflation, or malar descent. The bulging fat excision and/or CPF/septum hernia repair through transconjunctival approach is appropriate to correct the problem (**Fig 2**). However, with progression of aging process, the protruded intraorbital fat with tear trough and mild central V deformity owing to volume loss will happen. In this type III aging, skin is not redundant and aging malar is not descended, the herniated fat can be transferred to augment the tear trough deformity and central V deformity (**Fig 3**). Optional autologous fat grafting can be added to increase the fullness of anterior cheek if the herniated fat is not enough to fill the deformity. In type IV aging, the skin is redundant, the baggy lower eyelid is prominent, and the midface is drooping, but the volume deflation is not obvious. In this type of aging, a subciliary incision to excise the herniated fat with a CPF hernia repair procedure and SOOF lift is adequate to correct the deformity (**Fig 4**). On occasion, the baggy lower eyelid is not obvious and intraorbital fat removal is not required. The CPF is repaired to the arcus marginalis to prevent the anticipated herniation in the future. In type V aging, the skin is redundant, the midface is descending, and deflation is moderate to severe; fat transposition to cover the visible inferior orbital rim is indicated for obvious baggy lower eyelids with a simultaneous SOOF lift and autologous structural fat grafting (**Fig 5**). Alternatively, CPF repaired to the arcus marginalis is combined with a SOOF lift and autologous fat graft in type V aging, with not obviously herniated intraorbital fat. The choice of septum or CPF hernia repair depends on the strength of septum. If the septum is already degenerated into a thin, lax membranous structure, which is usually found in type IV or V aged patient, CPF hernia repair may be a good choice for preventing fat herniation in the future. If the septum structure is still strong and intact, septum hernia repair to arcus marginalis is first choice, usually in the type II or III (young) patient. However, the

Table 1
Surgical strategies according the aging type

	Type I	Type II	Type III	Type IV	Type V
Redundant lower eyelid skin	-	-	-	+	+
Baggy eyelid	-	+	+	+/–	+/–
Superficial/deep fat deflation	+	-	+	-	+
Malar fat descent	-	-	-	+	+
Surgical strategy	AFG or fillers	Bulging fat excision + CPF/septum hernia repair (transconjunctival incision)	1. Bulging fat excision + CPF/septum hernia repair and AFG 2. Fat transposition $\pm$ AFG (transconjunctival incision)	Bulging fat excision + CPF hernia repair and SOOF lift (subciliary incision)	1. Bulging fat excision + CPF repair and SOOF lift and AFG 2. Fat transposition + AFG and SOOF lift (subciliary incision)

Abbreviations: AFG, autologous fat grafting; SOOF, suborbicularis oculi fat; CPF, CPF.

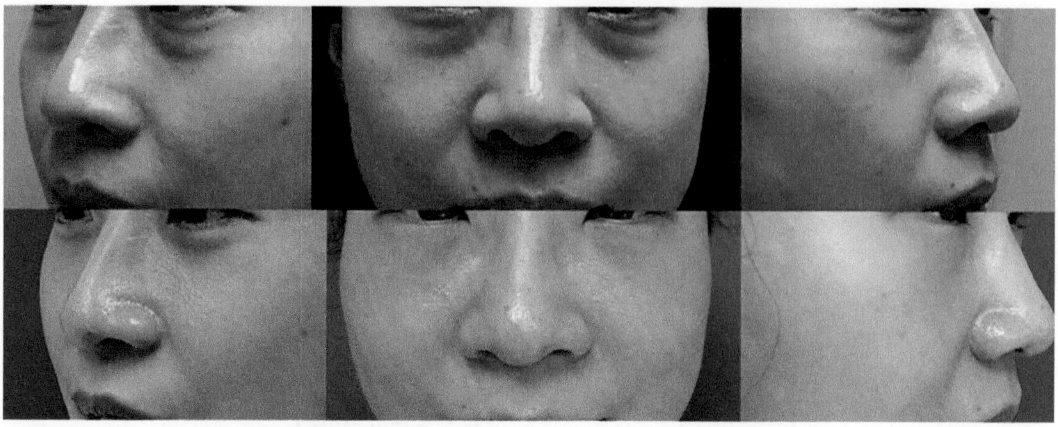

Fig. 2. The upper row figure showed the type II female who presented with medial and central herniated intraorbital fat with not obvious midface deflation. The lower row figure demonstrated the good outcome after transconjunctival approach with fat conservative excision and CPF repair.

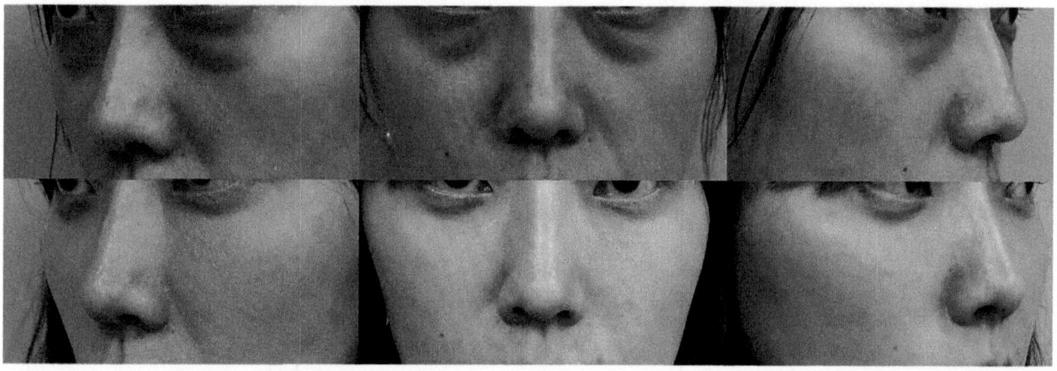

Fig. 3. The upper row figure shows a type III young female presented with prominent medial and central baggy lower eyelid with midface soft tissue deflation (tear trough, central V deformity, and midcheek groove). The lower part figures showed a good correction of the baggy lower eyelid and midface deficiency by transconjunctival approach with fat transposition to augment the tear trough and central V depression and additional autologous fat graft for a midface deficiency.

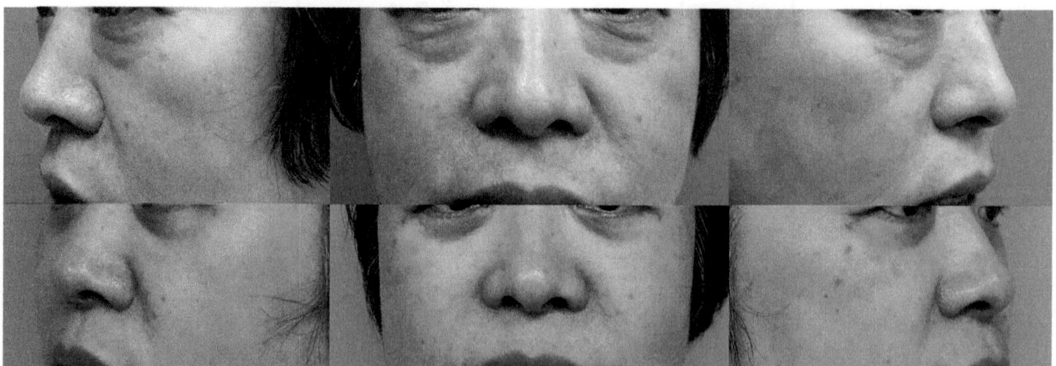

Fig. 4. The upper row figure shows a type IV deformity with redundant lower eyelid skin; the midface volume deficiency is mild. The herniated intraorbital fat is mild to moderate. Obvious lid–cheek junction and tear trough extended laterally to form a palpebral–malar groove owing to midface descent. The lower row figures demonstrate the good result from conservative fat removal and CPF hernia repair to strengthening the septum and SOOF lift to give the cheek more fullness and blend the lid–cheek junction. Shortening of vertical lid–cheek junction was also noted.

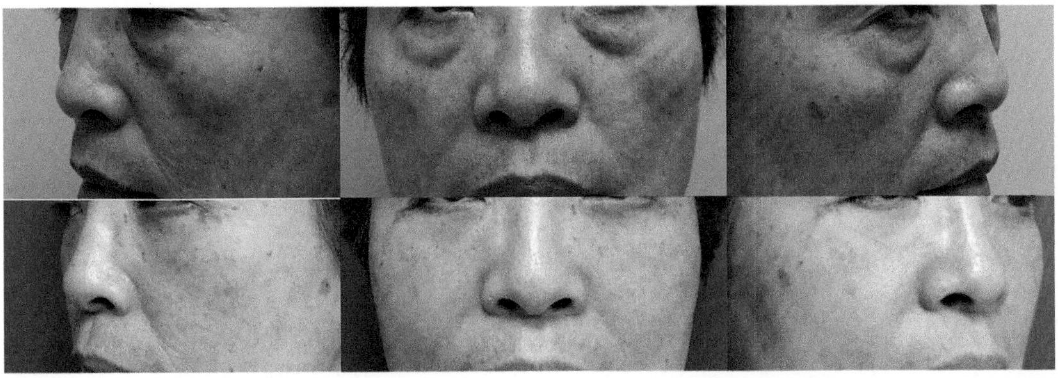

Fig. 5. The upper row figure shows a type V deformity with redundant lower eyelid skin, midface volume deficiency of the tear trough and palpebralmalar groove, V and Y deformities, midface descend, and prominent herniated intraorbital fat. The bottom row of figures demonstrates good results achieved by transposing intraorbital fat to the inferior orbital rim to blend the lid–cheek junction, a SOOF lift, and structure autologous fat grafting to give the cheek more fullness.

distinctions between the types are not always so straightforward. In addition, surgeon preference of surgical strategy differs. Surgeons should develop their own algorithm according to their experiences and adopt their familiar surgical strategies according to the aging types and the communications with patient.

AUTHOR'S PREFERENCE FOR A MIDFACE LIFT: OPERATIVE PROCEDURE FOR A SUBORBICULARIS OCULI FAT LIFT

The procedure usually can be performed under local anesthesia with infiltration of mixture of 10 mL 2% xylocaine and 1:100000 epinephrine. Usually, 4 to 5 mL is used at each side. A transcutaneous approach is used for lower blepharoplasty and midface SOOF lift simultaneously. A subciliary incision 1 to 2 mm from the eyelash following the lower eyelid curve with lateral extension following the crow's feet is made (**Fig 6**A). Then a skin flap is dissected for 5 to 7 mm to expose the pretarsal and preseptal OOM and then the interface between the pretarsal and preseptal OOM is opened (see **Figs. 6**B and C). Preservation of the pretarsal OOM is important for maintaining lower eyelid closure and support. Then the skin–OOM flap is elevated and dissected through the preseptal space down to the junction of the arcus marginalis and origin of the palpaberal OOM medially and the ORL laterally (see **Fig 6**D). Then, the origin of the OOM, tear trough ligament, orbital origin of the OOM, and the ORL are released completely and further dissected downward through the premaxillary space medially and the prezygomatic space laterally. The total release of the tear trough ligament is confirmed by seeing the floor of premaxillary space (levator labii superior) (**Fig 7**A). The prezygomatic space was dissection a further 1 cm lower than the ORL until the mobility of malar fat can be confirmed by forceps grasping the SOOF (see **Fig 7**B).

The key procedure for a successful midface lift is to completely release the tear trough–ORL ligament. Then the orbital septum is opened and the

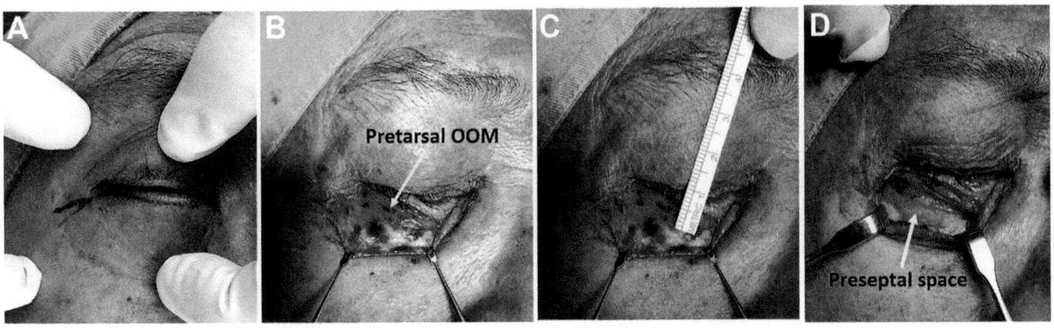

Fig. 6. The SOOF lift procedure (part 1). (*A*) Incision marking. (*B, C*) Skin flap elevation to expose the pretarsal and preseptal OOM. (*D*) Dissection of the preseptal space.

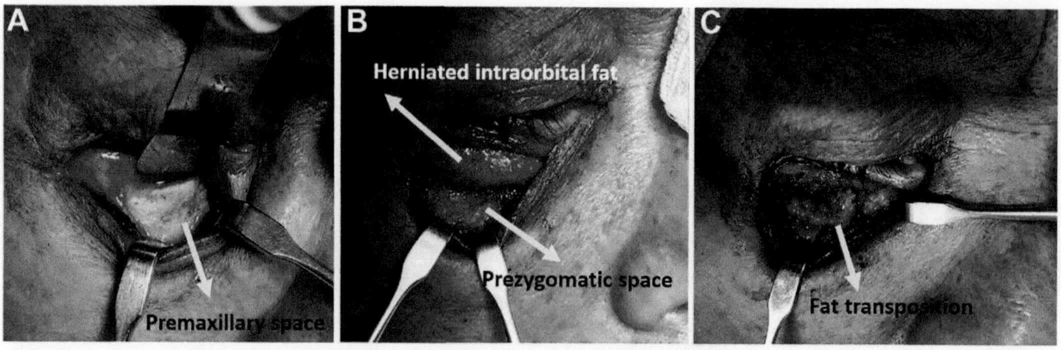

Fig. 7. The SOOF lift procedure (part 2). (*A*) Premaxillary space dissection. (*B*) Prezygomatic space dissection. (*C*) Intraorbital fat transposition to the inferior orbital rim.

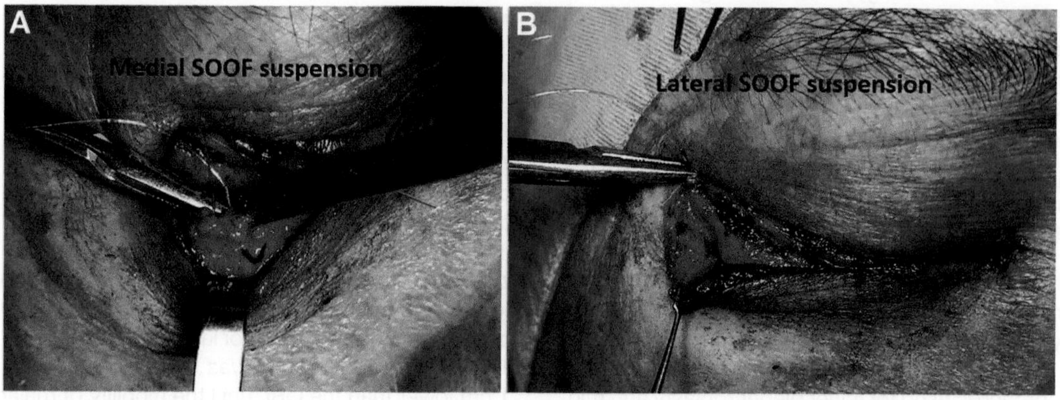

Fig. 8. The SOOF lift procedure (part 3). (*A*) Medial SOOF suspension. (*B*) Lateral SOOF suspension.

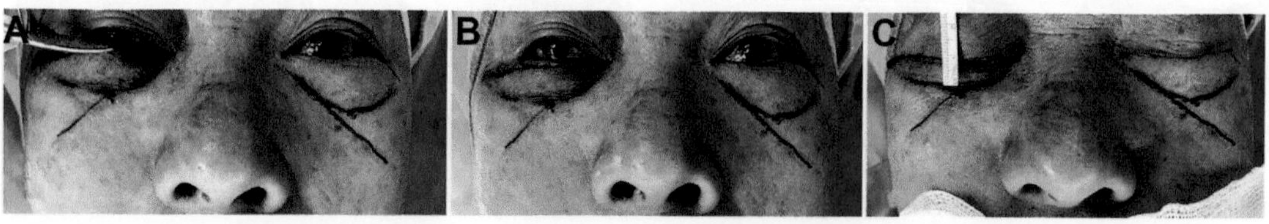

Fig. 9. The SOOF lift procedure (part 4). (*A*) Excessive skin–OOM flap excision. (*B*, *C*) The tear trough–ORL mark was raised by one-half compared with the contralateral side after SOOF a lift.

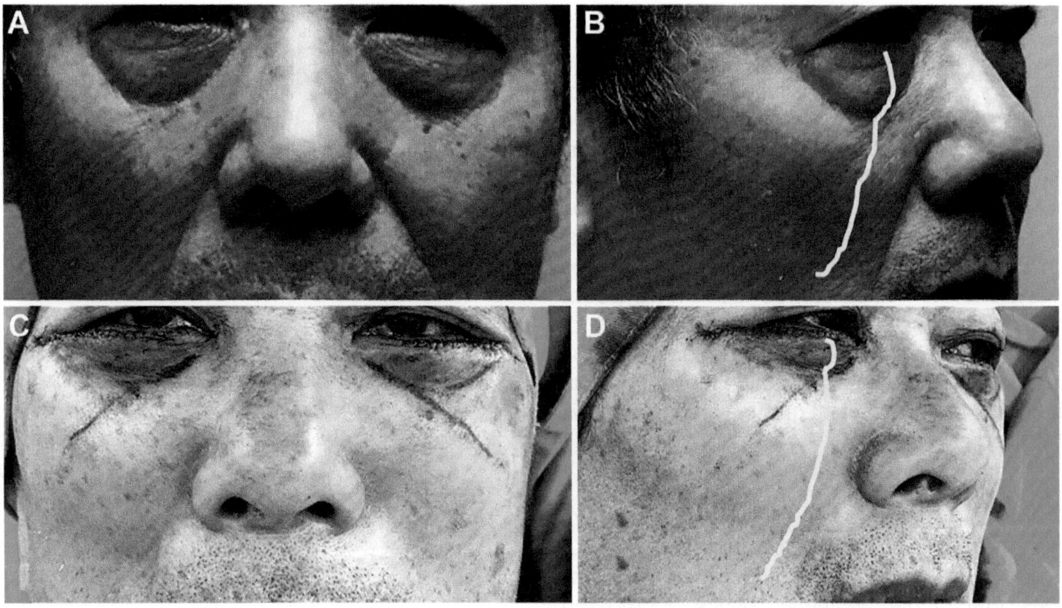

Fig. 10. Immediate outcome of a SOOF lift. (*A*) Before and (*C*) after the SOOF lift. Long and short lid–cheek junction (*B*) before and (*D*) after the SOOF lift with greater fullness of anterior cheek shown after fat transposition and SOOF lift.

herniated medial, central, and lateral intraorbital fat is either excised conservatively with CPF hernia repair or transposed to the inferior orbital rim for augmentation of the depressed area and cover the visible inferior orbital rim (see **Fig 7**C). For conservative fat excision, the CPF is repaired to the arcus marginalis with 5-0 Vicryl to form a new, strong septum and avoid intraorbital fat herniation. For fat preservation and transposition, the intraoribtal fat was transposed to tear through deformity and inferior orbital rim with fixation with 5-0 Vicryl to the floor of premaxillary and prezygomatic space. Then the SOOF lift is performed by fixed the medial SOOF to preperiosteal fat at lateral part of inferior orbital rim in a superolateral direction and lateral SOOF to periosteum at the lateral orbital thickening area in a vertical direction (**Figs. 8**A and B). Then the excess skin and OOM are excised conservatively when the patient's mouth and eyes are opened to the maximum degree. The OOM is vertically suspended and fixed to the lateral orbital thickening again and the skin was closed in layers (**Fig 9**A). After lifting the SOOF with 1 eye, it can be noticed that the tear trough–ORL mark is significantly raised by one-half, and more lower eyelid skin can be removed than with the traditional OOM suspension technique (see **Figs. 9**B and C). The vertical lid–cheek distance can be improved dramatically and shortened with fullness of anterior midcheek accordingly (**Fig 10**).

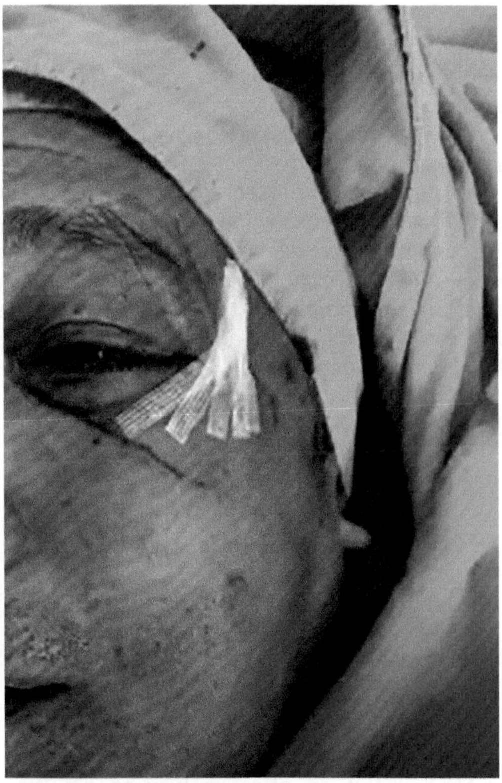

Fig. 11. The midcheek is further taped by the 3M Steri-Strips for support.

POSTOPERATIVE CARE

The midcheek is further supported by the 3M Steri-Strips for 7 days and the stiches are removed at 7 days postoperatively (**Fig 11**). The lower eyelid scar massage starts 1 week after stich removal. The massage is gently pushed along the subciliary incision from medial to lateral side and press on the lateral extension scar against the lateral orbital rim with some forces for 1 minute and 3 to 5 times a day. The Steri-strips can be taped for 2 weeks and the scar massage should take 3 months, or at least until the scar is soft and not obvious. The patient is informed not to massage the fat transposition side or structural fat grafting area before it is stabilized at 3 months.

SUMMARY

A graded approach to solve the aging lower eyelid/midface according to the different aging type provides predictable aesthetic results. Compared with the traditional OOM suspension, the SOOF lift can remove more redundant lower eyelid skin in a safer way. The herniated intraorbital fat can be transposed to cover the inferior orbital rim and augment the tear trough deformity and/or central V deformity if the protruded fat is enough. Fat preservation or conservative excision with CPF hernia repair is indicated if it is pseudoherniation or protruding without the sign of midface fat deflation or descent, respectively. A SOOF lift with a preperiosteal approach is an effective method to bring the drooping malar fat to cover visible inferior orbital rim and blend the lid–cheek junction. The complete release of the tear trough–ORL ligament and preperiosteal dissection through the premaxillary and prezygomatic spaces are key steps in a successful SOOF lift. Autologous fat grafting can be a touch-up procedure to further augment the deflation of deep fat compartment and contouring the superficial irregularity.

CLINICS CARE POINTS

- Preseptal, prezyogmatic and premaxillary spaces are avscular planes which are easily to be opened by blunt dissection.
- Releasing the tear-trough–orbital retaining ligament is the key point to lift the ptotic midface structure.
- SOOF lift is an effective way to lift the descend midface for covering the V and Y deformity and provide a safer way for removing more redundant lower eyelid skin.
- Autologous fat grafting is a touch-up procedure to further augment the midface deficiency.

REFERENCES

1. Stevens HP, Willemsen JC, Durani P, et al. Triple-layer midface lifting: long-term follow-up of an effective approach to aesthetic surgery of the lower eyelid and the midface. Aesthetic Plast Surg 2014;38(4):632–40.
2. Wong CH, Mendelson B. Facial soft-tissue spaces and retaining ligaments of the midcheek: defining the premaxillary space. Plast Reconstr Surg 2013;132(1):49–56.
3. Alghoul M, Codner MA. Retaining ligaments of the face: review of anatomy and clinical applications. Aesthet Surg J 2013;33(6):769–82.
4. Mendelson BC, Jacobson SR. Surgical anatomy of the midcheek: facial layers, spaces, and the midcheek segments. Clin Plast Surg 2008;35(3):395–404. discussion 393.
5. Mendelson BC, Muzaffar AR, Adams WP Jr. Surgical anatomy of the midcheek and malar mounds. Plast Reconstr Surg 2002;110(3):885–96. discussion 897-911.
6. Rohrich RJ, Pessa JE. The fat compartments of the face: anatomy and clinical implications for cosmetic surgery. Plast Reconstr Surg 2007;119(7):2219–27.
7. Gierloff M, Stohring C, Buder T, et al. Aging changes of the midfacial fat compartments: a computed tomographic study. Plast Reconstr Surg 2012;129(1):263–73.
8. Buchanan DR, Wulc AE. Contemporary thoughts on lower eyelid/midface aging. Clin Plast Surg 2015;42(1):1–15.
9. de la Plaza R, Arroyo JM. A new technique for the treatment of palpebral bags. Plast Reconstr Surg 1988;81(5):677–87.
10. Wong CH, Hsieh MKH, Mendelson B. The tear trough ligament: anatomical basis for the tear trough deformity. Plast Reconstr Surg 2012;129(6):1392–402.
11. Stutman RL, Codner MA. Tear trough deformity: review of anatomy and treatment options. Aesthet Surg J 2012;32(4):426–40.
12. Muzaffar AR, Mendelson BC, Adams WP Jr. Surgical anatomy of the ligamentous attachments of the lower lid and lateral canthus. Plast Reconstr Surg 2002;110(3):873–84. discussion 897-911.
13. Farkas JP, Pessa JE, Hubbard B, et al. The Science and Theory behind Facial Aging. Plast Reconstr Surg Glob Open 2013;1(1).

14. Varani J, Spearman D, Perone P, et al. Inhibition of type I procollagen synthesis by damaged collagen in photoaged skin and by collagenase-degraded collagen in vitro. Am J Pathol 2001;158(3):931–42.
15. Yin L, Morita A, Tsuji T. Skin aging induced by ultraviolet exposure and tobacco smoking: evidence from epidemiological and molecular studies. Photodermatol Photoimmunol Photomed 2001;17(4):178–83.
16. Paskhover B, Durand D, Kamen E, et al. Patterns of change in facial skeletal aging. JAMA Facial Plast Surg 2017;19(5):413–7.
17. Shaw RB Jr, Kahn DM. Aging of the midface bony elements: a three-dimensional computed tomographic study. Plast Reconstr Surg 2007;119(2):675–81. discussion 682-3.
18. Mendelson B, Wong CH. Changes in the facial skeleton with aging: implications and clinical applications in facial rejuvenation. Aesthetic Plast Surg 2012;36(4):753–60.
19. Wong CH, Mendelson B. Midcheek lift using facial soft-tissue spaces of the midcheek. Plast Reconstr Surg 2015;136(6):1155–65.
20. Lambros V. Observations on periorbital and midface aging. Plast Reconstr Surg 2007;120(5):1367–76.
21. Ramanadham SR, Costa CR, Narasimhan K, et al. Refining the anesthesia management of the face-lift patient: lessons learned from 1089 consecutive face lifts. Plast Reconstr Surg 2015;135(3):723–30.
22. Chen J, Zhang T, Zhu X, et al. Fat repositioning with a combination of internal fixation and external fixation in transconjunctival lower blepharoplasty. Aesthet Surg J 2021;41(8):893–902.
23. Majidian Ba M, Kolli Bs H, Moy Md RL. Transconjunctival lower eyelid blepharoplasty with fat transposition above the orbicularis muscle for improvement of the tear trough deformity. J Cosmet Dermatol 2021. [Epub ahead of print].
24. Parsa AA, Lye KD, Radcliffe N, et al. Lower blepharoplasty with capsulopalpebral fascia hernia repair for palpebral bags: a long-term prospective study. Plast Reconstr Surg 2008;121(4):1387–97.
25. Parsa FD, Miyashiro MJ, Elahi E, et al. Lower eyelid hernia repair for palpebral bags: a comparative study. Plast Reconstr Surg 1998;102(7):2459–65.
26. Quatela VC, Antunes MB. Transtemporal midface lifting to blend the lower eyelid-cheek junction. Clin Plast Surg 2015;42(1):103–14.
27. Chatel H, Hersant B, Bosc R, et al. Midface rejuvenation surgery combining preperiosteal midcheek lift, lower blepharoplasty with orbital fat preservation and autologous fat grafting. J Stomatol Oral Maxillofac Surg 2017;118(5):283–8.
28. de la Plaza R, de la Cruz L. Lifting of the upper two-thirds of the face: supraperiosteal-subSMAS versus subperiosteal approach. The quest for physiologic surgery. Plast Reconstr Surg 1998;102(6):2178–89.
29. De La Plaza R, Valiente E, Arroyo JM. Supraperiosteal lifting of the upper two-thirds of the face. Br J Plast Surg 1991;44(5):325–32.

Incisional Blepharoplasty for the Asian Eye

Hyung Min Song, MD, MS*, Khanh Ngoc Tran, MBBS, FRACS

KEYWORDS

• Asian blepharoplasty • Supratarsal crease • Epicanthoplasty • Orbital fat • Eyebrow

KEY POINTS

- Soft tissue work in blepharoplasty is even more critical in Asians than in whites, for long-term sustainability of the eyelid crease.
- During the evaluation, always check the position of the eyebrows. When compensated brow ptosis is anticipated, a preoperative explanation of the relationship between eyebrow change and the double eyelid should be given.
- Orbital fat manipulation is an important consideration in double eyelid surgery, because the shape and height of double eyelids change according to the amount of orbital fat.

INTRODUCTION

Asian blepharoplasty (double eyelid surgery, supratarsal crease [STC] surgery) refers to the surgical creation of a STC in Asians and should be distinguished from the traditional upper blepharoplasty for persons of Western descent.[1] The most obvious characteristic of the Asian eyelid is the absent or very low lid crease and fuller upper eyelid. White eyelids typically have a double eyelid; however, Asian eyelids can be categorized into 3 types: single eyelid, low eyelid crease, and double eyelid.[2] The presence, position, and depth of the STC are highly variable in Asians (usually lower than that of whites, in the range of 2–5 mm from the eyelid margin), and it is absent in approximately 50% of Asians.[1] Most single eyelid eyes look swollen and heavy because of the prominent fat pads and the thick skin of the upper eyelid, and the pupils are less exposed, making the eye appear less fresh (**Fig. 1**A).

THE ANATOMIC DIFFERENCE FROM WHITES EYELID

Less Cantilevered Orbital Bone/Transition Area

The most important anatomic differences between the eyes of whites versus Asians are that the former possess cantilevered orbital rims with deeper set globes, which results in the formation of an eyelid crease.[2] In contrast, Asian eyes typically have shallow orbits and supraorbital ridges with minimal to no cantilevering, resulting in there being a transition area between the orbital rim and STC, a characteristic that is absent in non-Asians[1,2] (**Fig. 2**A). The white upper lid crease coincides with the orbital rim, whereas the Asian crease typically arises a fair distance below the orbital rim, owing to the flat supraorbital ridge. If a double eyelid is made without a transition area in Asians, it becomes a very unnatural and awkward double eyelid, not a Westernized eye (see **Fig. 2**B, C).

Epicanthal Fold

Although the epicanthal fold can manifest across a range of ethnicities, it is a major anatomic feature of the Asian upper eyelid, occurring at frequencies of 60% to 90%.[3] The epicanthus represents a remnant fibromuscular volume on the upper medial canthal region, that often obscures the medial canthus and is characterized by vertical skin shortage and tension that causes difficulty in horizontal skin folding.[2,3] It acts as a major hindrance to double eyelid formation in Asian blepharoplasty.[3]

Drsong4u Aesthetic Plastic Surgery Clinic, 2-3 Floors, Dosandaero 37gil 6, Gangnam-gu, Seoul 06026, Korea
* Corresponding author.
E-mail address: drsong4u@naver.com

Facial Plast Surg Clin N Am 29 (2021) 511–522
https://doi.org/10.1016/j.fsc.2021.06.004

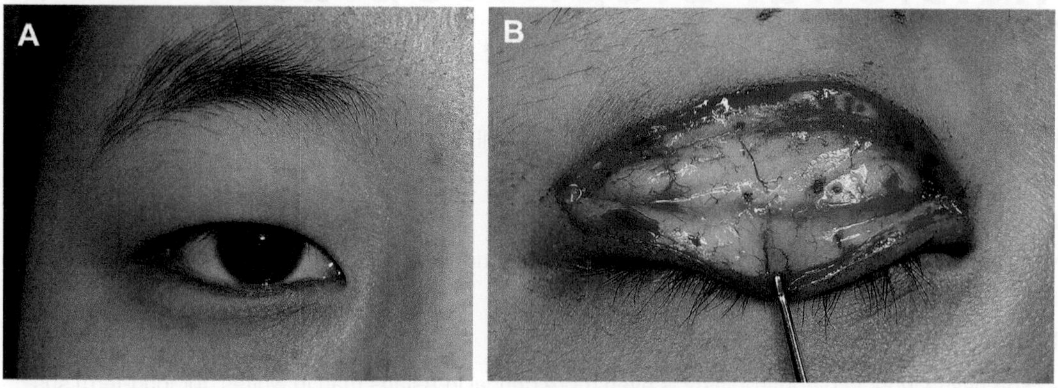

Fig. 1. Single eyelid (*A*) and thick skin and bulky fat pad (*B*). As the Asian upper eyelid contains more prominent preseptal fat resulting in greater lid fullness, the soft tissue work in blepharoplasty is even more diverse and essential in Asian eyes than in white eyes, in order for there to be sustainability of the eyelid crease. Asian eyelid surgery is not about Westernizing the eyes. Instead, the goal is to create a lid crease configuration that resembles the natural-appearing crease found in other Asians. Asian blepharoplasty should therefore be performed specifically following the orbital anatomy of Asians. This article details the incisional method of blepharoplasty to create natural-appearing creases for Asians with single eyelids.

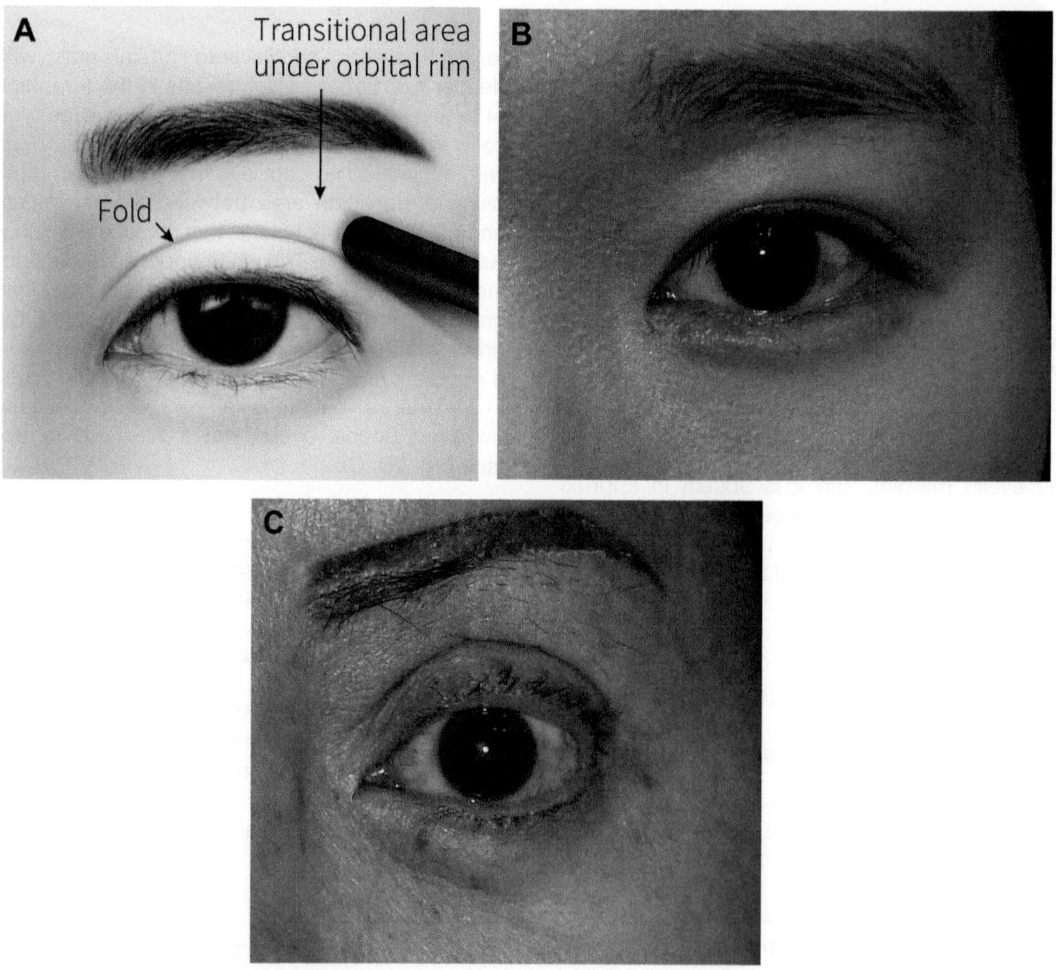

Fig. 2. (*A*) The transition area under the orbital rim is situated above the crease fold in the typical Asian eye. (*B*) A natural STC with a transition area present. (*C*) There is an unnatural STC located directly below the orbital rim without a transition area present, which appears very awkward.

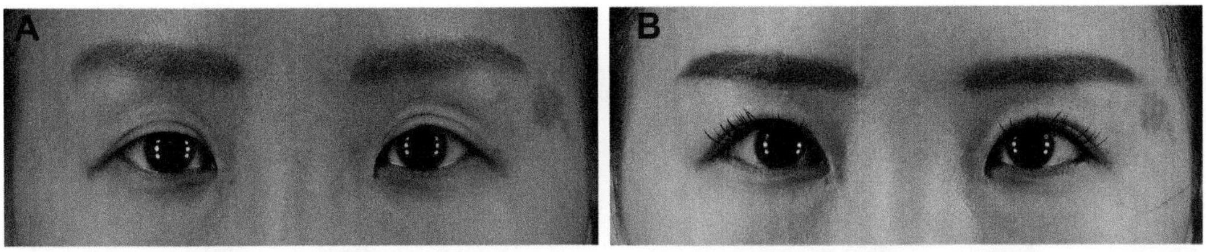

Fig. 3. Failed upper lid incisional blepharoplasty with loss of the crease line in the setting of severe epicanthal folds (*A*) and following revision surgery with epicanthoplasty (*B*). The severe epicanthal fold is a common cause of STC loss.

Although the standards of the beauty of the East and the West differ, even in the East there is a preference for large eyes with narrow interepicanthal distance.[4] Because the epicanthal fold can cause telecanthus, epicanthoplasty is often used to make a larger horizontal palpebral fissure.

In patients with severe epicanthal fold, surgery results are often poor if double eyelid surgery alone is performed without also addressing the epicanthus. Severe epicanthal folds are a common cause of STC loss after blepharoplasty (**Fig. 3**), as the preexisting vertical skin tension caused by the epicanthal fold acts as tensional stress on the newly formed surgical crease.[3] In such cases, medial epicanthoplasty is necessary in order to remove this vertical tension, so that the newly created STC cannot be easily undone.

Orbital Fat Pads

The amount of orbital fat (OF) varies according to race and gender. There may also be variability between an individuals' left and right eye (**Fig. 4**). OF manipulation is very important because the shape and height of the double eyelids will change according to the amount of OF present. In Asians, OF protrudes downward to the front of the tarsal plate in an apronlike configuration, resulting in a somewhat puffy upper eyelid. The OF sac is a very delicate structure, and numbness of the upper eyelid following blepharoplasty may represent injury to the terminal branches of the ophthalmic division of the trigeminal nerve, which pass superiorly and superomedially to the fat in the upper OF compartments.[5] To prevent this complication, the OF sac should not be removed along with the fat. Instead, the OF sac must be opened to remove the fat. As the OF pad is a critical structure that forms the glide zone between the levator aponeurosis (LA) and the septum, one should be very conservative with its removal.[2,5] Excessive fat removal is not recommended in Asian blepharoplasty, as it may result in unsightly deep folds, extra creases, or a sunken appearance.

Fibrous Structures on the Levator Aponeurosis

When the orbital septum is incised, the OF pads that herniate outwards are retracted to reveal within the lower aspect of the preaponeurotic fat space a transverse fibrous structure, that differs from the higher positioned Whitnall ligament, called the lower-positioned transverse ligament (LPTL) (**Fig. 5**A).[6] This loose yet inelastic structure spans superomedially to inferolaterally and can be identified in almost every upper eyelid.[6] Although Whitnall ligament is located on the levator muscle, the LPTL is located just above the fusional line between the orbital septum and the LA.[6,7] Within the preaponeurotic space, the superficial expansion of the LA turns up around the LPTL to become the orbital septum. Hence, contraction of the levator muscle leads to retraction of the preaponeurotic fat against the LPTL.[6] The LPTL is thought to determine the low position of the preaponeurotic fat and can restrict the vertical width of the palpebral fissure.[6,7]

In addition, on the upper aspect of the smooth, fascia-like surface of the LA, fatty tissue as well

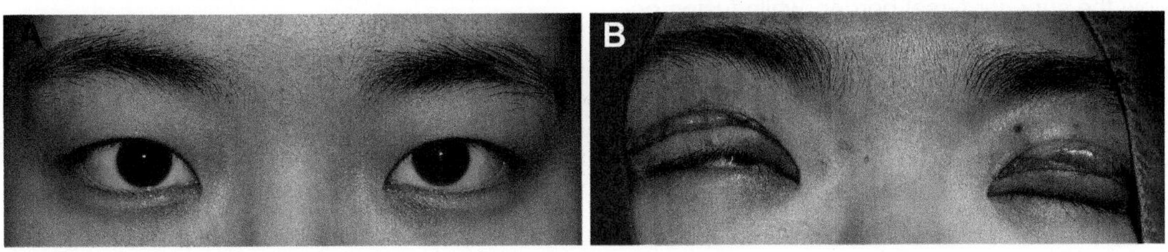

Fig. 4. There is a difference in OF volume between the left and right eye (*A, B*). Note that the more OF there is, the puffier the upper eyelid will appear.

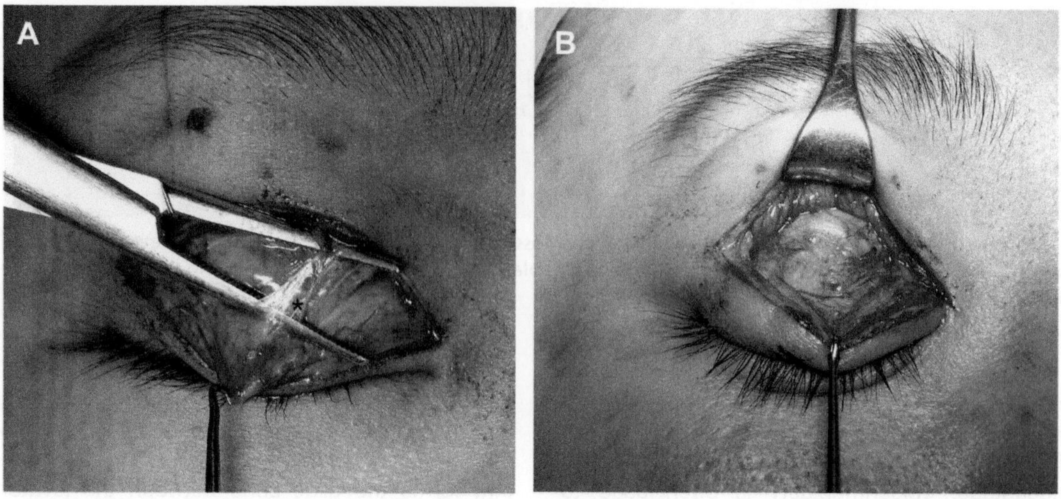

Fig. 5. (*A*) The LPTL (*) and (*B*) fibrous web bands on the LA. These 2 structures can restrict the vertical width of the palpebral fissure and should be released.

as tough fibrous web bands are commonly encountered (see **Fig. 5**B).[7] These fibrous web bands between the LA and OF can limit movement of the LA, which is a cause of eye-opening limitation. Subclinical and mild blepharoptosis can be corrected by releasing these fibrous bands without manipulating the LA or the Müller muscle.[7,8]

THE ANATOMICAL PRINCIPLES OF THE DOUBLE EYELID

Although the exact mechanism remains controversial,[2,8] the STC is thought to be an anatomic invagination of the eyelid skin along the superior tarsal border. There exists a superficial fascia beneath the orbicularis oculi muscle (OOM), which fuses with the LA at the lid fold level. Below the fold, these fasciae remain fused or "conjoined." Thus, the external fold in the upper eyelid reflects this internal fascial union (conjoined fascia) and is not simply a result of the LA inserting into the skin.[8]

The STC is formed at the fused height of the orbital septum and LA. This fusion can be as low as the lower anterior portion of the tarsus near the lid margin. In the Asian single eyelid, the point of fusion of the orbital septum to the LA is typically below the superior tarsal border, while fusion occurs above the superior tarsal border in whites (see **Fig. 4**).[1,8] A pretarsal fat pad is also identified in the Asian single eyelid. Because of these anatomic differences, in the Asian eye the STC is smaller or is entirely absent and creates an impression of a fuller and thicker eyelid.[8]

The eyelid consists of 5 main layers (superficial to deep).[2,8] In order to surgically create an STC, a component of the anterior lamella (skin and OOM) must be fixated to an element of the posterior lamella (LA).[1,2] Asian double eyelid surgery removes the factors (descending preaponeurotic fat pad, pretarsal fat) that prevent the bonding between the 2 lamellas, as well as creates adhesion between them[1,2] (**Fig. 6**).

PREOPERATIVE CONSULTATION FOR BLEPHAROPLASTY

The preoperative consultation begins with a thorough assessment and documentation of the patient's eye condition, including whether

- The eyes and eyebrows are left to right symmetric
- The eyes are of equal size
- The power to open the eyes the same
- One eye is more protruded than the other
- There is a difference in the degree of skin sagging

The most common sources of lid asymmetry include the following[3]:

- A difference in brow position
- Inequality of globe exposure
- Orbital position posture
- Lateral canthus posture
- Lower lid posture

Brow and eyelid asymmetry is common in patients being evaluated for upper eyelid blepharoplasty.[9] Because there is a high likelihood that asymmetric eyes will have asymmetric STC after blepharoplasty, the patient should be made aware of the preexisting eye and facial asymmetry beforehand. Preoperative

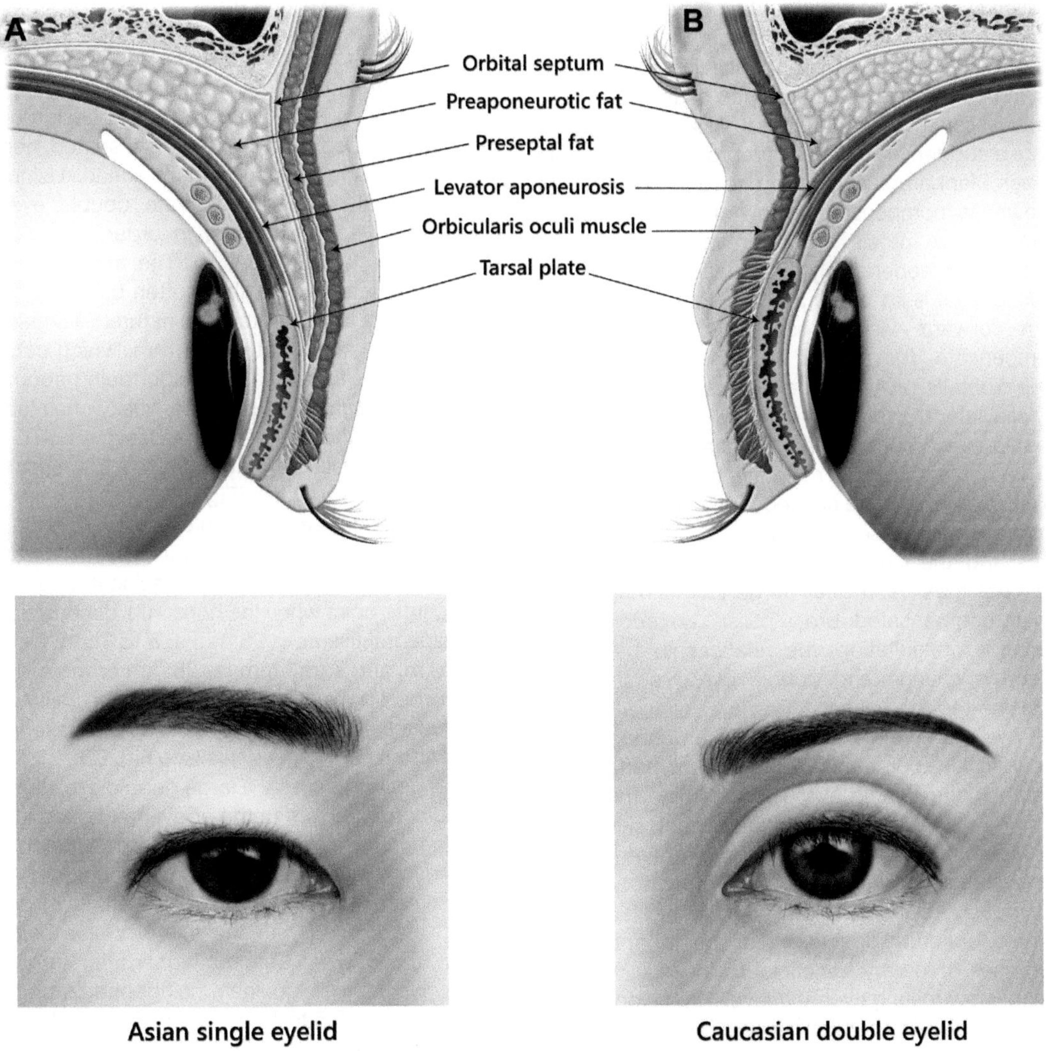

Fig. 6. Anatomic differences between the eyelids in Asians and whites. Asian single eyelid shows the fusion of the orbital septum to the LA below the superior tarsal border (*A*), whereas fusion is above the superior tarsal border in whites (*B*).

counseling includes discussions about the anatomic limitations imposed by their periorbital tissues and expected surgical results.

The next step is to determine the patient's desired height for the double eyelid crease. The level and shape of the planned eyelid fold should be individualized and discussed with each patient. Teenage patients usually request a lower, more subtle double eyelid crease. As they get older, they generally want a larger double eyelid.

The peak level of growth in the vertical dimension of the palpebral fissure is reached between ages 10 and 13 years, that of the intercanthal distance between ages 14 and 16 years, and that of the horizontal dimension of the palpebral fissure between ages 17 and 19 years.[10] Therefore, for teenage patients, a nonincisional method is recommended first, reserving the option of having a higher crease created with the incisional method later, if desired. If a patient's skin is thick, the eye-to-eyebrow distance is close, or the eye size is small, a small crease looks more natural than a high crease. However, if the patient's skin is thin and the eye size is large, the STC height can be tailored to the patient's desire. In the case of single eyelids, oftentimes the eyes will have a swollen appearance. Whether this is due to the fat or the thickness of the skin itself, or a combination, should be identified.

THE IMPORTANCE OF EYEBROW POSITION IN ASIAN UPPER BLEPHAROPLASTY

It is extremely important to check the brow position during the initial evaluation. Postoperative crease asymmetry is a common source of dissatisfaction after double eyelid surgery, occurring in 13% to 35% of Asian blepharoplasties.[11] Eyebrow asymmetry is one of the common causes. It is not unusual for even youthful East Asians to experience a sudden drop in their eyebrow position after upper blepharoplasty, owing to a phenomenon known as compensated brow ptosis. Compensated brow ptosis is a prevalent condition whereby, preoperatively, the patient's eyebrow resting level is so ptotic and low that it interferes with forward vision, especially laterally. To compensate, the patient subconsciously forces their frontalis muscles into constant contraction, to alleviate the obstructed view.[12,13] Following double eyelid surgery, the forehead muscles are no longer required to maintain their contraction to aid with vision, and consequently, the eyebrows drop. In such cases, the distance between the eyes and the eyebrows reduces, and the eyes may not look fresh after surgery.[12,13] Therefore, when compensated brow ptosis is recognized during a consultation, the relationship between eyebrow change and double eyelid should be explained to the patient.

If there is eyebrow asymmetry, an endoscopic brow lift is recommended first. If not performed together, the double eyelid incision line must be designed a little higher, or additional skin and OOM should be excised, in order to prevent double eyelid asymmetry following surgery.

In young Asians, an endoscopic brow lift is performed for natural double eyelids, not for antiaging purposes. It is very beneficial to those with profoundly low resting eyebrow levels with significant frontalis activated compensated brow ptosis. If the distance between the eyes and eyebrows is narrow, the creation of double eyelids will appear unnatural. However, if the eye-to-eyebrow distance is increased by performing an endoscopic brow lift, it is then possible to create a fresher and more pleasing STC. To evaluate for this preoperatively, lift the eyebrows by hand. If by doing so the hidden double eyelids are exposed and their size and shape are also good, an endoscopic brow lift alone may be sufficient without the need for double eyelid surgery (**Fig. 7**).

DESIGN OF DOUBLE EYELID SURGERY

The design of the double eyelid crease is the most important step in surgery. Postoperative asymmetry is usually caused by poor surgical design and markings. To begin, have the patient seated, holding a mirror and looking straight ahead. Using a bougie, create and demonstrate double eyelid creases of varying heights, in order to choose the desired size (**Fig. 8**A, B). The measurement of the double eyelid height is often based on the experience of the operator. The natural STC height in East Asians is about 6 to 8 mm, which corresponds to the tarsal plate's height being about 6 to 8 mm.[1,2] High STC are anatomically unsuitable for Asians. If the height of the designed STC is higher than the tarsal plate's height, it is easy to create secondary ptosis (**Fig. 9**A, B).[12]

To introduce the authors' criteria, the height of the incision line for making natural STC in Korean women is 6 mm from the point passing through the pupil center point when the horizontal dimension of the palpebral fissure is 25 mm, 6.5 to 7 mm for 26 to 27 mm, and 7 to 8 mm for 28 mm or more. The outer orbital rim's height determines the maximum height of the double eyelid, and the STC's maximum height should not exceed this (see **Fig. 8**B).

If the goal is to create a large double eyelid, add an additional 0.5 mm to the abovementioned incision line. In the case of men who want small STC or inside creases, the incision line's height is at approximately 5 to 6 mm. In the setting of protruded eyes, even with the same crease height design, the STC will become higher after surgery. Therefore, the incision line's height should be set a little lower by 0.5 to 1 mm, depending on the degree of eye protrusion.

The horizontal dimension of the palpebral fissures is another factor that influences the STC height design. In the case of small eyes, if the incision line is set high, it will create the optical illusion of smaller and swollen-appearing eyes (**Fig. 10**A, B). Before concluding the crease design, turn the lid over and measure the height of the tarsus. Measuring the height of the tarsus will confirm that the planned pretarsal skin segment height aligns with the tarsal height.

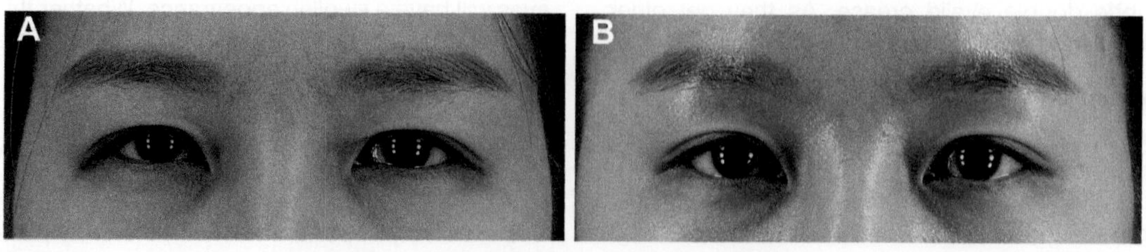

Fig. 7. Endoscopic brow lift. Preoperative photograph (*A*) and postoperative photograph at 7 months (*B*).

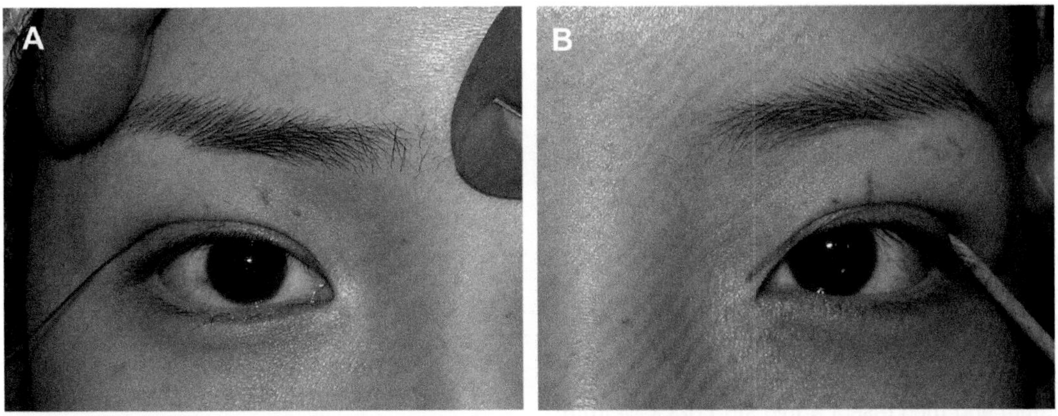

Fig. 8. Determination of STC height using a bougie. Show the patient several double eyelid crease heights and have them decide (*A*). The height of the outer orbital rim determines the maximum height of the double eyelid. STCs should not exceed this height (*B*).

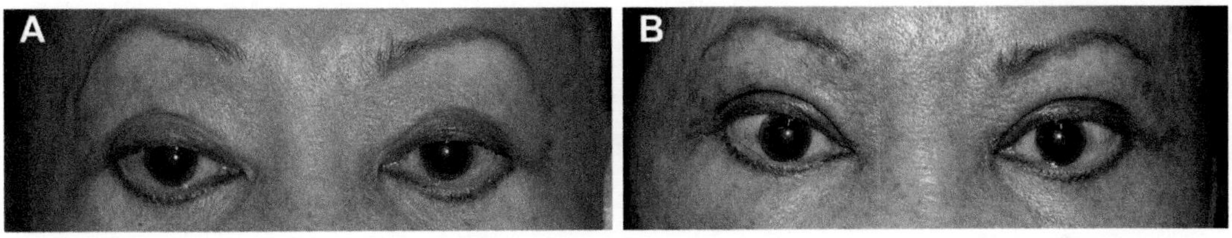

Fig. 9. Secondary ptosis because of high fold. Preoperative photograph (*A*) and postoperative photograph (*B*). Ptotic eyes were corrected by lowering the STCs during revision surgery.

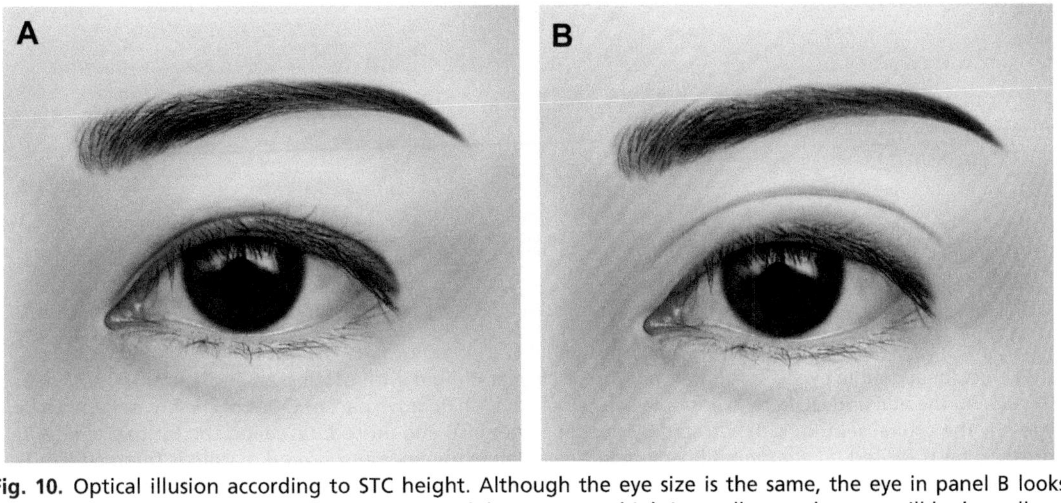

Fig. 10. Optical illusion according to STC height. Although the eye size is the same, the eye in panel B looks smaller than the eye in panel A. If the upper eyelid crease is set high in small eyes, the eyes will look smaller.

SURGICAL TECHNIQUE OF INCISIONAL SUPRATARSAL CREASE SURGERY

Lidocaine 1% mixed with 1:100,000 epinephrine at a volume of approximately 2 cc is injected along the design line, avoiding visible blood vessels. Ten minutes are allowed to transpire for optimal hemostasis. Using a no. 15 blade, an incision is made along the designed line (**Fig. 11**A, B). When the OOM is exposed, retract using skin hooks and incise the OOM horizontally with a Bovie electrocautery device (Bovie Medical Corporation, Clearwater, FL, USA) to reveal the orbital septum directly beneath. Fully expose the orbital septum and then resect a thin strip of OOM from the lower skin flap by aligning it with the outer skin edge (see **Fig. 11**C). The authors caution the operator to be conservative with this step, as excessive OOM trimming can result in an incisional scar that is hollow along the length of the incision line and remains severe. Hemostasis is performed.

Next, the orbital septum is incised horizontally to expose the fat pad. The OF is detached along the smooth upper surface of the LA (see **Fig. 11**D, E). Remove any LPTL fibers and separate the fibrous bands between the septum surface and LA, up until Whitnall ligament. Manipulation of the OF should be performed from outside the orbital septum, to avoid damaging the LA. When removing OF, it is first injected with local anesthetic; the segment to be removed is then clamped using a fine mosquito clip, cut with scissors, and cauterized with the Bovie for hemostasis. The clamp is then partially eased and the fat edge recauterized to prevent late bleeding. In double eyelid surgery, the medial OF pad is hardly touched. Only a limited segment of herniated middle OF that has descended below the upper border of the tarsal

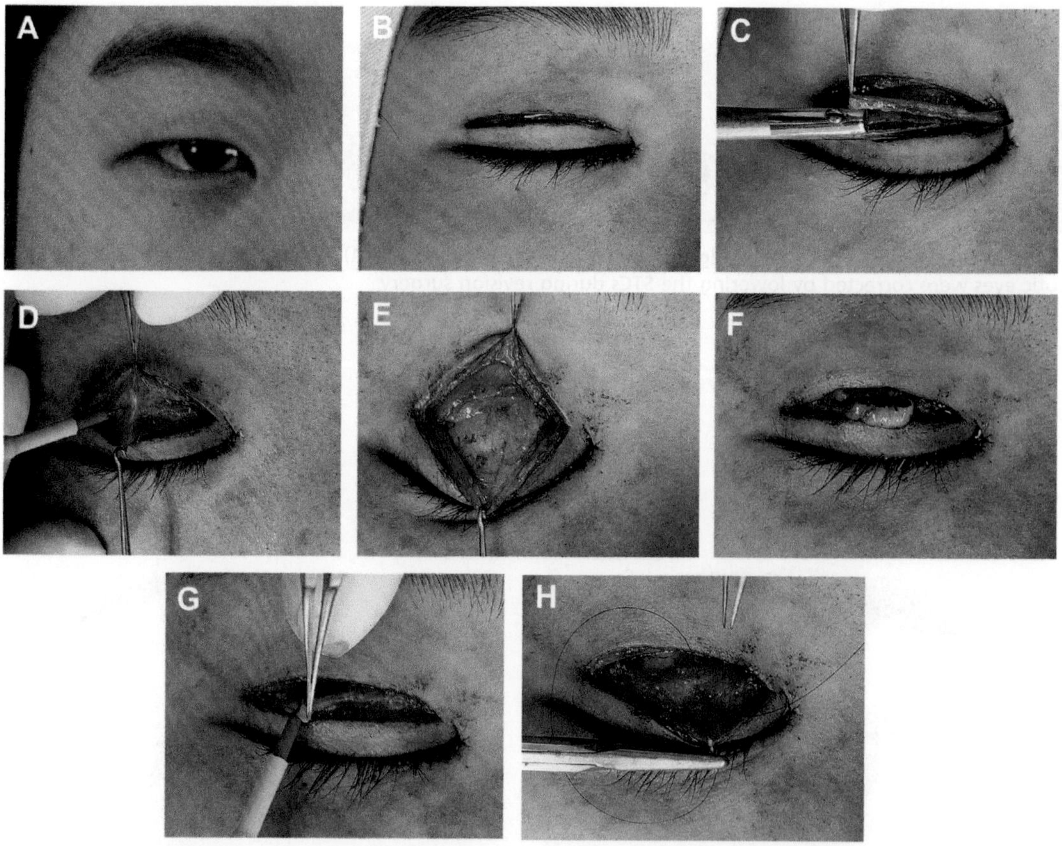

Fig. 11. Incisional double eyelid surgery technique. A 20-year-old girl with ptotic eyes and epicanthus (*A*). Make an incision in the skin and OOM to expose the orbital septum (*B*). Remove part of OOM of the lower flap in a belt shape (*C*). The orbital septum is penetrated by needle cautery (*D*) and incised, revealing the fat pad and LA (*E*). Any excess fat is excised (*F*). Redundant conjoined tissue below the aponeurosis end margin is trimmed (*G*). The lower flap's muscle and dermis are fixed to the tissue (conjoined fascia), where the orbital septum and LA meet (*H*).

plate is removed (see **Fig. 11**F). In instances whereby the eyelid has a slightly sunken appearance because of an insufficient medial fat pad, a segment of middle fat pad can be transposed to fill in that region, thereby creating a smoother and fuller double eyelid.[14]

Following OF removal, the patient's eyes are opened to determine pupil symmetry. If left-to-right symmetry is not correct, additional LA advancement is performed. Once pupil symmetry is confirmed, remove any redundant conjoined tissue below the LA's end margin and fix the lower flap into place (see **Fig. 11**G).

There are various ways to fix the lower skin to make an STC:

- Directly to the tarsal plate
- To the tissue (conjoined fascia) where the orbital septum and LA meet (see **Fig. 11**H)
- To the tarsal plate and the LA together

The eyes are briefly opened during lower skin flap fixation (internal fixation) to check for crease height symmetry. Next, the upper skin flap is redraped, and any excess skin overlapping the lower flap is excised. In single Asian eyelids, skin sagging is often present; hence, extra skin is often excised. After adjusting both eyes to optimize symmetry, if it is observed that the skin is thin and the operator is concerned about triple folds, or in cases of reoperation, then permanent fixation sutures may be placed in a buried manner between the inferior incision flap dermis, the LA, and the upper flap dermis, at 3 points (the level of the mid pupil, lateral and medial limbus). To lower the double eyelids, reduce the amount of resected skin and OOM, set the incision line low, or fix it lower than the tarsal plate's upper edge. To make the double eyelid shallower rather than deep, fix it to the LA without firmly fixing it to the tarsal plate, or reduce the number of fixation sutures.

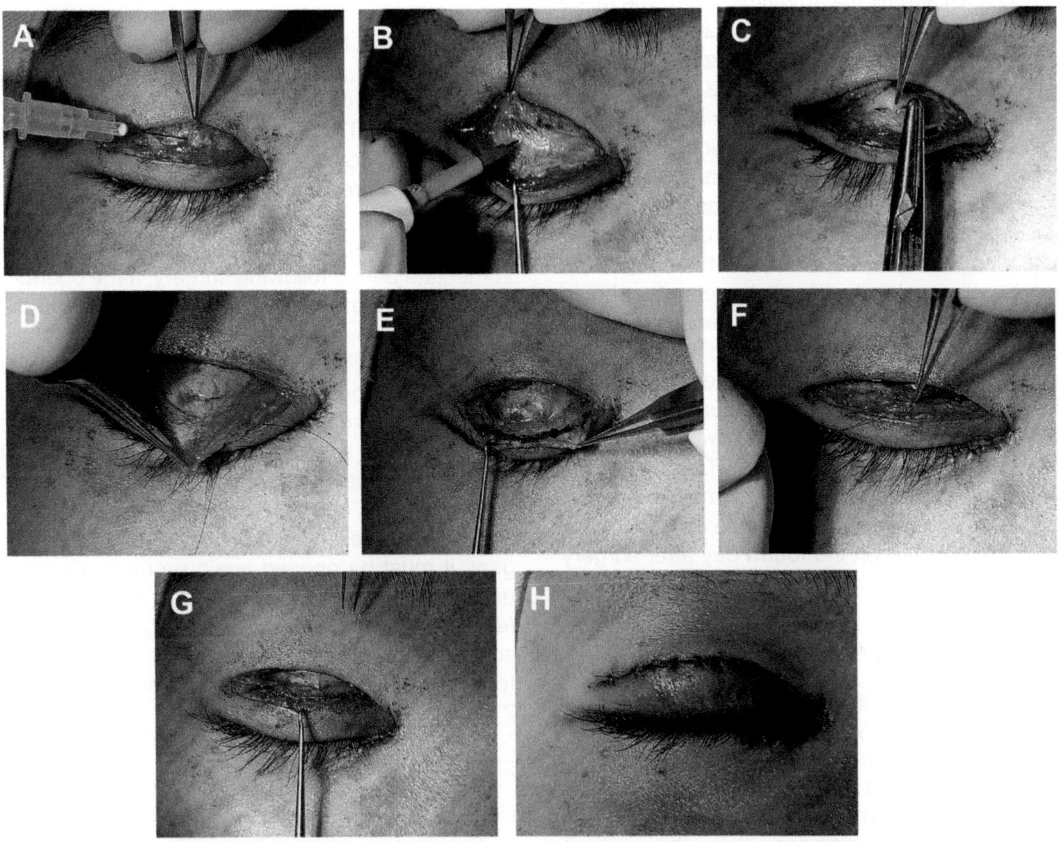

Fig. 12. LA advancement. Carefully separate the LA from the tarsal plate (*A, B*). A horizontal mattress fixation suture is performed. A view of a partway penetrating 7-0 nylon needle at 1.5 mm from the top of the tarsal plate (*C*) that pierces through the LA at 2 horizontal points and comes down to tie the thread (*C, D*). After suture fixation, cut off the advanced LA, leaving a 1.5-mm margin from the fixed suture (*E*). The aponeurosis' end connects with the lower flap muscle and dermis to form a double eyelid (*F, G*). The skin of the lower flap and the muscle and skin of the upper flap are sutured with 7-0 nylon (*H*).

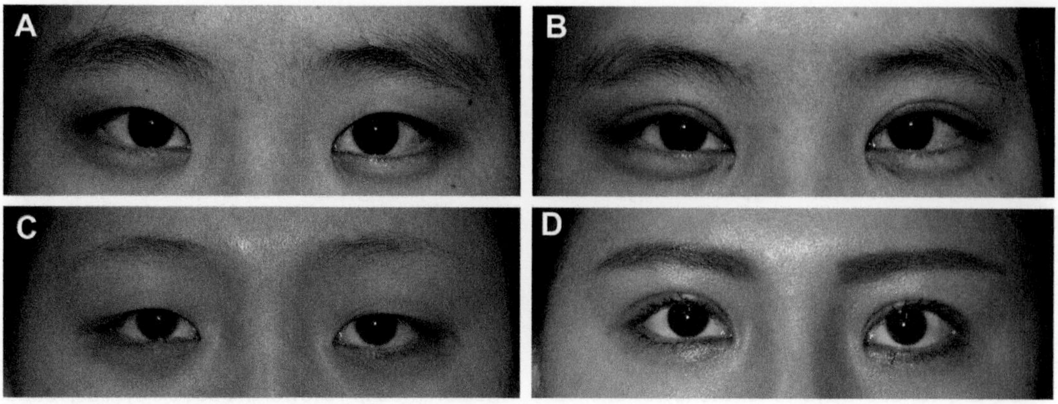

Fig. 13. Double eyelid surgery only, preoperatively (*A*) and postoperatively (*B*). Double eyelid surgery with levator advancement, preoperatively (*C*) and postoperatively (*D*). The patient in panels C, D had a more attractive eye shape than the patient in panels A, B because the eyelid fissure was increased compared with before surgery.

LEVATOR APONEUROSIS ADVANCEMENT

In LA advancement with double eyelid surgery, carefully separate the LA from the tarsal plate (**Fig. 12**A, B) and fix the advanced LA to the tarsal plate's upper end using a horizontal mattress suture (**Fig.12**C, D). After the first fixation suture is placed on both eyes and crease symmetry is confirmed, additional fixation is made on either side, with a similar degree of tension as with the first suture. Following fixation, any remaining aponeurotic tissue below the anchor point is excised, taking care to leave a margin of approximately 1.5 mm (see **Fig. 12**E), as trimming it too closely may make it difficult to release, should there be overcorrection requiring reoperation at a later stage. The process following LA advancement is the same as with double eyelid surgery. The aponeurosis' end margin is sutured to connect with the dermis and OOM of the lower flap to form a double eyelid (see **Fig. 12**F, G). The skin of the lower flap and the OOM and skin of the upper flap are sutured with 7-0 nylon (see **Fig. 12**H). Sutures are removed on the fourth day after surgery (**Fig. 13**A–D).

POSTOPERATIVE CARE

Patients may experience temporary dry eye after double eyelid surgery[15] and should be advised of this preoperatively as well as educated about the use of artificial tears or eye ointments to prevent possible corneal damage.

The authors recommend that the patient perform ice massage intermittently for the first half day following surgery. It is recognized that ice massage reduces pain on the first day after surgery, although there is no correlation with reduction of postoperative swelling or bruising hematoma.[16] Patients are encouraged to continue their daily activities. They are also instructed to practice eye opening exercises, using a specific method that involves the patient stabilizing their leveled forehead with one hand while holding a hand mirror in front of them with the other. The hand mirror is slowly raised, with the patient's gaze following it until the mirror passes the forehead's height. The patient then stops, closes their eyes, counts to 3, and then reopens their eyes. This cycle is repeated several times a day for 1 week.

In cases whereby asymmetry is identified in the immediate period following surgery, if the operator is confident that the symmetry was correct in the operating room, a wait-and-see approach is taken. However, if the asymmetry has not self-corrected by 1 week, reoperation is performed. If the incision line is the same height, the most common cause of postoperative asymmetry is the presence of differing quantities of sagging skin. The second most common cause is original eye asymmetry. If the eye is swollen because of bleeding after surgery, it must be opened again promptly to evacuate the hematoma, relieve ocular pressure, and facilitate quick recovery. After surgery, a prescribed antibiotic ointment is to be applied lightly to the suture line. Eye makeup can be applied after 2 weeks.

SUMMARY

Upper lid blepharoplasty in the Asian eye is a procedure that requires a thorough grasp of Asian orbital anatomy and meticulous management of the eyelid soft tissue, including OF manipulation, in order to create an aesthetically pleasing, natural-appearing and long-lasting STC. It is critical during the initial evaluation process to assess for and identify factors that may contribute to the fold-resistant eyelid, in order to appropriately address them intraoperatively and hence maximize the surgical outcome. It is also important to evaluate the position of the eyebrows, and if compensated brow ptosis is anticipated, the patient must be counseled accordingly, in order to establish appropriate postsurgery expectations.

CLINICS CARE POINTS

Pearls

- The outer orbital rim's height determines the maximum height of the double eyelid, and the supratarsal creases' maximum height should not exceed this.
- Before concluding the crease design, turn the lid over and measure the height of the tarsus. This is to confirm that the planned pretarsal skin segment height aligns with the tarsal height.
- To prevent late bleeding when excising orbital fat, cauterize the cut fat edge twice, once after cutting and again after first partially loosening the mosquito clip clamp.
- The lower-positioned transverse ligament or fibrous web bands on the levator aponeurosis are commonly encountered in Asian blepharoplasty and can limit movement of the levator aponeurosis. Subclinical and mild blepharoptosis can be corrected by releasing these structures.
- If there is eyebrow asymmetry, an endoscopic brow lift is recommended first. If not performed together, the double eyelid incision line must be designed a little higher, or additional skin and muscle should be excised, in order to prevent double eyelid asymmetry following surgery.
- After adjusting both eyes to optimize symmetry, if it is observed that the skin is thin and the operator is concerned about triple folds, or in cases of reoperation, then a permanent fixation suture may be placed in a buried manner.

Pitfalls

- Failure to address severe epicanthal folds is the most common cause of failure to sustain a created supratarsal crease.
- High supratarsal creases are anatomically unsuitable for Asians. If the height of the designed supratarsal crease is higher than the tarsal plate's height, it is easy to create secondary ptosis.
- Exercise caution to avoid excessive trimming of the lower flap's orbicularis oculi muscle, as this can result in unsightly long-term hollowing along the length of the incision line scar.
- Numbness of the upper eyelid following double eyelid surgery may represent injury of the sensory nerve branches. To prevent this complication, the orbital fat sac should not be removed along with the fat.
- Avoid excessive orbital fat pad removal to prevent undesirable cosmetic outcomes.
- In levator aponeurosis advancement, when aponeurotic tissue below the fixed anchor points is excised, take care to leave a margin of approximately 1.5 mm, as trimming it too closely may make it difficult to release should the patient require reoperation at a later stage because of overcorrection.

DISCLOSURE STATEMENT

The authors have nothing to disclose.

REFERENCES

1. Chen WP. Asian blepharoplasty. Update on anatomy and techniques. Ophthal Plast Reconstr Surg 1987; 3:135–40.
2. Saonanon P. Update on Asian eyelid anatomy and clinical relevance. Curr Opin Ophthalmol 2014; 25(5):436–42.
3. Kwon BS, Anh HN. Reconsideration of the epicanthus: evolution of the eyelid and the devolutional concept of Asian blepharoplasty. Semin Plast Surg 2015;29:171–83.
4. Kim YC, Kwon JG, Kim SC, et al. Comparison of periorbital anthropometry between beauty pageant contestants and ordinary young women with Korean ethnicity: a three-dimensional photogrammetric analysis. Aesthetic Plast Surg 2018;42(2):479–90.
5. Klatsky S, Manson PN. Numbness after blepharoplasty: the relation of the upper orbital fat to sensory nerves. Plast Reconstr Surg 1981;67(1):20–2.
6. Yasuhiro T, Hirohiko K, Shinsuke K, et al. Histological analysis of the lower-positioned transverse ligament. Open Ophthalmol J 2007;1:17–9.
7. Kim JH, Lee IJ, Park MC, et al. Aesthetic blepharoptosis correction with release of fibrous web bands between the levator aponeurosis and orbital fat. J Craniofac Surg 2012;23(1):e52–5.
8. Siegel R. Surgical anatomy of the upper eyelid fascia. Ann Plast Surg 1984;13(4):263–73.
9. Macdonald KI, Mendez AI, Hart RD, et al. Eyelid and brow asymmetry in patients evaluated for upper lid

blepharoplasty. J Otolaryngol Head Neck Surg 2014;43(1):36.

10. Park DH, Choi WS, Yoon SH, et al. Anthropometry of Asian eyelids by age. Plast Reconstr Surg 2008; 121(4):1405–13.
11. Kim YW, Park HJ, Kim S. Secondary correction of unsatisfactory blepharoplasty: removing multilaminated septal structures and grafting of preaponeurotic fat. Plast Reconstr Surg 2000;106(6):1399–404.
12. Flowers RS, Duval C. Blepharoplasty and periorbital aesthetic surgery. In: Aston SJ, Beasley RW, Thorne CHM, editors. Grabb and Smith's plastic surgery. 5th edn. Philadelphia: Lippincott-Raven Publishers; 1997. p. 612.
13. Karlin JN, Rootman DB. Brow height asymmetry before and after eyelid ptosis surgery. J Plast Reconstr Aesthet Surg 2020;73(2):357–62.
14. Lee W, Kwon SB, Oh SK, et al. Correction of sunken upper eyelid with orbital fat transposition flap and dermofat graft. J Plast Reconstr Aesthet Surg 2017;70(12):1768–75.
15. Watanabe A, Selva D, Kakizaki H. Long-term tear volume changes after blepharoptosis surgery and blepharoplasty. Invest Ophthalmol Vis Sci 2014; 56(1):54–8.
16. Pool SM, van Exsel DC, Melenhorst WB, et al. The effect of eyelid cooling on pain, edema, erythema, and hematoma after upper blepharoplasty: a randomized, controlled, observer-blinded evaluation study. Plast Reconstr Surg 2015;135(2):277e.

Nonincisional Blepharoplasty for Asians

Kyoung Hwa Bae, MD, Ji Sun Baek, MD, Jae Woo Jang, MD, PhD*

KEYWORDS

• Asian eyelid • Asian blepharoplasty • Double eyelid • Nonincisional blepharoplasty • Suture method

KEY POINTS

- Nonincisional blepharoplasty (suture method) is the preferred method for double eyelid creation because it provides a more natural appearance, is a simple and easy technique, causes only mild swelling and less scarring postoperatively, and enables fast recovery.
- Proper selection of patients for double eyelid creation using the suture method yields a good cosmetic result with long-lasting double folds.
- Medial epicanthoplasty is usually performed simultaneously with double eyelid surgery for larger and more attractive eyelid creases, especially in patients with an epicanthal fold.

INTRODUCTION

Upper eyelid blepharoplasty is one of the most frequently performed esthetic procedures in Asia. Asian blepharoplasty, also known as double eyelid surgery, involves the surgical creation of a supratarsal crease.

It is generally agreed that approximately 50% of Asians are born with upper eyelid creases; however, the height of the double eyelid crease is low in many of them. Moreover, well-defined double eyelids are present in only approximately 10% of Asian men and 33% of Asian women.

The goal of blepharoplasty for Asians is to achieve fresh, youthful, and attractive eyes, while retaining their ethnic appearance. The Asian upper eyelid has several distinct anatomic characteristics, such as a low, poorly defined, or absent eyelid crease; a narrow palpebral fissure; and/or an epicanthal fold. The upper eyelid margin of a single eyelid in East Asians is, in most cases, covered by the upper eyelid skin. Therefore, after double eyelid surgery, in which the upper eyelid skin is pulled upward, an apparent increase in the size of the eyes is noted. East Asians consider that double eyelid surgery makes the eye appear larger and more esthetically pleasing.[1]

Double eyelid surgery is performed not only for cosmetic purposes but also for the correction of problems such as entropion, lash ptosis, and ptosis (**Fig. 1**).[2] Most patients prefer that the correction of these problems and double eyelid surgery be performed simultaneously. Furthermore, when patients with blepharoptosis undergo double eyelid surgery, the palpebral fissures become wider, resulting in a more pleasing eye shape (**Fig. 2**).[3]

The primary goal of double eyelid surgery is to create a supratarsal crease that is consistent with the natural configuration present in the general Asian population and not that in the Western population.

ANATOMY OF THE ASIAN EYELID

An absent or exceptionally low eyelid crease and a puffy upper eyelid are the most obvious characteristics of Asian eyelids. Asian eyelids with no eyelid crease are referred to as single eyelids. Asian eyelids can be divided into 3 types: single eyelid, low eyelid crease (double eyelid structurally, but apparently single eyelid), and double eyelid. Although not visible, a small fold commonly exists under the overhanging eyelid skin.

Department of Ophthalmic Plastic and Reconstructive Surgery, Kim's Eye Hospital, 136 Yeongshin-ro, Yeongdeungpo-gu, Seoul 07301, Republic of Korea
* Corresponding author.
E-mail address: jjw@kimeye.com

Facial Plast Surg Clin N Am 29 (2021) 523–532
https://doi.org/10.1016/j.fsc.2021.06.005

facialplastic.theclinics.com

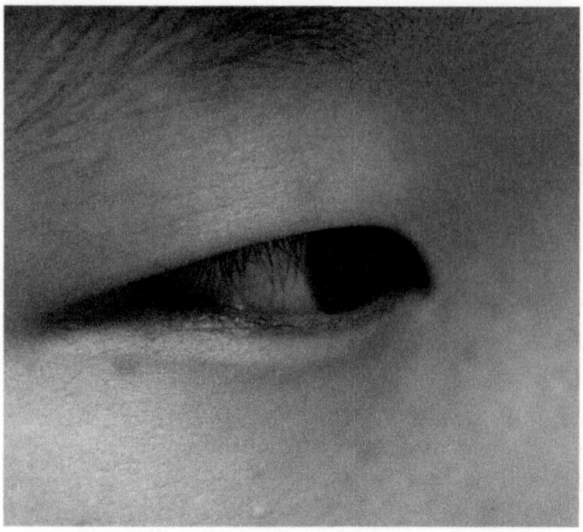

Fig. 1. Lash ptosis or entropion in the single eyelid in Asian patients.

The reasons for an absent or a low eyelid crease in an Asian upper eyelid are as follows: (1) fusion of the orbital septum and levator aponeurosis below the superior tarsal border; (2) extension of the preaponeurotic fat pad and a thick subcutaneous fat layer prevent the fusion of the levator fibers toward the skin near the superior tarsal border; and (3) the primary insertion of the levator aponeurosis into the orbicularis muscle and upper eyelid skin near the eyelid margin.[4,5]

CANDIDATES OF THE NONINCISIONAL TECHNIQUE FOR DOUBLE EYELID SURGERY

There are 3 types of double eyelid surgery: the nonincisional technique, the partial incisional technique, and the incisional technique. The choice of technique is based on the preference, skin quality, and volume of orbital fat in the upper eyelid of the patient.[6]

The incisional and nonincisional techniques have their own advantages and disadvantages. The nonincisional technique (suture method) is preferred over the incisional technique because it provides a more natural appearance, is a simple and easy technique, causes only mild swelling and less scarring postoperatively, and enables a fast recovery. The disadvantages of the nonincisional technique are the inability to completely deal with preaponeurotic fat and soft tissue, which leads to the possibility of disappearance of the double eyelid crease, and development of inclusion cyst or exposure of a knot because of a buried suture (**Fig. 3**).[7]

Patient selection is important for successful double eyelid creation with the nonincisional technique to achieve a good cosmetic result with long-lasting double folds. The indications for the suture technique are as follows: (1) relatively thinner skin and nonredundant or mild redundant skin; (2) little orbicularis muscle bulk or orbital fat; (3) disappearance of the eyelid crease after the incisional technique or partial incisional technique; and (4) reoperation owing to various complications after eyelid crease surgery (**Figs. 4–7**).

NONINCISIONAL TECHNIQUE WITH MEDIAL EPICANTHOPLASTY

The epicanthal fold in Asian eyelids is a unique feature in combination with the single eyelid. The prevalence of epicanthal folds ranges from 50% to 80%.[8,9] The epicanthal fold, which is common in Asians, is characterized by a curved skin fold that partially hides the caruncle and lacrimal lake. The epicanthal fold may cause weakening of the esthetic appearance after blepharoplasty because it reduces the height and horizontal length of the palpebral fissure.

Medial epicanthoplasty is a procedure to release the epicanthal fold. This operation is generally performed with double eyelid surgery and has 2 important aspects.[10] First, the released epicanthal fold lengthens and modifies the medial corner of the palpebral fissure. Medial epicanthoplasty reveals a more nasal scleral triangle and simultaneously decreases the interepicanthal

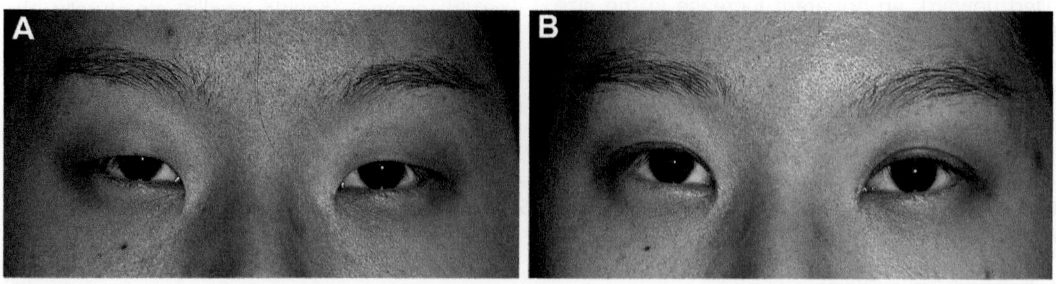

Fig. 2. (*A*) Preoperative photographs and (*B*) postoperative photographs after simultaneous levator resection, double eyelid surgery, and medial epicanthoplasty.

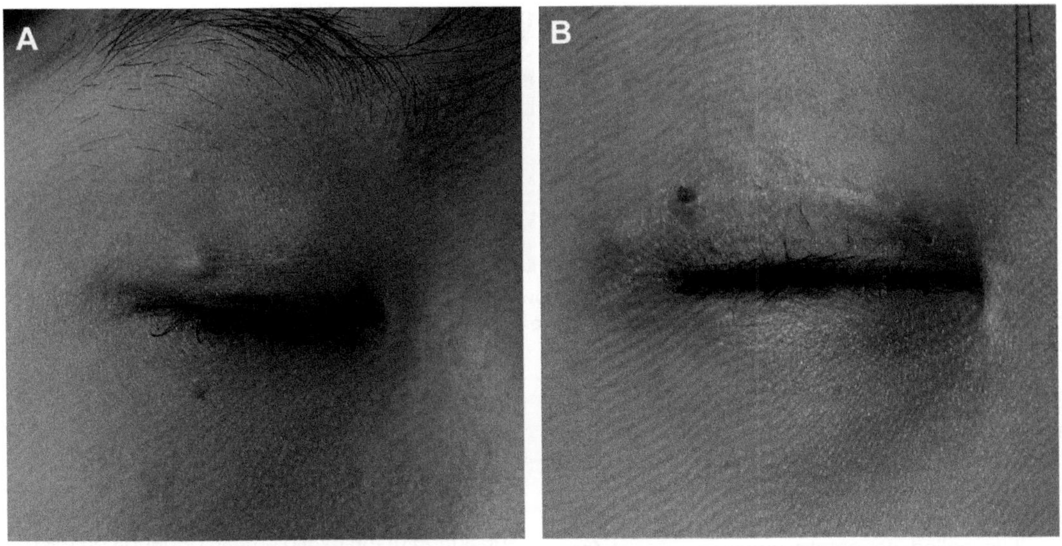

Fig. 3. Complications after performing the buried suture method. (*A*) Inclusion cyst and (*B*) exposure of knots.

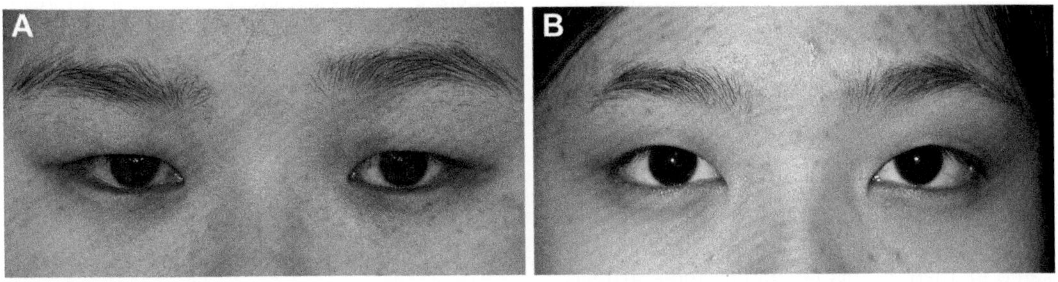

Fig. 4. The typical shapes of eyelids, which are indications for (*A*) incisional method or (*B*) nonincisional method in double eyelid surgery.

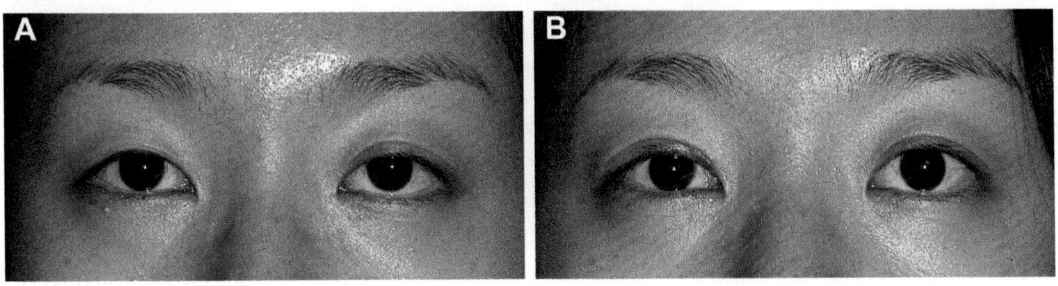

Fig. 5. (*A*) Loss of the double eyelid fold in the right eye after performing the incisional method. (*B*) Double eyelid creation using the buried single continuous suture method.

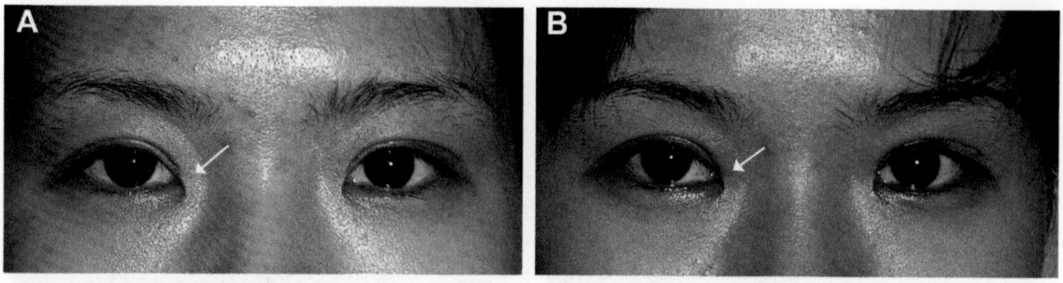

Fig. 6. (*A*) The right eye had an outside fold (*white arrow*), and the left eye had an inside fold. (*B*) The change from the outside to inside fold (*white arrow*) with one-point suture between the medial limbus and medial canthus using the 6-0 Vicryl suture.

distance. Thus, it creates a balance between the nasal and lateral scleral triangles by exposing the obscured caruncle. Second, the shape of the eyelid crease depends on the shape of the epicanthal folds. If the crease line meets the epicanthal fold, it is called an onfold (outside crease: fan type). If the crease line lies above the epicanthal fold, it is called an outfold (outside crease: mixed or parallel crease). If the crease lies below the epicanthal fold, it is called an infold (inside crease).

The tendency to create an infold is higher in patients with an epicanthal fold. The creation of an onfold or outfold requires modification or removal of the epicanthal fold.[6] Medial epicanthoplasty is usually performed simultaneously with double eyelid surgery for larger and more attractive eyelid creases, especially in patients with an epicanthal fold (**Fig. 8**).

SURGICAL PROCEDURES

The nonincisional technique was first described by Mikamo in 1896. In this technique, three 4-0 silk sutures were passed through the full thickness of the eyelid from the conjunctiva to the outer layer of the skin to create adhesions between the levator aponeurosis and the overlying subdermal tissue at the superior tarsal margin.[11] Subsequently, others have described various nonincisional techniques: (1) single continuous or multiple interrupted, buried suture method, and (2) skin–levator suture or skin–tarsus suture method (**Fig. 9**).

Design of the Double Eyelid Crease

The shape of the eyelid crease depends on the degree of the epicanthal fold and the height of the eyelid crease. The height and shape of the eyelid crease usually depend on the interpalpebral fissure and the tarsus of the eyelid. The eyelid crease height is 6 to 8 mm in Asian women and slightly lower in Asian men. In general, a high-set crease results in an outside crease, whereas a moderate- to low-set crease results in an inside crease. The inside crease is usually natural in patients with an epicanthal fold.

The important point is not the height of the designed crease line during eye closing, but the width of the double eyelid during eye opening, called the "pretarsal show." In East Asians, the appropriate height of the pretarsal show is 2 to 3 mm or 20% to 30% of the interpalpebral fissure. The double eyelid crease line in the nonincisional method was designed to be 1 to 2 mm higher than that in the incisional method because it did not involve skin removal.

Mikamo Method

The eyelid crease was designed to be 6 to 8 mm above the ciliary margin. Three 4-0 silk sutures

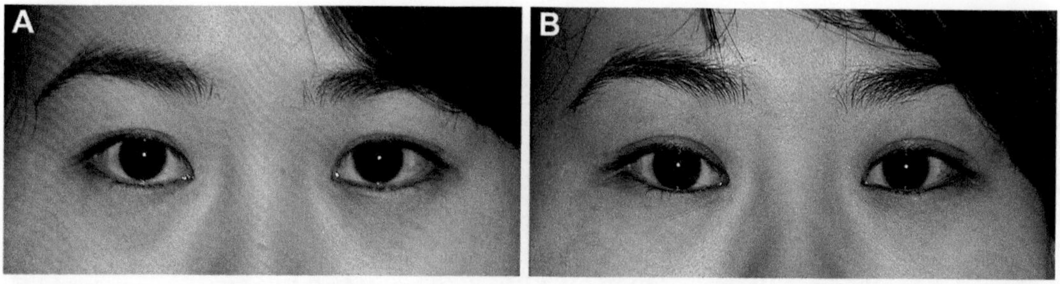

Fig. 7. (*A*) The patient desired a higher and clearer double eyelid after correction with the incisional method. (*B*) Postoperative photograph after single continuous buried suture method showed the change in the double eyelid (from low fold to high fold).

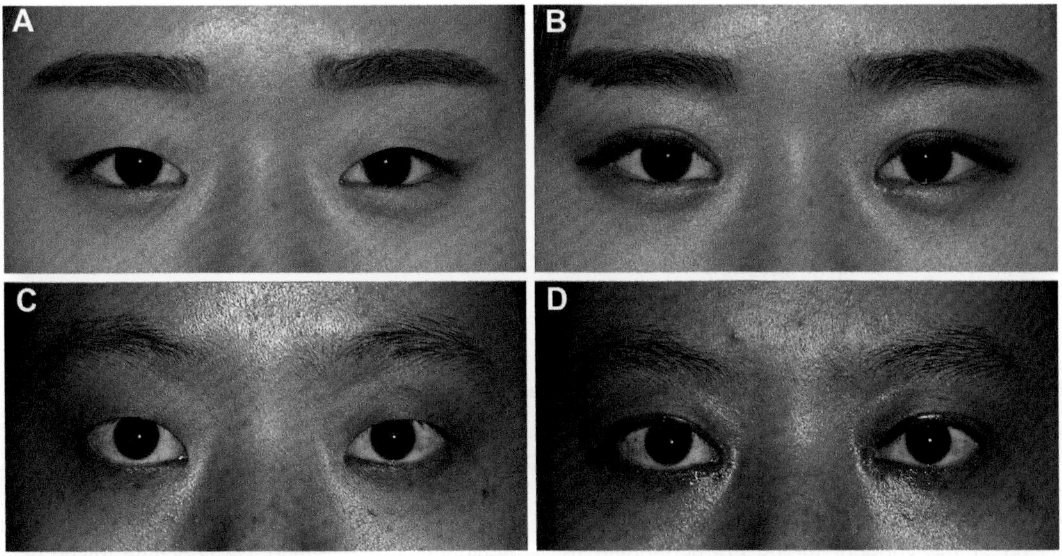

Fig. 8. Preoperative and postoperative photographs after single continuous suture method with redraping medial epicanthoplasty. (*A, C*) preoperative photographs, and (*B, D*) postoperative photographs.

were used; the suture needle was passed through the full thickness of the lid from the conjunctiva to the skin. The depth of the double fold depended on the time of suture removal (2–6 days postoperatively) because the knot was not buried in this technique (**Fig. 10**).

Until recently, ophthalmologists have been using 3 interrupted full-thickness 6-0 Vicryl sutures similar to the Mikamo method, except for buried knots, to correct child entropion.[2]

Maruo Method

Maruo reported a 2-way continuous buried suture method.[12] Each double-armed needle with 5-0 or 6-0 thread was introduced through 1 end of the proposed double eyelid crease line. Five stab incisions were made along the designed crease line. One needle was passed from a to b through the half-thickness tarsus (not penetrating), b to c through the subcutaneous tissue, c to d through the tarsus, and d to e through the tarsus. The other needle was passed in the opposite direction and exteriorized at e. The 2 ends of the suture thread were tied (**Fig. 11**).

Jung Method

The center dot was marked on the proposed crease line, as suggested by the vertical

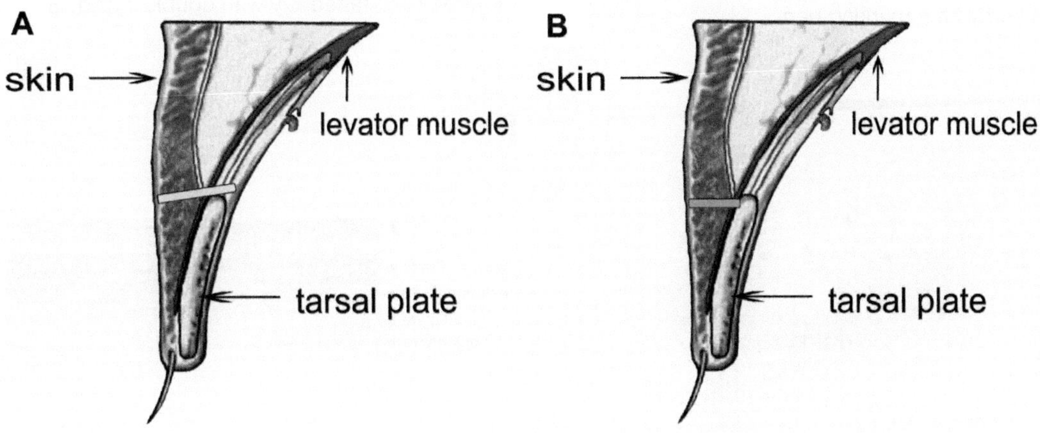

Fig. 9. The 2 ways of suture fixation in the buried suture method. (*A*) Skin-levator suture method and (*B*) skin-tarsus suture method.

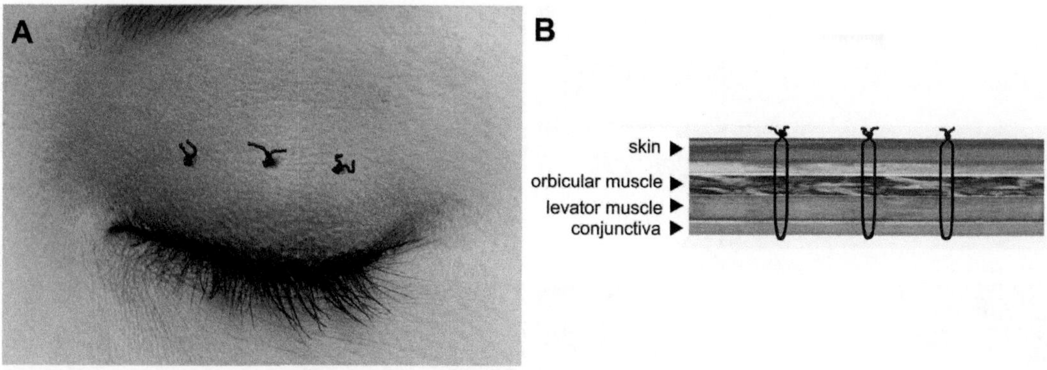

Fig. 10. Mikamo method (*A, B*). Full-thickness interrupted suture method.

midpupillary line. Two additional dots were marked 7 to 8 mm laterally and medially. After everting the eyelid, the conjunctiva (1–2 mm) was incised at the superior tarsus corresponding to the central dot. One end of the 7-0 nylon double-armed suture was passed through the levator aponeurosis to the subcutaneous plane along the superior tarsal border without puncturing the skin. The needle was kept in the subcutaneous plane, and the suture arm was reversed through the same tissue and exteriorized through the conjunctiva. The 2 threads were tied together with a knot and buried within the central conjunctival incision (**Fig. 12**).

The Authors' Preferred Method

The design of the double eyelid was based on the preference of the patient, and the shape and height of the eyelid crease were determined during the consultation. Usually, the authors determined the natural crease by simply pushing the eyelid using forceps or a lacrimal probe in the sitting position. After determining the shape and height of the eyelid crease, the proposed crease line was marked with a marking pen.

A 0.5% ophthalmic solution of proparacaine hydrochloride was used to anesthetize the cornea. Local anesthesia was induced in the eyelid and conjunctiva by injecting 2% lidocaine mixed with 1:100,000 epinephrine using a 30-gauge needle.

A 2-mm stab incision was made laterally, and 2-point stab incisions were made centrally and medially using a no. 11 blade. A 24-mm round needle of a double-armed 7-0 nylon suture was passed through the same point through the upper tarsus margin from the conjunctiva to the skin. Thereafter, this suture was threaded in 1 direction through the skin and upper part of the tarsus alternately through each of the point incisions. At the medial end, the suture was passed through the subcutaneous tissue to the lateral end, as presented in the diagram in **Fig. 13** (light blue line). A knot was tied over the lacrimal probe for easy adjustment of the suture tension and prevention of knot slippage (**Fig. 14**). The knot was buried within the lateral stab incision without skin suture (**Fig. 15**).

If a larger and more pleasing eyelid crease is sought, medial epicanthoplasty is usually performed simultaneously with double eyelid surgery.

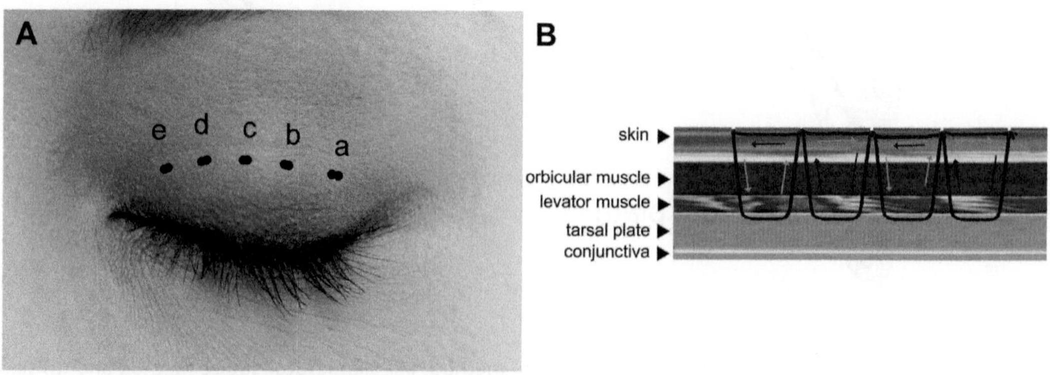

Fig. 11. Maruo method: (A, B) transcutaneous intradermal and intratarsal suture method.

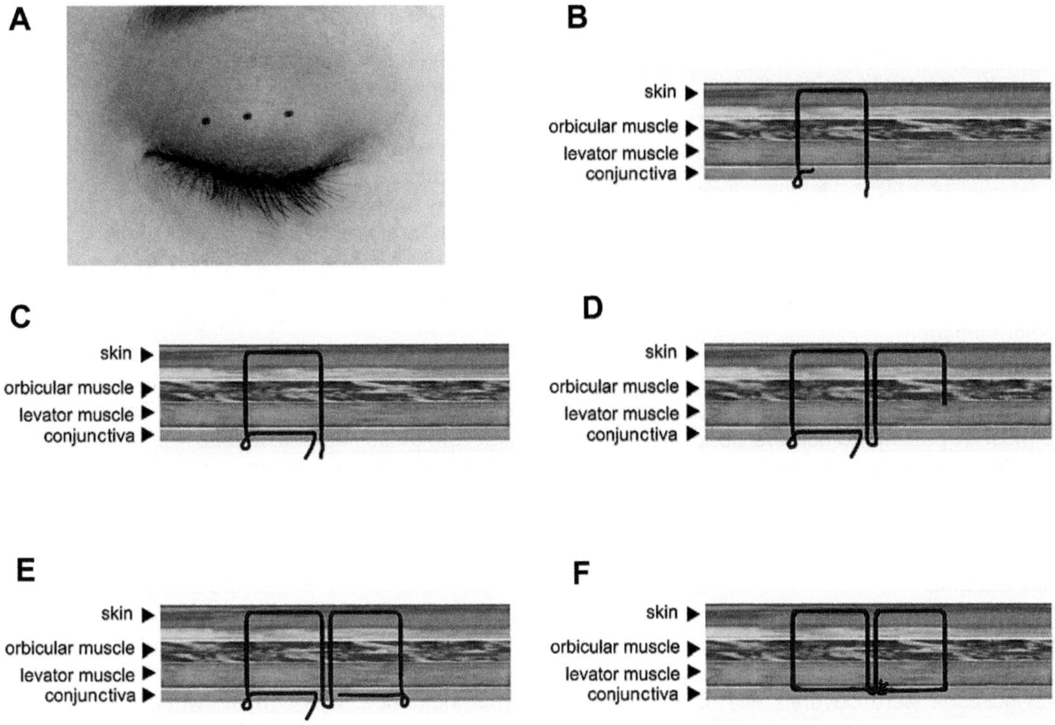

Fig. 12. Jung method: (A to F) Transconjunctival intramuscular suture method. (F) Knotting in the subconjunctiva tissue.

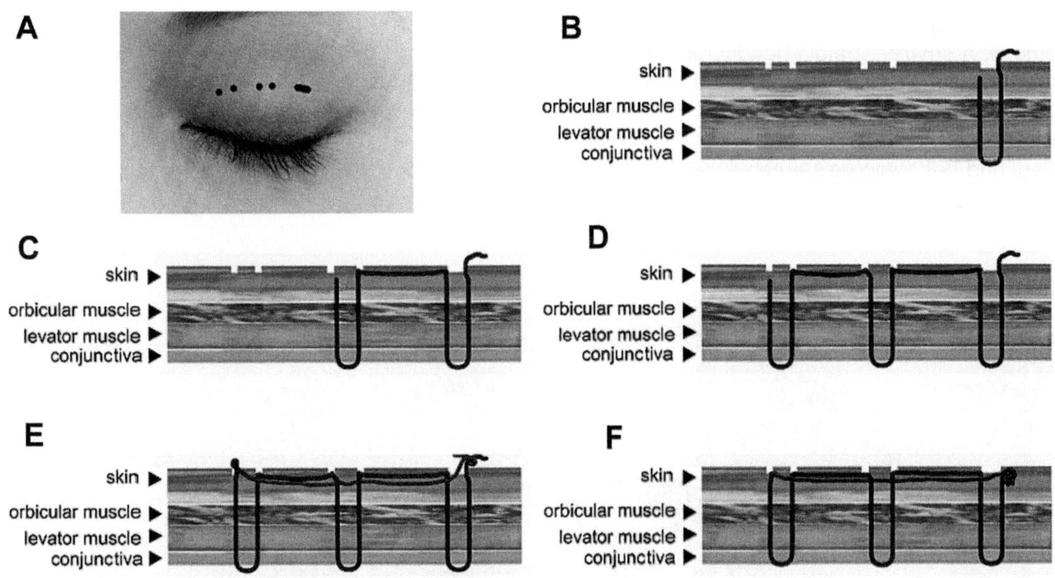

Fig. 13. The authors' preferred method: single continuous buried suture technique. (A) A 2-mm stab incision laterally, and 2-point stab incisions are made centrally and medially. (B, C, D) The 3 loops of full-thickness suture at the upper tarsus margin were made from the lateral to medial portion of eyelid. (E) At the medial end, suture passed through the subcutaneous tissue to the lateral end (*light blue*). (F) The suture knot was buried within the stab incision.

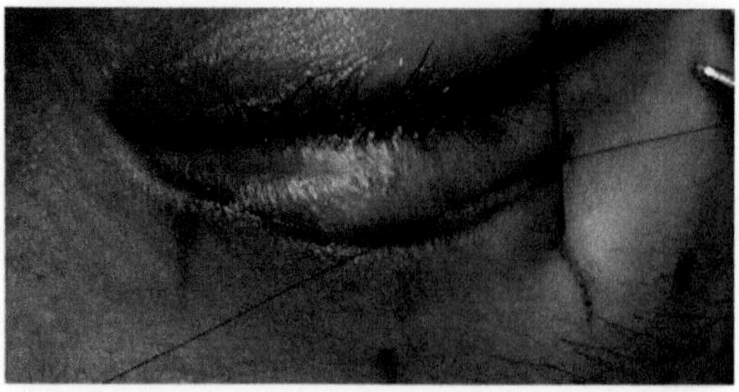

Fig. 14. The knot was tied over the lacrimal probe for easy adjustment of the suture tension and prevention of knot slippage.

The authors usually use the skin redraping method in almost all patients to achieve good results, that is, a mild to moderate epicanthal fold. In addition, entropion and epiblepharon are corrected simultaneously using epicanthoplasty because they require the same incision line below the lower lid ciliary margin.[10]

Patients were instructed to open the eyes to check the shape, height, and symmetry of the double eyelid creases under local anesthesia. The stab incisions were covered with eye ointment, and the eyelid was compressed gently with sterile gauze at the end of the surgery.

In the full-thickness suture method from the skin to the conjunctiva of the superior tarsal margin, the long round needle (24 mm, 3/8 circle round needle, double armed 7-0 nylon suture) is convenient (**Fig. 16**). A triangular cutting needle can damage the vessel and cause bleeding. However, for the transcutaneous intradermal and intratarsal suture methods, a smaller spatula needle may be better than the cutting needle. The cutting needle can damage the tarsus during the biting of the partial thickness of the tarsus and result in cheese-wiring, and not a secure suture.

DISCUSSION

In the suture method, the goal is to create adhesion between the levator aponeurosis or tarsus and the overlying subdermal tissue without a large skin incision. This method is fast and convenient for creating a double fold, usually causes minimal swelling postoperatively, and enables fast recovery. Although this method is usually used for cosmetic reasons, it was found to be useful in everting the lashes in mild upper lid entropion.[13] However, this method has common complications, such as loosening or loss of double fold and development of inclusion cyst or knot exposure owing to the buried stitch. To reduce the risk of these complications, various modified methods have been reported in the literature.[7,9,11,14–18]

The main problem of the nonincisional technique is the loosening or disappearance of the double fold. The reported rate of loss of the double fold ranges from 1.31% to 16.8%. Homma and colleagues[7] reported that the incidence rate of loss of double fold varied in the number of stitches. The incidence was 1.31% when the 2-suture method was used and 3.43% when the 1-suture method was used. However, Ko and colleagues[19] reported that there was no difference in the reoperation rate because of the loss of the double eyelid among patients treated with the 1-, 2-, and 3-suture methods. In the authors' study, the rate of loss of the double eyelid crease was 19.3% in the full-thickness 3 interrupted buried method group and 8.6% in the full-thickness single continuous buried method group.[2] The success rate, considering the persistency of double eyelid crease, was significantly higher in the continuous group than in the interrupted group. The adhesion between the dermis and the tarsus or levator

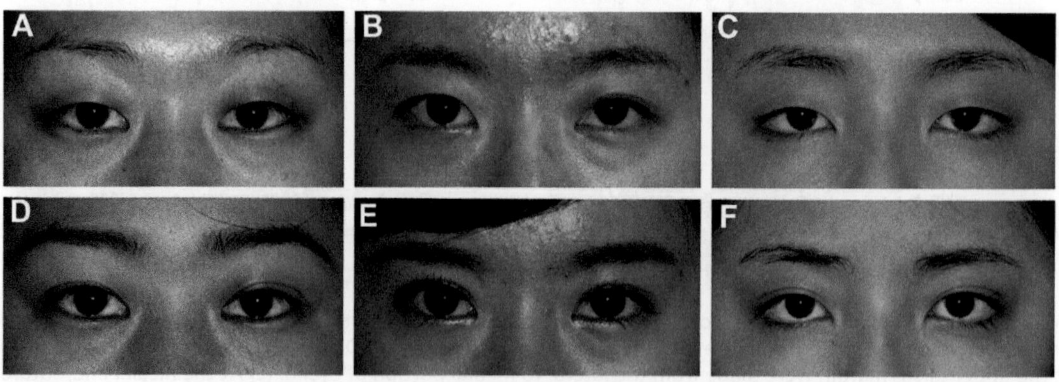

Fig. 15. (*A, B, C*) Preoperative and (*D, E, F*) postoperative photographs after the single continuous buried suture method. The shape of eyelid crease: (*D*) infold, (*E*) onfold, (*F*) outfold, fan-type.

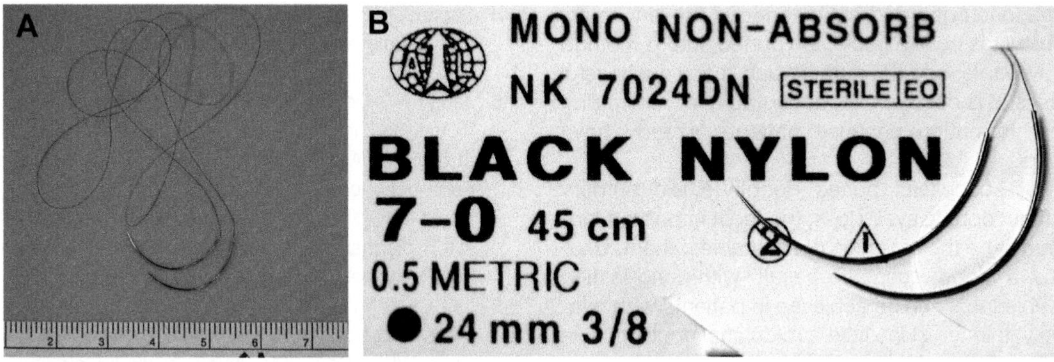

Fig. 16. (A, B) Special design for the full-thickness suture method: a 24-mm round (tapered) needle, double-armed 7-0 nylon suture.

muscle is probably enhanced by alternative running sutures from the dermis to the superior tarsus margin in the continuous group. This effect was further enhanced by running the suture back through the subcutaneous tissues, creating a stronger and lasting adhesion, enabling comprehensive eyelid manipulation under the skin. The number of stitches and the method used might influence the disappearance of double eyelid crease after nonincisional double eyelid surgery. However, no consistent results regarding the double fold loss rate associated with the number of sutures in the buried suture method were found in the literature.

In addition, complications such as inclusion cyst and exposure of suture knot may occur after performing the buried suture method. Homma and colleagues[7] reported that the incidence of inclusion cysts was 3.2% when the 2-suture method was performed and 1.7% when the 1-suture method was performed. In the authors' study,[2] these complications were significantly less common in the continuous group than in the interrupted group. The number of buried suture knots could be attributed to the result. In summary, the incidence of double fold loss did not differ between the single and multiple buried suture methods; however, the incidence of inclusion cyst and knot exposure was considerably lower in the single suture method than in the multiple suture method. Currently, surgeons prefer the single continuous buried suture method for double eyelid surgery. They aim for minimum number and proper placement (deep intradermal or in the orbicularis oculi muscle) of knots.

However, other suture-related complications, such as an uncomfortable pulling sensation, mild pain, corneal irritation, and foreign body sensation, should be considered when performing the suture method for double eyelid surgery. A study reported that patients with an uncomfortable pulling sensation had developed a linear scar or depressed deformity of the conjunctiva without inflammation or depressed deformity of the levator muscle.[20] These symptoms were relieved after suture removal. In the buried suture method, the fixation points include the levator muscle and tarsal plate. Levator muscle fixation involves levator and muller muscle–intradermal fixation of the eyelid skin. Tarsal fixation can be performed by 2 methods: the intratarsal-intradermal fixation (the needle is passed through the half thickness of the tarsus) or the penetration of the conjunctival tarsus.[21] In the penetration of conjunctival tarsus method, various chronic inflammations at the conjunctival site along the tarsal plate can cause corneal irritation, foreign body sensation, mucus production, and deformity of the tarsal plate.[20] Moreover, late-onset suture exposure at the conjunctival site can cause sudden severe pain because of corneal erosion or abrasion. Hence, to prevent these complications, the tarsal fixation point was changed from the conjunctival tarsal surface to the anterior surface of the tarsus.

In the levator muscle fixation method, it is difficult to adjust the suture level because supportive tissues, such as the tarsal plate, and a larger volume of soft tissues are not available for fixation. The higher chance of strangulation or levator aponeurosis deformity because of tighter fixation may result in temporary postoperative ptosis. In addition, loose suture tension would result in the loosening of the double eyelid. The authors commend that suture tying over the lacrimal probe may be helpful for the adjustment of suture tension.

It is known that the incisional technique should be performed in the case of recurrence after incision or partial incision surgery. In these cases, the patient had already removed proper preaponeurotic and subcutaneous fat, and puffy orbicularis oculi muscle, the buried suture method is available, and the authors had many successful cases. It is cosmetically acceptable for minimizing scar formation because patients already have scars.

For successful buried double eyelid surgery without double eyelid loss, the most important factor may be the selection of a suitable patient. Usually, a good cosmetic result with long-lasting double folds can be achieved in patients with relatively thinner skin, little orbicularis oculi muscle bulk or fat, and no excess skin.

SUMMARY

Various nonincisional techniques for double eyelid surgery have been introduced in the past. They are simple, noninvasive, and efficient techniques to create a double eyelid. The authors prefer the full-thickness single continuous method using the 7-0 nylon, round long needle. Appropriate choice of the patients and surgical method results in a natural, esthetically pleasing eyelid and decreases the loss of eyelid crease.

CLINICS CARE POINTS

> In Asian double eyelid surgery, a single continuous suture method provides a more natural appearance when the appropriate patient is selected, but otherwise the loss of the double eyelid can occur.

DISCLOSURE STATEMENT

The authors indicate no financial support or conflict of interest.

REFERENCES

1. Scawn R, Joshi N, Kim YD. Upper lid blepharoplasty in Asian eyes. Facial Plast Surg 2010;26:86–92.
2. Baek JS, Ahn JH, Jang SY, et al. Comparison between continuous buried suture and interrupted buried suture methods for double eyelid blepharoplasty. Craniofac Surg 2015;26:2174–6.
3. Park DH, Kim CW, Shim JS. Strategies for simultaneous double eyelid blepharoplasty in Asian patients with congenital blepharoptosis. Aesthetic Plast Surg 2008;32:66–71.
4. Jeong SK, Lemke BN, Dortzbach R, et al. The Asian upper eyelid: an anatomical study with comparison to the Caucasian eyelid. Arch Ophthalmol 1999;117:907–12.
5. Saonanon P. Update on Asian eyelid anatomy and clinical relevance. Curr Opin Ophthalmol 2014;25:436–42.
6. Jang JW. Double-eyelid surgery: incisional techniques. In: Jin HR, editor. Aesthetic plastic surgery of the East Asian face. New York: Thieme Medical Publisher, Inc; 2016. p. 162–72.
7. Homma K, Mutou Y, Mutou H, et al. Intradermal stitch blepharoplasty for Orientals: does it disappear? Aesthetic Plast Surg 2000;24:289–91.
8. Lee CK, Ahn ST, Kim N. Asian upper lid blepharoplasty surgery. Clin Plast Surg 2013;40:167–78.
9. Chen WPD, Park JDJ. Asian upper lid blepharoplasty: an update on indications and technique. Facial Plast Surg 2013;29:26–31.
10. Baek JS, Choi YJ, Jang JW. Medial epicanthoplasty: what works and what does not. Facial Plast Surg 2020;36:584–91.
11. Shirakabe Y, Kinugasa T, Kawata M, et al. The double-eyelid operation in Japan: its evolution as related to cultural changes. Ann Plast Surg 1985;15:224–41.
12. Wu W. A two-way continuous buried-suture approach. Aesthetic Plast Surg 2009;33:426–9.
13. Lew H, Yu SB, Yun YS, et al. Correction of epiblepharon of the upper eyelid by the buried suture technique: correlation with morphological features of the upper eyelid. Ophthalmologica 2008;222:100–4.
14. McCurdy JA. Upper blepharoplasty in the Asian patient: the "double eyelid" operation. Facial Plast Surg Clin North Am 2005;13:47–64.
15. Wong JK. A method in creation of the superior palpebral fold in Asians using a continuous buried tarsal stitch (CBTS). Facial Plast Surg Clin North Am 2007;15:337–42.
16. Choi AK. Oriental blepharoplasty: nonincisional suture technique versus conventional incisional technique. Facial Plast Surg 1994;10:67–83.
17. Hiraga Y. The double eyelid operation and augmentation rhinoplasty in the oriental patient. Clin Plast Surg 1980;7:553–67.
18. Fan J, Low DW. A two-way continuous buried-suture approach to the creation of the long-lasting double eyelid: surgical technique and long-term follow-up in 51 patients. Aesthetic Plast Surg 2009;33:421–5.
19. Ko RY, Baek RM, Oh KS, et al. Complication of non-incision oriental blepharoplasty: is disappearance of the lid crease a fearful complication? J Korean Soc Plast Reconstr Surg 2000;27:199–203.
20. Mizuno T. Treatment of suture-related complications of buried-suture double-eyelid blepharoplasty in Asians. Plast Reconstr Surg Glob Open 2016;4:e839.
21. Kure K, Minami A. A simple and durable way to create a supratarsal fold (double eyelid) in Asian patients. Aesthet surg J 2001;21:227–32.

Cosmetic Bone-Contouring Surgery for Asians

Sanghoon Park, MD, PhD

KEYWORDS

• Facial bone contouring • Zygoma reduction • Mandible reduction • High-L osteotomy
• Maximal malar projection (MMP)

KEY POINTS

- Zygoma reduction decreases the width of cheekbones in order to achieve slim, smooth, and feminine facial aesthetic lines. The purpose of mandible reduction is to make the lower face appear slim, oval, and have a smooth contour.
- The 2 surgical methods in this article (L-shaped osteotomy of the zygoma and intraoral mandible reduction) are the most widely used and accepted surgical methods.
- The zygomatic body and arch are usually moved posteromedially during surgery; the point of maximal malar projection should be evaluated and transposed to a new ideal position.
- Mandible reduction does not simply mean angle reduction but making the overall frontal jaw line slim and natural.

INTRODUCTION

Many investigators have emphasized the difference between white people and Asians, and the facial bone is one of the major factors that create differences in those groups.[1–3] For example, most caucasians are dolichocephalic, whereas most Asians are brachycephalic (**Fig. 1**). Facial shape in the frontal view also differs. The faces of caucasians tend to be long and narrow, whereas the faces of Asians tend to be wide and short. Consequently, Asian faces usually give a square impression.

What Is the Ideal Face?

A study showed there is a huge difference between Asians and caucasians in terms of the ideal face.[4] Regarding the vertical proportion of the face, Asians prefer a short chin compared with white people because it gives a more feminine and soft impression. Asians usually regard a broad face as unattractive and aesthetically unpleasing, especially in women, because it gives the face a masculine appearance.[5–8] Prominent cheekbones are a trademark of strong personality, which is not desired in Asian regions. Recently, size of the face is the issue, and Asian people prefer a small face in proportion with the whole body. It is extremely important for surgeons to understand each patient's end-image of the surgery as well as the motivation for considering facial bone surgery.

Facial bone surgery has evolved for more than 100 years but has only recently been applied to cosmetic fields.[2,3] It is still a minor portion of Western cosmetic surgery, whereas it may be more popular in Asians. Aesthetic facial bone surgery can be divided into the surgery of the middle face, lower face, and chin, but this article focuses more on the middle and lower face.

PATIENT ASSESSMENT AND CONSULTATION

Analysis of the individual's entire face should come from a thorough understanding of facial skeletal types, and establishment of proper surgical indications for each technique is mandatory in order to achieve aesthetically pleasing results. Direct physical examination is most important when collaborating with the patient's aesthetic concerns and establishing a surgical plan. A

The author has no financial conflicts of interest in any materials described in this article.
Department of Facial Bone Surgery, ID Hospital, 142 Dosan-daero, Gangnam-gu, Seoul 06039, South Korea
E-mail address: spark@idhospital.com

Facial Plast Surg Clin N Am 29 (2021) 533–548
https://doi.org/10.1016/j.fsc.2021.07.001

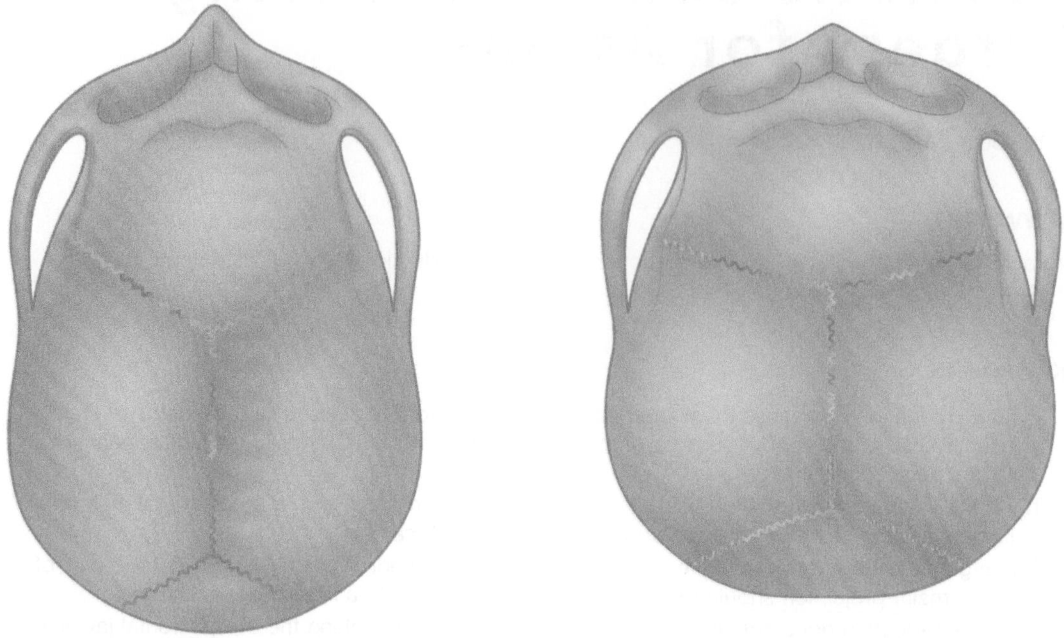

Fig. 1. Bony facial morphology seen from above. Compare the (*left*) dolichocephalic white face and the (*right*) brachycephalic Asian face.

computed tomography (CT) scan with three-dimensional reconstruction is essential to evaluate the shape of the facial bone precisely to plan surgery.

Frontal Evaluation

Frontal evaluation can be simplified by visualizing an anterior and posterior facial plane. The anterior facial plane is defined by the superior temporal line, lateral border of the lateral orbital rim, malar prominence, midface, and mentum (**Fig. 2**, blue line). The posterior facial plane is defined by the contour line of the head and zygomatic arch (see **Fig. 2**, red line). A combination of variable forms of these 2 planes defines the variety of facial shapes encountered in clinical practice. Anterior and posterior facial lines that are wide and parallel to each other in the midface area lead to a wide facial appearance. Severity of zygoma protrusion is usually determined by bizygomatic distance. In patients in whom the cheek bones protrude outward, the facial line connecting the temple-zygoma-cheek-mandible angle becomes convoluted and gives a harsh look to the face (see **Fig. 2**). In patients in whom the mandible angle flares out, the facial shape forms a square and gives a masculine impression.

The length and shape of the chin should be examined. The chin plays a key role in overall facial impression (**Fig. 3**).

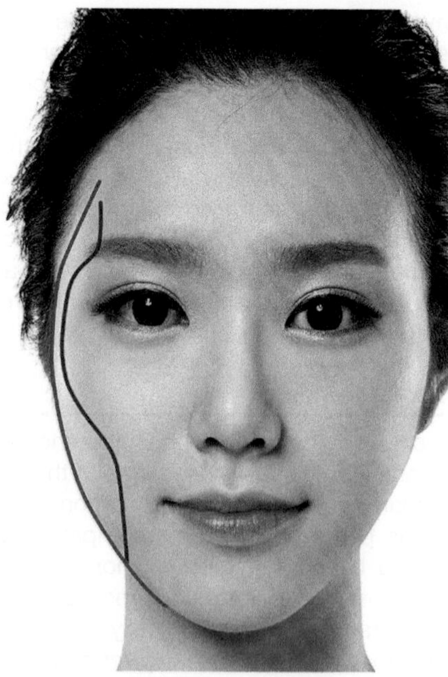

Fig. 2. Anterior and posterior facial contour lines. The anterior facial contour line connects the temple, zygomatic body, cheek, and mandible body (*blue line*), whereas the posterior facial contour line connects the temple, zygomatic arch, mandible angle, and chin (*red line*). If the anterior contour line is too convoluted, the patient gives a strong, offensive, old, tired, masculine impression. The posterior contour line reflects the facial width and facial size.

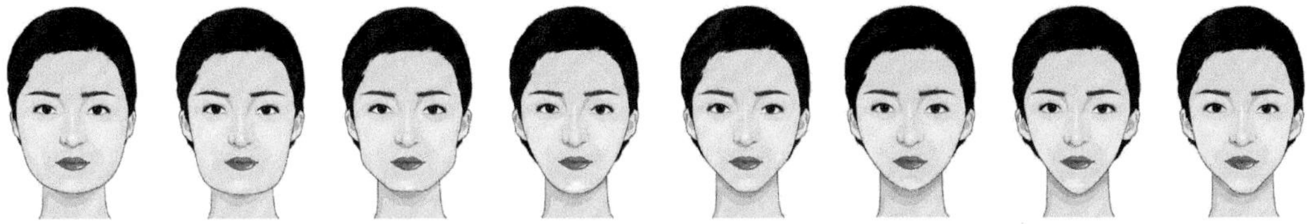

Fig. 3. Classification of the chin shape in the frontal view. From left to right: round, broad, blunt, angular, trapezoid, triangular, pointed, and pear-shaped chin types. Round chin gives a feminine impression, whereas angular chin gives a masculine impression. The difference in chin shape gives a different facial impression.

Three-Quarter Oblique Evaluation

The zygomatic body is most clearly appreciated in the three-quarter oblique view, exposing the shape of zygoma as well as the degree and location of zygomatic body protrusion. Severity of zygomatic protrusion is usually determined with the point of maximal malar projection (MMP). The MMP is the most protruded portion of the outer contour of the zygomatic complex in the three-quarter views. Shape and position vary among patients, thus altering the projection, and position of the MMP point placed precisely in the patient's aesthetically ideal position, is the key to a successful postoperative result.

The ideal MMP point may vary among different ethnicities and patients' needs; however, patients who desire zygoma reduction want the MMP to be medial to the lateral canthus in the horizontal dimension, and not too high or too close to the lateral canthus in the vertical dimension[9,10] (**Fig. 4**).

Lateral Evaluation

The gonial angle and the mandibular plane should be identified using the lateral cephalogram. If the gonial angle is less than 100°, the facial shape looks square. If the gonial angle is located too low or the mandibular plane is too flat (<30°), the lateral face also looks square[11] (**Fig. 5**).

Facial profile should be evaluated and understood in lateral evaluation. In class III profile, mandible surgery should be done cautiously in order to not exacerbate the prognathic look. In contrast, in class II profile patients, zygomatic reduction should be done cautiously to exacerbate a long face.

Basal Evaluation

When viewed from below, the degree of projection in the suborbital area and protruding zygomatic arch can be evaluated. This view helps in

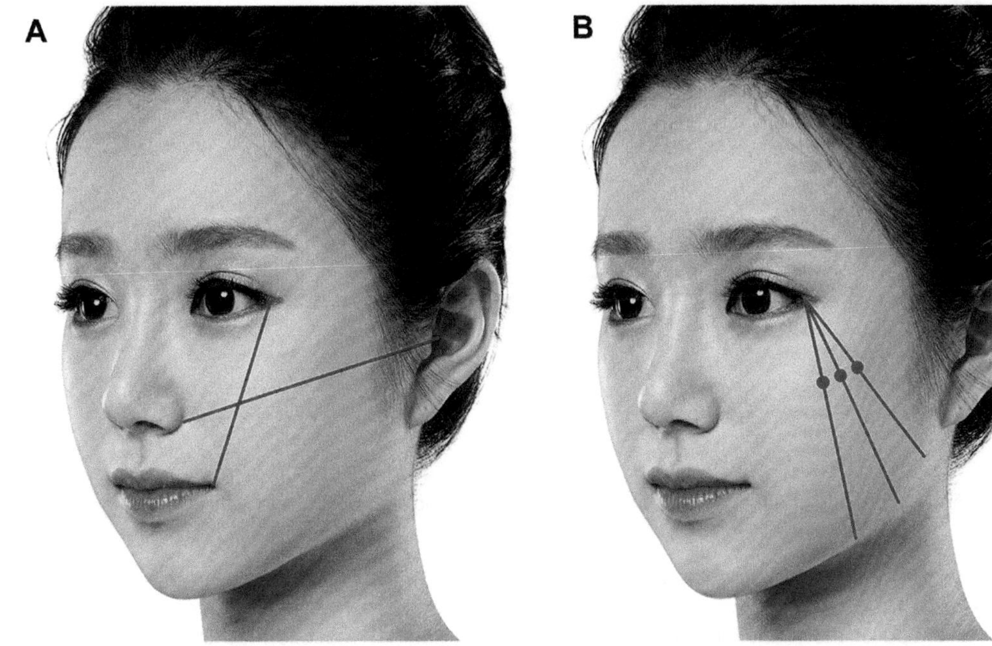

Fig. 4. Determining the ideal position of the MMP. (*A*) Hinderer analysis. (*B*) Wilkinson analysis.

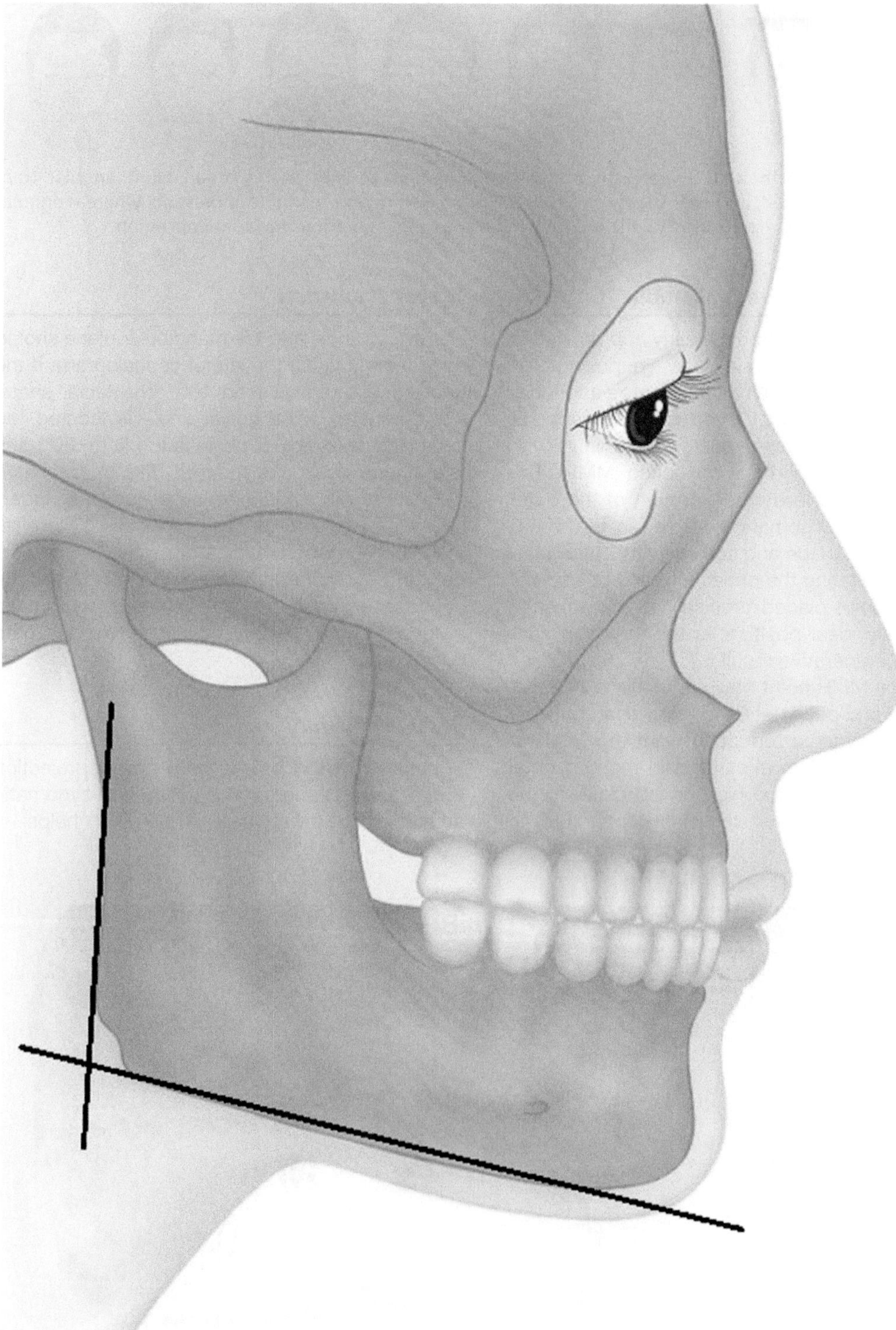

Fig. 5. The gonial angle and the mandibular plane determine the facial impression in lateral view.

evaluating symmetry and facilitates evaluation of the zygomatic arch.

Transverse shape of the mandible can also be evaluated (**Fig. 6**). The angle of divergence and convexity of the mandible are observed. In patients with an inward curled angle with convex transverse shape, sagittal resection at the body helps to reduce the width of the mandible more effectively.

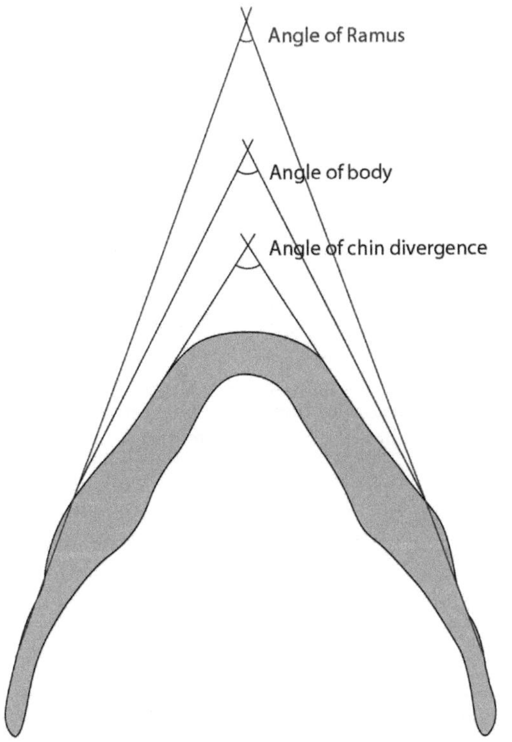

Fig. 6. Let patients raise the chin and the transverse shape of the mandible is evaluated. The angle of chin divergence and convexity of the mandible (angle of ramus and body divergence) is observed. A patient with wide angle of chin divergence may require combined chin surgery. Wide angle of ramus and body usually predicts big change and satisfaction after mandible reduction.

Soft Tissue Evaluation

Because facial soft tissue is also an important component in zygoma reduction, it should be given due consideration to achieve a satisfactory aesthetic result. If the patient has thin skin with minimal soft cheek tissue, changes following zygoma reduction will be obvious with minimal prospect of soft tissue drooping. Such patients are ideal candidates for zygoma reduction.

In contrast, the risk of cheek drooping increases if the patient has abundant soft tissues or thick skin. Surgeons should discuss the possibility of cheek drooping with the patient during the informed consent process and contemplate appropriate additional procedures, such as liposuction or lifting, to counter this possibility.

SURGICAL TECHNIQUES

Zygomatic Reduction

An L-shaped osteotomy of the zygomatic body is the preferred method for patients with moderate to severe malar protrusion caused by wide zygomatic arch and prominent body.[12] An L-shaped osteotomy is made in the anterior part of the zygomatic body and a separate osteotomy is made in the posterior part of the zygomatic arch. The L-shaped osteotomy technique can change both the zygomatic body and arch; it also has the advantage of controlling the degree of reduction as well as the shape after reduction.

General anesthesia is recommended for all zygoma reduction surgeries. Either nasotracheal or endotracheal intubation can be used.

For the zygomatic approach, a standard upper labiobuccal vestibular incision is made on each side of the maxilla.[12] The soft tissues are elevated superiorly and laterally. Dissection is done subperiosteally to the area of the zygomatic body, the anterior wall of the maxillary sinus, and the lateral and inferior orbital rim. As the dissection extends superolaterally over the malar eminence, a portion of the origin of the zygomatic major and zygomatic-cutaneous ligaments may be partially divided from the bony surface.

The course of the frontal branch of the facial nerve and the zygomatic arch is marked on the facial skin. About a 1-cm vertical incision is made within the sideburn, 2 to 3 cm anterior to the tragus.[13,14] This incision should lie posterior to the course of the facial nerve. The arch is identified after the dissection of the periosteum, and fine elevators are passed over the top and behind the arch and as far posteriorly as possible to ensure that the osteotomy is still anterior to the temporomandibular joint.

An L-shaped osteotomy line is marked over the malar eminence (**Fig. 7**). This line generally extends medially from the lateral border of the orbital rim to just below the infraorbital foramen. The surgeon should be careful not to start the osteotomy too low from where the arch changes from a vertical to a horizontal direction, because this may result in insufficient volume reduction at the zygomatic body. The short limb of the osteotomy then turns at about a 90° angle toward the zygomaticomaxillary buttress. Great attention must be paid to avoid injury to the orbital contents or infraorbital nerve. A second, parallel line is drawn lateral to the first line to represent the strip of bone to be resected, allowing inset of the fragment. The distance of the second line from the first line depends on the patient's preference and the width of the zygomatic body (see **Fig. 7**). A wider parallel osteotomy can be made for greater reduction; however, the usual width of the strip is 3 to 5 mm. A double-blade reciprocating saw with a distance of 2, 3, 4, 5, 6, or 7 mm between the 2 blades (**Fig. 8**) was designed at our clinic and

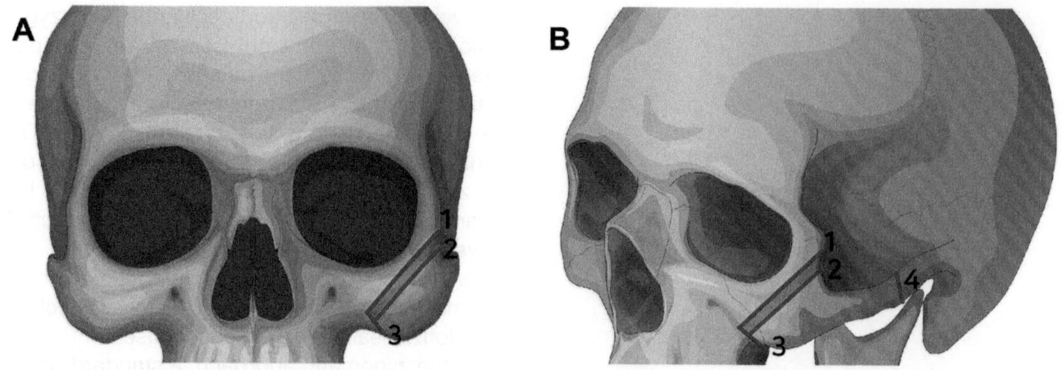

Fig. 7. Design of bone cuts in zygoma reduction. An L-shaped osteotomy line is marked over the malar eminence. A second, parallel line is drawn lateral to the first line to represent the strip of bone to be resected. A posterior bone cut is made 2 to 3 cm anterior to the tragus. Numbers in the figures are order of osteotomy.

has proved to be very useful in achieving this goal. A simple osteotomy and repositioning of the zygomatic body alone usually cannot successfully reduce the size of the zygoma, which necessitates ostectomy and removal of bone.[14,15] Careful dissection is required in the zygomatic-pterygoid space to prevent injury to vessels, which may lead to profuse bleeding and postoperative bruising.

A reciprocating saw is used to make the vertical osteotomy on the zygomatic arch[14](see **Fig. 8**). When the posterior osteotomy is completed, the zygomatic segment should be free to move while remaining attached to the masseter. Additional bone distal to the osteotomy may be burred if necessary.

The osteotomized body and arch are positioned posteriorly and medially after the osteotomy and the intervening segment is removed. While making sure that there is good contact between bony surfaces, 6-hole miniplates with screws are placed to fix the anterior portion of the bony segment

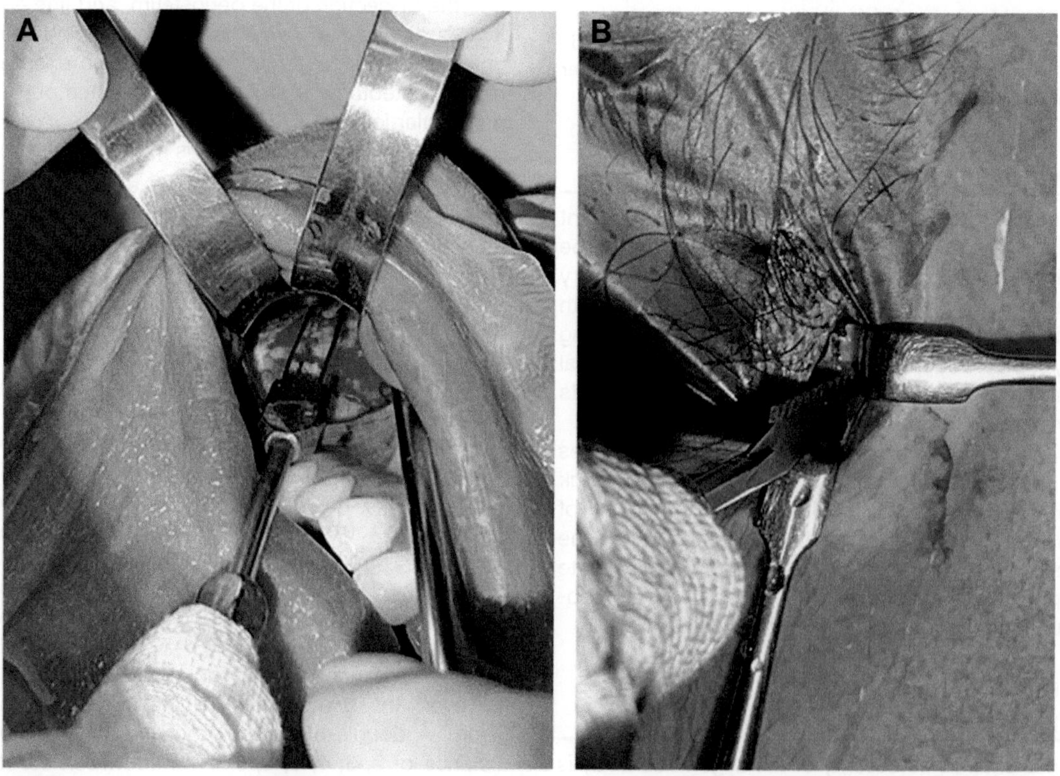

Fig. 8. Position of the saw (double-bladed reciprocating saw) for anterior (*A*) and posterior (*B*) osteotomy.

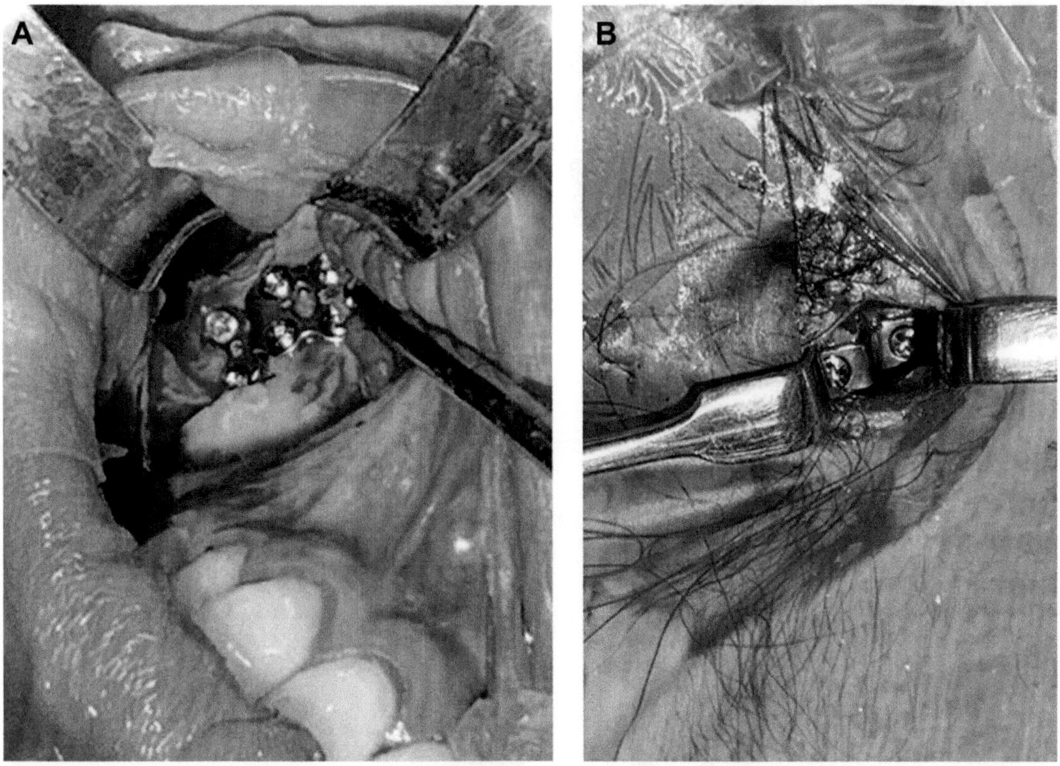

Fig. 9. Rigid fixation of malar complex. (*A*) Applying a prebent double-square miniplate to the zygoma body. (*B*) Applying a prebent miniplate to the zygomatic arch.

(**Fig. 9**). It is important to prevent three-dimensional rotation of the segment.[13] A 3-hole miniplate with screws is used to fix the posterior zygomatic arch (see **Fig. 9**). Prebent titanium plates are extremely useful during this step because the bony segments are mobile and three-dimensional positioning is difficult because of the limited surgical exposure. Positioning of the osteotomized segment is the most critical step for satisfactory postoperative results.

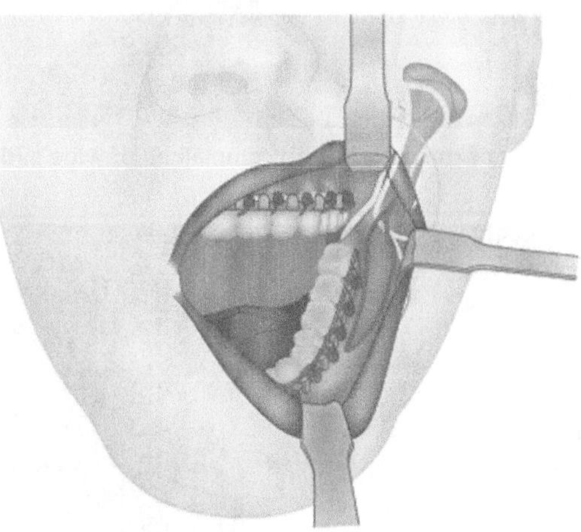

Fig. 10. Mandibular buccal vestibular approach. Visualization and access is possible without leaving external scars and without violating the facial motor and sensory nerves.

Mandible Reduction

Intraoral mandible reduction with an oscillating saw is the standard technique for mandible reduction.[16] For patients who require a combination of chin surgery together with mandible reduction, the so-called V-line surgery is performed. However, genioplasty or V-line surgery are beyond the

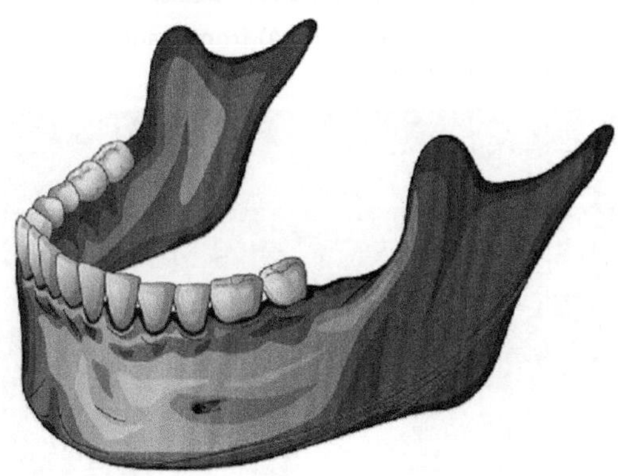

Fig. 11. The osteotomy line of the mandible reduction. Osteotomy line should not be too short and not too vertical.

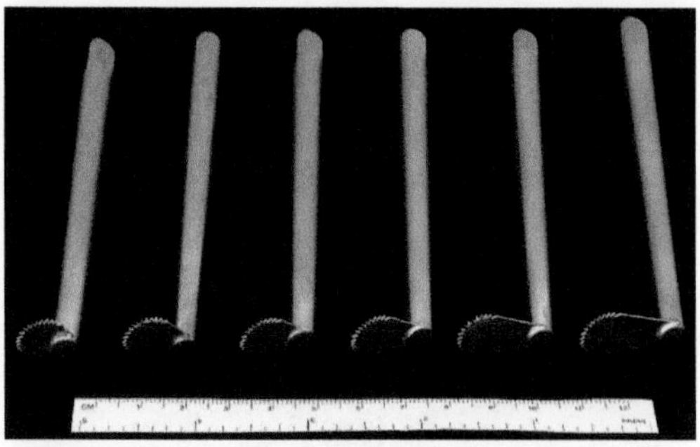

Fig. 12. Serially larger oscillating saws were prepared and used to complete the bone resection.

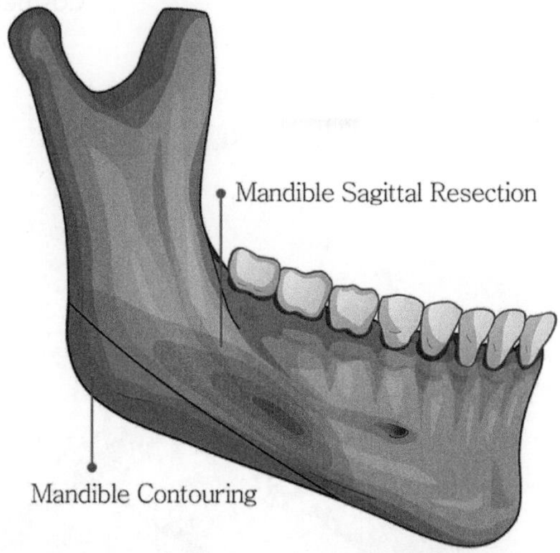

Fig. 13. Areas of bone resection in the lateral cortex to maximize the slimming effect and smooth shape.

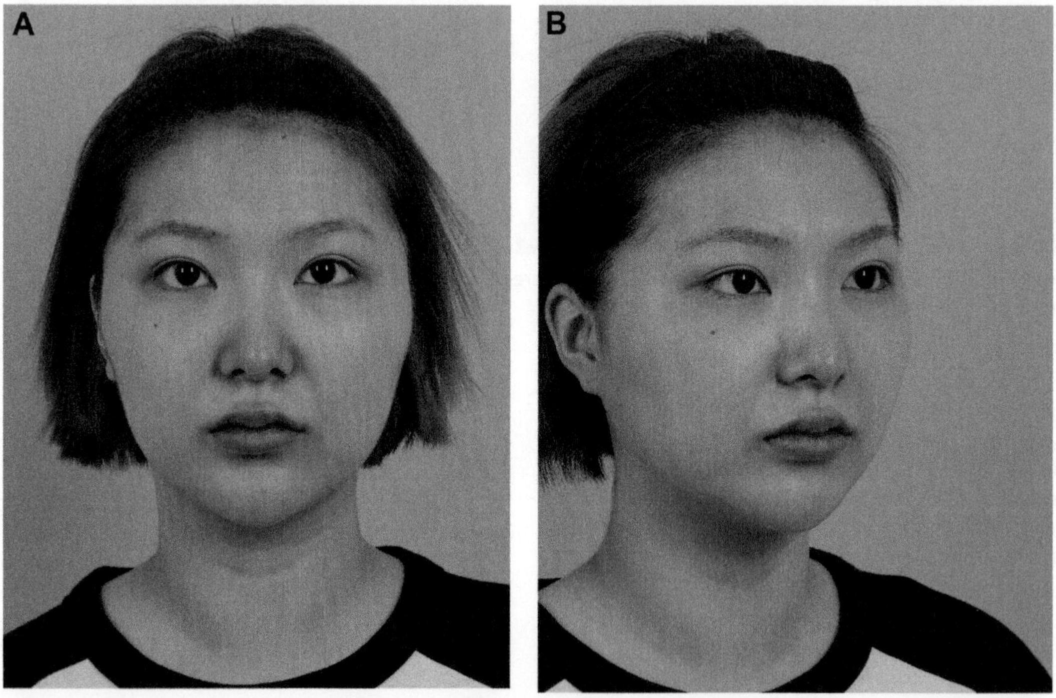

Fig. 14. Case 1. Preoperative (*A*) frontal and (*B*) three-quarter views of the patient who complained of wide mid-face and malar protrusion.

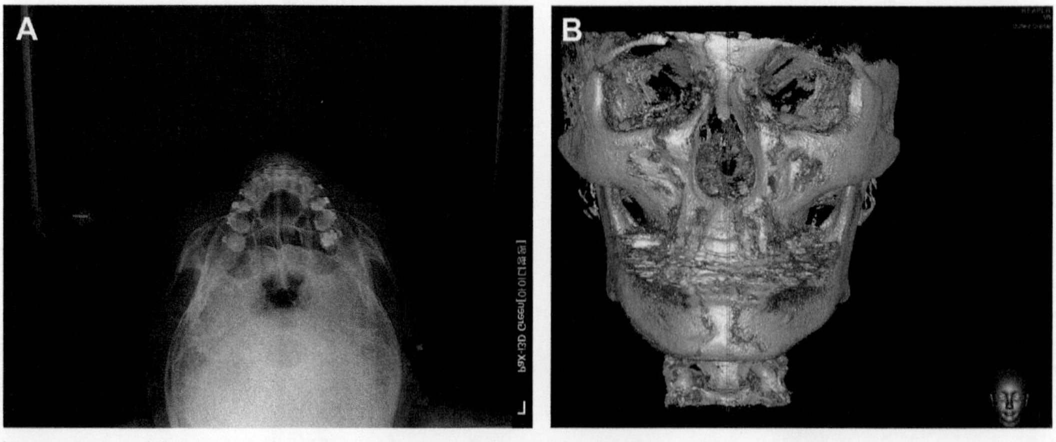

Fig. 15. Case 1. (*A*) Preoperative submentovertex radiography. (*B*) CT.

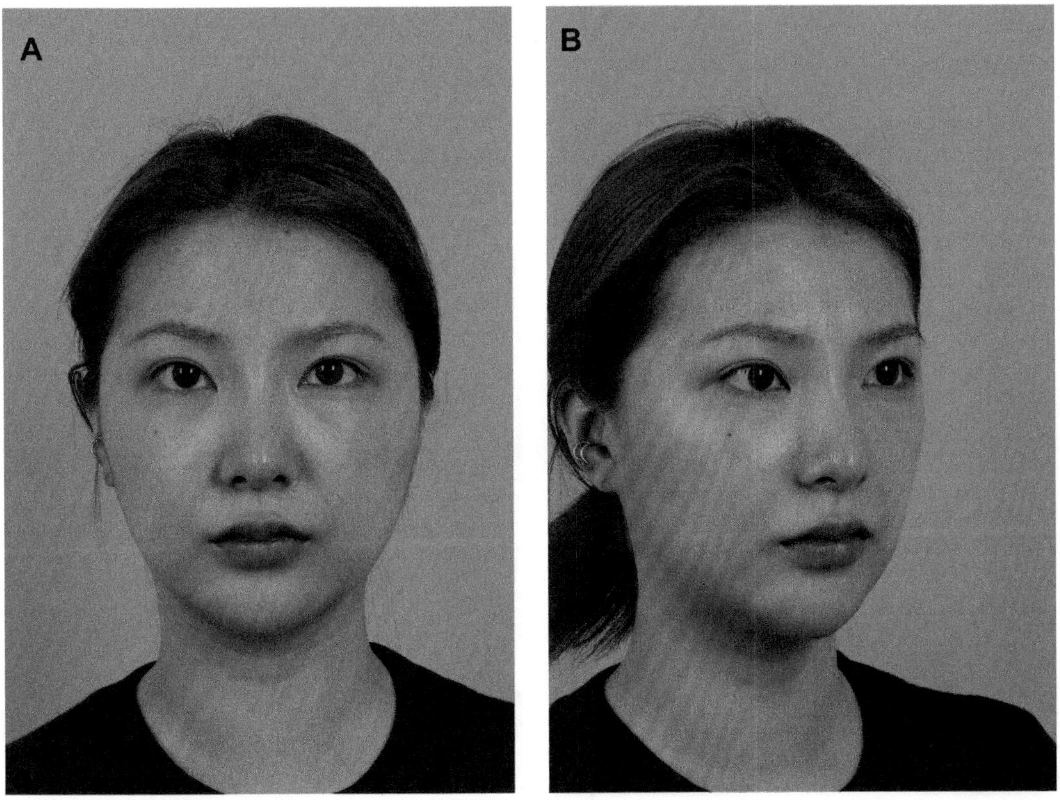

Fig. 16. Case 1. Postoperative (*A*) frontal and (*B*) three-quarter views. The malar prominence and midfacial width were reduced markedly.

scope of this article and are discussed elsewhere in this issue.

For the mandibular approach, a standard buccal vestibular incision is made (**Fig. 10**). Through subperiosteal elevation, the masseter muscle fibers are stripped from the lower border of the body, angle, and posterior border of the ramus with an angle stripper to secure a good operative field. During the dissection, the mental nerve, the marginal mandibular branch of the facial nerve, the retromandibular vein, and the facial artery should be protected.

After the surgical field is exposed by the abovementioned procedure, the mandibular angle is hooked by using a specialized angle retractor, and the desired level of the osteotomy line is marked on the bone with gentian violet solution. The marked line is then checked with dental

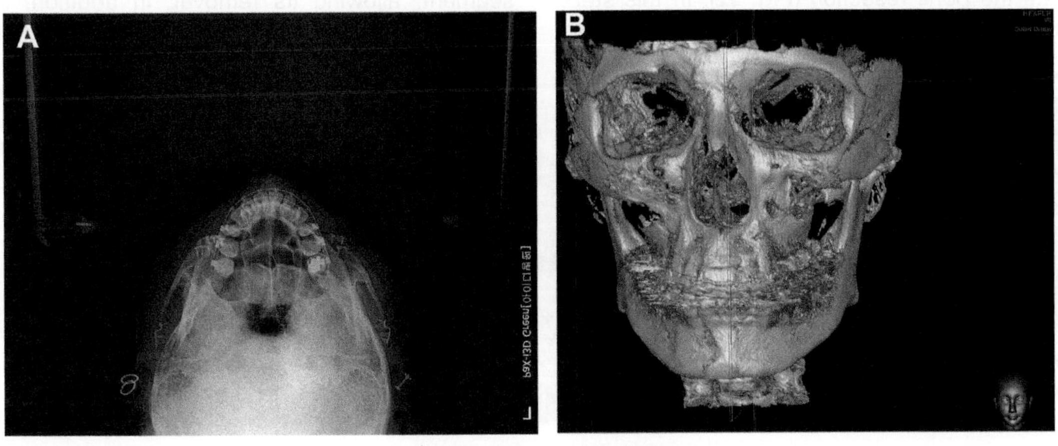

Fig. 17. Case 1. (*A*) Postoperative submentovertex radiography. (*B*) CT.

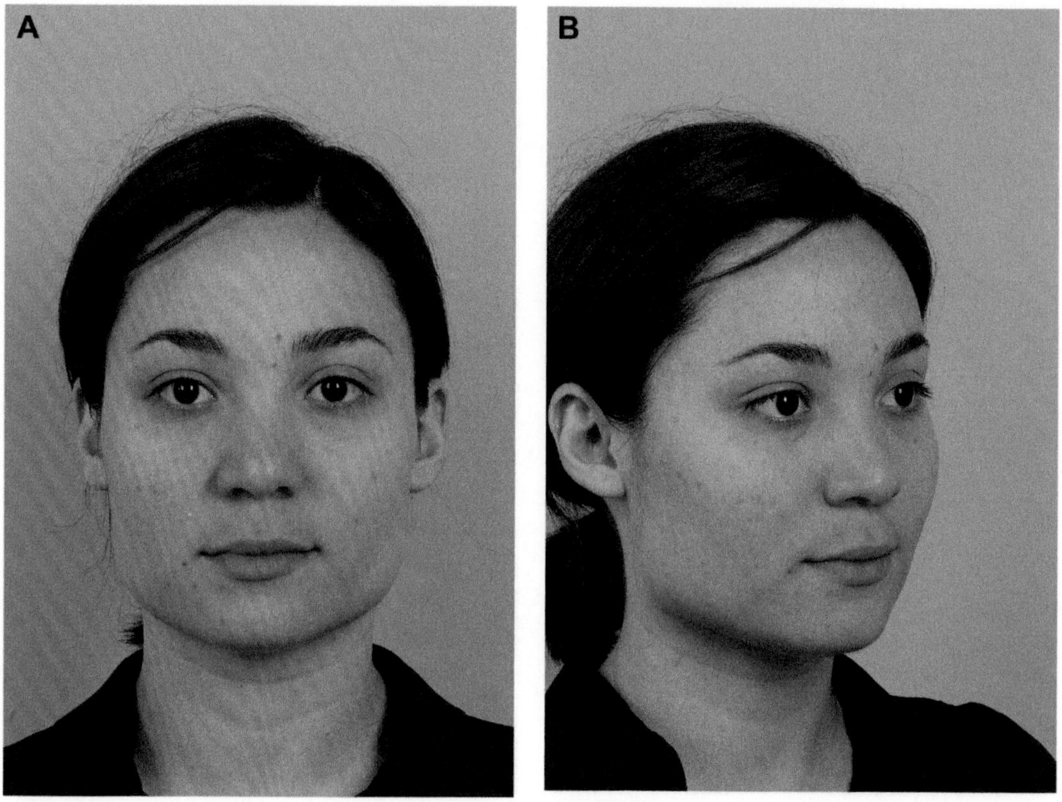

Fig. 18. Case 2. Preoperative (*A*) frontal and (*B*) three-quarter photographs of a 27-year-old white patient who complained of broad and angular lower face. She also complained of asymmetry of lower jaw line with canting of occlusal plane and asymmetric chin shape.

mirrors. In general, the upper limit of osteotomy should not be beyond the occlusal plane and the anterior limit should not violate the chin (**Fig. 11**). Usually, the anterior limit is immediately under the mental foramen. However, the upper and anterior limit of osteotomy can be adjusted case by case.

Serially larger oscillating saws are used to complete the bone resection (**Fig. 12**). In this step, thorough full-thickness ostectomy can cause soft tissue injury in the medial surface of the mandible, so surgeons should pay attention in order to not place the oscillating saw too deeply.[16] After ostectomy, the attachment of muscle to the medial part of the mandible usually remains. A large elevator or electrocautery is used to divide any remaining medial pterygoid muscle fibers from the medial surface of the osteotomized segment, allowing its removal. In addition, a high-speed bur is used to remove any additional

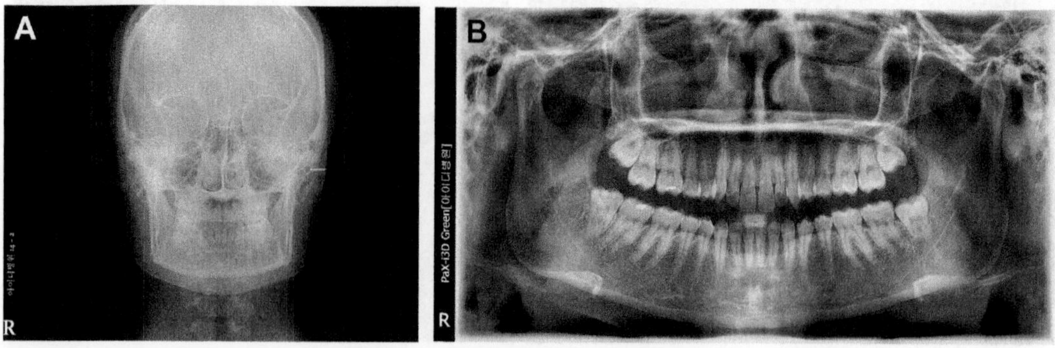

Fig. 19. Case 2. Preoperative (*A*) frontal and (*B*) panoramic radiography.

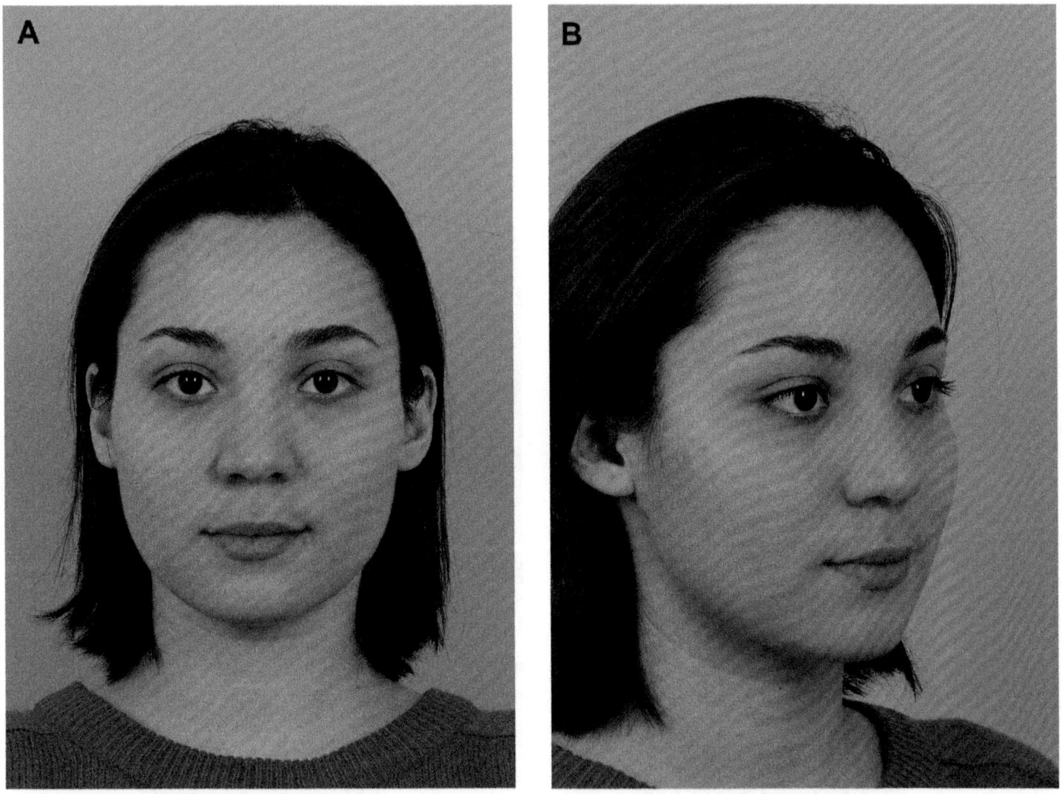

Fig. 20. Case 2. Postoperative (*A*) frontal and (*B*) three-quarter photographs. Her lower face converted from square shape to smooth contour and asymmetry also improved.

bone from the lateral cortex and to make a smooth transition (**Fig. 13**).

CASE STUDIES

Case 1

A 25-year-old woman complained of wide midface and malar protrusion (**Figs. 14** and **15**). Via intraoral approach, an L-shaped osteotomy with a 5-mm reduction of zygoma was performed to reduce the projection of her zygoma. The posterior part of the zygomatic arch was divided with complete osteotomy. The zygoma was repositioned medially and posteriorly and fixed with miniplates and screws (**Figs. 16** and **17**). The malar prominence and midfacial width reduced markedly at 11 months postoperatively.

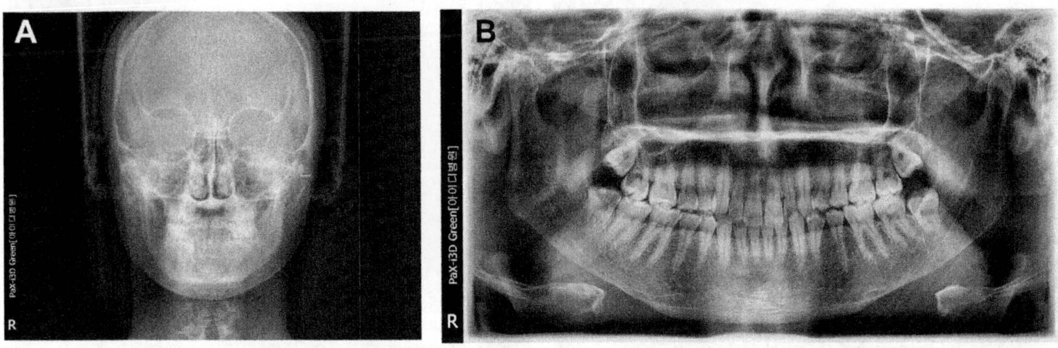

Fig. 21. Case 2. Preoperative (*A*) frontal and (*B*) panoramic radiography. Bilateral osteotomies are asymmetric to balance the asymmetric face.

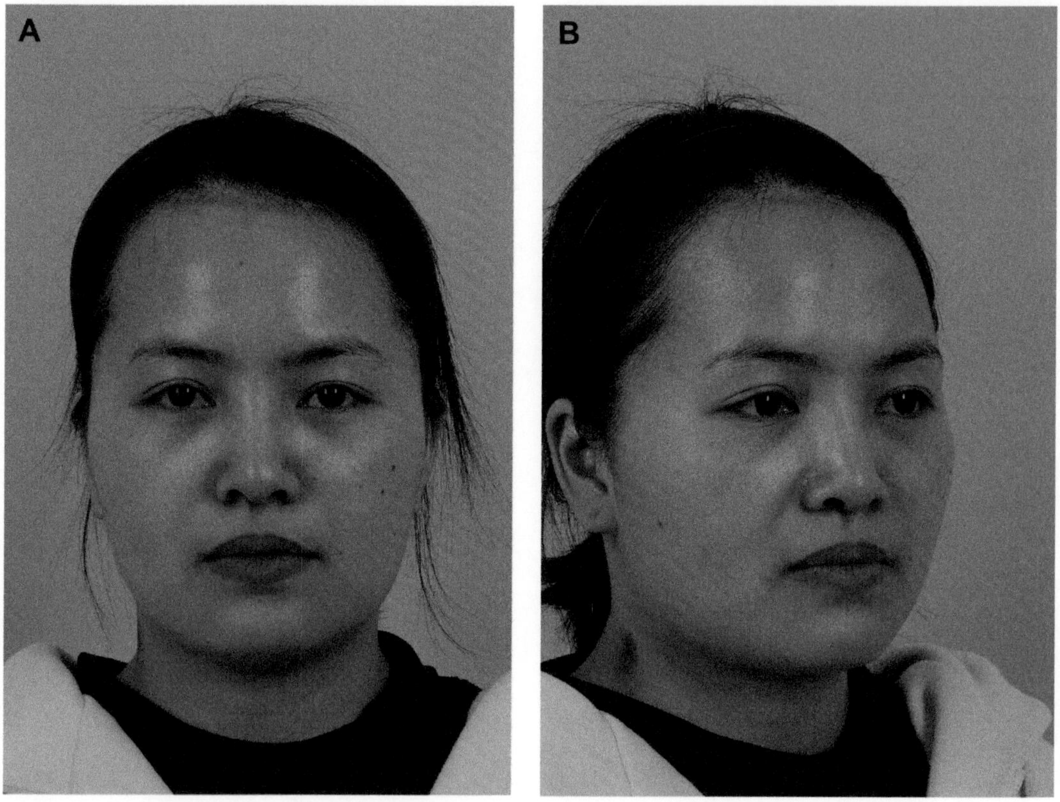

Fig. 22. Case 3. Preoperative (*A*) frontal and (*B*) three-quarter views of a 28-year-old Vietnamese woman who complained of wide face.

Case 2

A 27-year-old white woman had a broad and angular lower face contour and desired slimming and softening of the lower face. She wanted to have a more feminine appearance (**Figs. 18** and **19**). She also complained of asymmetry of lower jaw line with canting of occlusal plane and asymmetric chin shape. However, after consultation for her asymmetry, she decided to get neither 2-jaw surgery nor chin correction. With an intraoral approach, asymmetric resection of the lower mandibular border to the angle was done. Sagittal resection of the mandibular cortex was shaved as

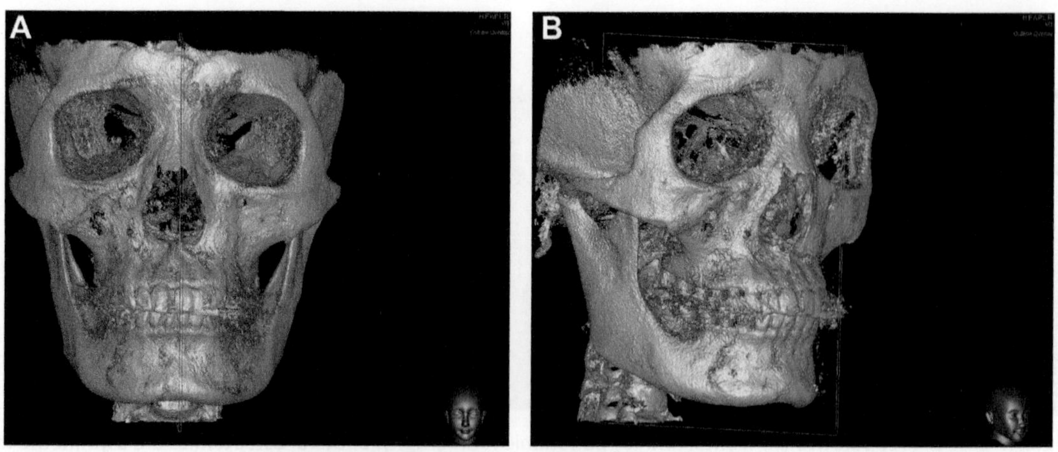

Fig. 23. Case 3. Preoperative (*A*) frontal CT view and (*B*) and 3-quarter CT view.

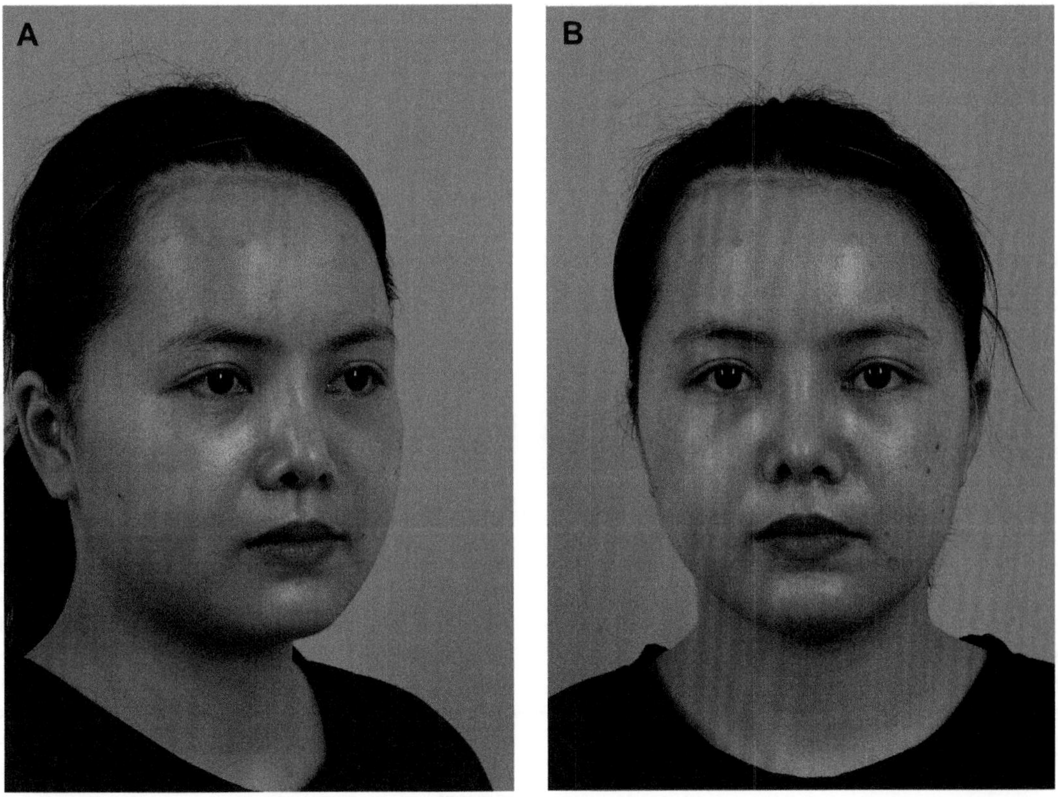

Fig. 24. Case 3. Postoperative (*A*) frontal and (*B*) three-quarter views. She underwent zygoma reduction and mandible-contouring surgery. Her whole facial contour appears slim and contoured.

much as possible to balance the bilateral shape. Her square-shaped lower face was converted to a smooth-contoured face and asymmetry improved (**Figs. 20** and **21**). Even though her asymmetry was not fully corrected, she was happy with the result.

Case 3

A 28-year-old Vietnamese woman complained of malar protrusion and wide lower face (**Figs. 22** and **23**). She underwent zygoma reduction and mandible-contouring surgery (see **Fig. 13**; **Figs.**

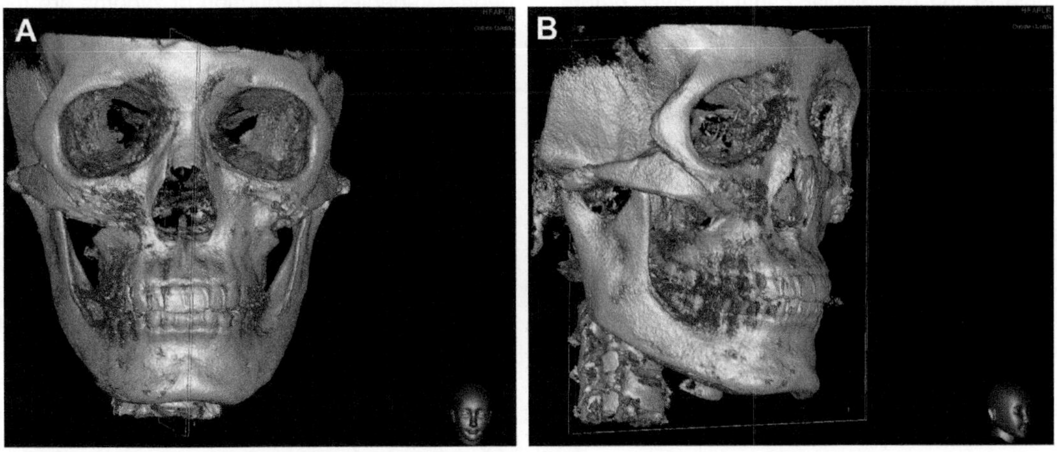

Fig. 25. Case 3. Preoperative (*A*) frontal CT view and (*B*) and three-quarter CT view.

24 and 25). Complete osteotomy was performed on the anterior and posterior parts of the zygoma and it was repositioned posteriorly and medially. Mandible-contouring surgery was performed to correct her square lower face concomitantly. Five months after the operation, the patient's facial contour appears slim and contoured.

COMPLICATIONS AND MANAGEMENT

Hemorrhage and Hematoma

A hemorrhage used to be the most life-threatening complication after mandibular contouring, because a hematoma extending into the floor of the mouth may result in airway obstruction. Inadvertent injury to a facial vessel was the most common cause of major bleeding.

Other hemorrhages can be prevented with meticulous hemostasis of the soft tissues and bone. Hypotensive anesthesia coupled with injection of local anesthetics with a vasoconstrictor may also help minimize blood loss and increases visualization of the operative field during the surgery. If the hematoma rapidly expands, the airway must be controlled with a nasopharyngeal airway or occasionally with endotracheal intubation.

Neurosensory Deficits

Neurosensory loss of the lower lip is a common postoperative complication after facial bone surgery. The transient neurosensory deficits around the lower lip after mandibular contouring usually result from neurapraxia of the mental nerve during retraction. The paresthesia around the upper lip or midface result from neurapraxia of the infraorbital nerve after zygoma reduction. This kind of complication can be reduced by minimizing dissection and exposure near the mental foramen or infraorbital foramen. Surgeons should be aware that the course of the mandibular canal is lower before the nerve comes out of the mental foramen.

Surgical Site Infection

Although wound infection following the surgery is uncommon, problematic issues may arise with preoperative conditions such as poor oral hygiene, periodontal disease, or sinusitis, and these should be screened for and the patient warned as part of informed consent.

Operative conditions such as improperly sealed wounds, insufficient saline irrigation, bone fragments or dust left behind in the wound, and damaged salivary glands should be carefully prevented. In order to prevent the risk of postoperative infections, intravenous antibiotics are administered during the admission. After discharge, prophylactic oral antibiotics are given for an additional week.

Nonunion

Symptoms and signs of nonunion for zygomatic reduction are pain, cheek drooping, and clicking sounds; however, some patients have no symptoms. Possible causes of nonunion are excessive resection of bone, unstable fixation, excessive movement (eg, caused by chewing), muscle pull, and trauma in the immediate postoperative period. Conservative treatment can be tried initially to relieve the pain and camouflage soft tissue depression. Malunion of the osteotomized segment may be corrected with revisional surgery.

DISCUSSION

Two surgical methods in this article, L-shaped osteotomy of the zygoma and intraoral mandible reduction, are the most widely used and accepted surgical methods. Some variations and combinations of surgeries are possible. Selection of surgical method or the extent of surgery is established by the surgeon from the characteristics of the facial bone as well as the patient's request.

Minimally invasive minizygoma reduction surgery can be performed under local anesthesia in patients with a wide zygomatic arch with minimal body protrusion. The surgery has the advantages of short operative time, fast recovery, and minimal postoperative swelling but also has limitations in terms of the result.

A combination of mandible reduction and zygomatic reduction, or even genioplasty, should be considered and discussed with the patient.

There are key variables to be determined before the surgery, especially for beginner surgeons. Variables in reduction of zygoma are the amount of ostectomy, medialization, setback, vertical repositioning, and the amount of arch medialization. Variables in mandible reduction are the amount of resection and extent of anterior osteotomy.

The most common reason for unsatisfactory aesthetic results following zygoma reduction is undercorrection of the zygomatic body. The main reason for this undercorrection is an overly low osteotomy that fails to move the MMP medially. Beginner surgeons may be afraid of injuring orbital contents under limited vision and put the osteotomy too low or too horizontal and fail to include the MMP. In contrast, too much resection of the zygomatic body may result in a visible bony step in thin-skinned patients.

The most common unfavorable results of mandible reduction for beginner surgeons are osteotomy problems, such as irregular jaw line, secondary angle, and excessive resection. If osteotomy falls too short and abruptly, a so-called secondary angle may result in the patient's complaint. When osteotomy goes too high posteriorly, there is a catastrophic risk of condyle injury, so care needs to be taken. Osteotomy problems may be treated with secondary surgery after consultation with the patient, but they should be carefully prevented with practice and supervision.

The angle resection was an old misnomer of the mandible reduction, because it began as cutting the angle. Mandible reduction should include the whole jawline to make the lower face slim and natural.

SUMMARY

Through advances in facial bone surgery techniques, surgeons have control over the width and line of the midface and lower face for aesthetic needs.

Two surgical methods in this article, L-shaped osteotomy of the zygoma and intraoral mandible reduction, are the most widely used and accepted surgical techniques.

On planning and executing facial bone surgery, surgeons should consider that ideal facial shape may be different based on various preferences. Hard and soft facial tissues should also be in good harmony.

Surgical complications and unfavorable results should be studied and carefully prevented.

CLINICS CARE POINTS

- Key variables in reduction of zygoma are the amount of ostectomy, medialization, setback, vertical repositioning, and the amount of arch medialization. Variables in mandible reduction are the amount of resection and extent of anterior osteotomy. These variables should be planned before surgery, and the accuracy of execution should be carefully confirmed during the surgery.
- The most common reason for unsatisfactory aesthetic results following zygoma reduction is undercorrection of the zygomatic body. The main reason for this undercorrection is an overly low osteotomy that fails to move the MMP medially. Make sure the osteotomy lies in the right position and angle.
- The most common unfavorable results of mandible reduction are osteotomy problems, such as irregular jaw line, secondary angle, and excessive resection. To prevent these problems, the osteotomy line is first marked with short-blade saw and then carefully deepened with longer-blade saw.
- Soft tissue swelling usually peaks in 3 to 4 days and reduces within 2 weeks. Soft tissue infection is rare but should be ruled out if swelling continues longer than this period or spreads to the neck or eye region.

REFERENCES

1. Park CG, Lee ET, Lee JS. Facial form analysis of the lower and middle face in young Korean women. J Korean Soc Plast Reconstr Surg 1998; 96:7–13.
2. Whitaker LA, Bartlett SP. Aesthetic surgery of the facial skeleton. Persp Plast Surg 1988;1:23–69.
3. Whitaker LA. Aesthetic contouring of the facial support system. Clin Plast Surg 1989;16:815–23.
4. Larrabee WF, Makielski KH. Variations in Facial anatomy with race, sex, and age. Surgical anatomy of the face. 2nd edition. Lippincott Williams & Wilkins; 2004.
5. Kim YH, Seul JH. Reduction malarplasty through an intra-oral incision: a new method. Plast Reconstr Surg 2000;106(7):1514–9.
6. Morris DE, Moaveni Z, Lo LJ. Aesthetic facial skeletal contouring in the Asian patient. Clin Plast Surg 2007;34(3):547–56.
7. Baek SM, Kim SS, Bindiger A. The prominent mandibular angle: Preoperative management, operative technique, and results in 42 patients. Plast Reconstr Surg 1989;83:272–80.
8. Yang DB, Park CG. Mandibular contouring surgery for purely aesthetic reasons. Aesth Plast Surg 1991;15:53–60.
9. Hinderer UT. Malar implants for improvement of the facial appearance. Plast Reconstr Surg 1975;56(2): 157–65.
10. Wilkinson TS. Complications in aesthetic malar augmentation. Plast Reconstr Surg 1983;71(5): 643–9.
11. Li J, Hsu Y, Khadka A, et al. Surgical designs and techniques for mandibular contouring based on categorization of square face with low gonial angle in Orientals. J Plast Reconstr Aesthet Surg 2012;65:1.
12. Cho BC. Reduction malarplasty using osteotomy and repositioning of the malar complex: clinical review and comparison of two techniques. J Craniofac Surg 2003;14(3):383–92.

13. Lee TS. Standard surgical instruments for facial bone surgery. In: Park S, editor. Facial bone contouring surgery. Singapore: Springer; 2017. p. 23–8.
14. Park S. Standard zygomatic reduction with intra-oral approach. In: Park S, editor. Facial bone contouring surgery. Singapore: Springer; 2017. p. 145–58.
15. Chung SE, Park S. Aesthetic midface analysis. In: Park S, editor. Facial bone contouring surgery. Singapore: Springer; 2017. p. 135–43.
16. Park S. Standard mandible reduction with intra-oral approach. In: Park S, editor. Facial bone contouring surgery. Singapore: Springer; 2017. p. 41–51.

Recent Trends in Orthognathic Surgery in Asia

Yoon-Ji Kim, DDS, MS, PhD[a], Bu-Kyu Lee, DDS, MS, PhD[b,*]

KEYWORDS

• Orthognathic surgery • Asian • Face • Esthetics • Jaw deformity

KEY POINTS

- Asian women prefer to have slimmer and softer faces compared with white women.
- The Le Fort I and bilateral sagittal split osteotomy short lingual techniques are the most popular surgical techniques.
- Diverse adjuvant jaw surgeries, such as malarplasty, lateral corticotomy, mandibular angle reduction, and genioplasty, are performed commonly during orthognathic surgery.
- The surgery-first approach is now accepted (recognized) as a reliable option for orthognathic surgery.
- The use of cutting-edge technologies has become popular for more precise and safer orthognathic surgery.

INTRODUCTION

Orthognathic surgery (OGS) for jaw deformities has seen a leap since Hullien first introduced jaw deformity surgeries back in 1849[1] and has recently become a safe and effective surgical method that improves the functional and esthetic aspects of the patient.[2] Over the last century, the technical developments in jaw deformity surgery could be categorized into the development of various effective mandible and maxillary surgery methods, the development of orthodontic treatment methods before and after surgery, and the development of surgical materials and devices. In this article, the latest trends in OGS currently being performed in Asia, especially in Korea, are detailed, with a focus on the unique features that differ among Western patients.

DIFFERENT FACTORS OF ASIAN AND WESTERNERS FOR ORTHOGNATHIC SURGERY

The standards of beauty are quite subjective and are influenced greatly by culture. In general, Western women think that an angular and distinct jaw shape is attractive, whereas Asian women prefer a small, slim, and soft face shape, which is more feminine.[3] In addition, the shape of the jaw itself differs between Westerners and Asians. Westerners have characteristics such as a narrow and long face, a high nose, a prominent tip of the chin, and relatively less protrusion of the maxilla and cheekbones. In contrast, Asians have a relatively wide face, a low nose, and a more protrusive maxilla and cheekbone. One of the main purposes of jaw-correction surgery is to improve esthetics that the patients prefer. Therefore, to achieve this

[a] Department of Orthodontics, Asan Medical Center, College of Medicine, University of Ulsan, 88, Olympic-ro 43-gil, Songpa-gu, Seoul 05505, Republic of Korea; [b] Department of Oral and Maxillofacial Surgery, Asan Medical Center, College of Medicine, University of Ulsan, 88, Olympic-ro 43-gil, Songpa-gu, Seoul 05505, Republic of Korea
* Corresponding author.
E-mail address: bukyu.lee@gmail.com

Facial Plast Surg Clin N Am 29 (2021) 549–566
https://doi.org/10.1016/j.fsc.2021.06.006
1064-7406/21/

goal, the surgical plan and surgical method selected differ significantly from those in the West.

CHARACTERISTICS OF SURGERY PLANNING IN ASIANS

In general, Asian women prefer a slim and smooth mandibular angle and jawline. With respect to the maxilla, they prefer it not to be too protrusive, an approximately 90° nasolabial angle, so that a low nose could be compensated. Regarding the chin, the preferences are that it should not be too big, but somewhat prominent. Overall, they wish to have the so-called oval or V-shaped face.[4] Therefore, during OGS in Asia, additional jaw plastic surgeries, such as mandibular contouring surgery, malarplasty (of the cheekbone), mandibular angle reduction, and various types of genioplasty, are often conducted simultaneously.

However, repositioning the jawbone only for esthetic purposes can cause serious jaw dysfunctions, such as difficulties in chewing and opening the mouth, sensory loss, relapse of jaw deformities, and even fatal side effects, so functional aspects of the jaw after OGS should be considered during surgical planning. To this end, the role of preoperative orthodontic treatment is important, and the ideal surgical planning of OGS is to consult (collaborate) with an orthodontist and a surgeon from the beginning to establish an adequate preoperative orthodontic treatment plan considering the final location of the jawbones.

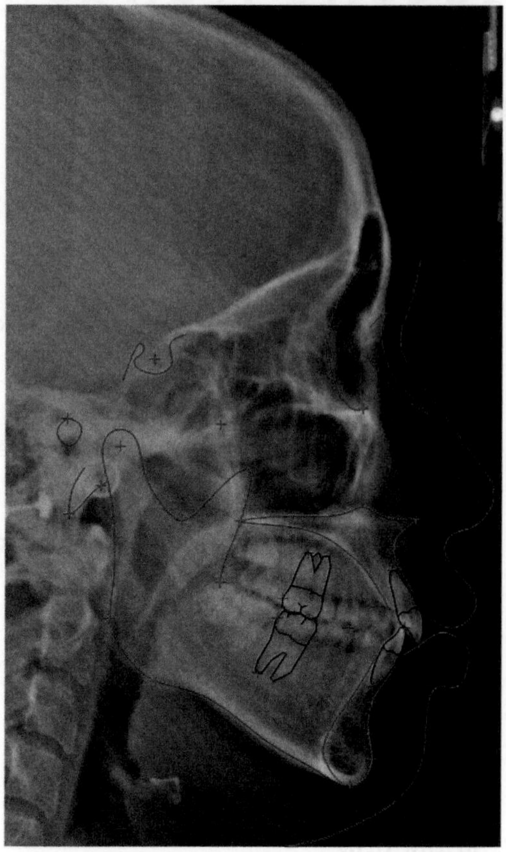

Fig. 1. Lateral cephalometric analysis is performed by identifying the anatomic landmarks.

DIAGNOSIS

The lateral cephalogram is the method used most commonly to analyze the malocclusion. Anatomic landmarks are identified, and linear and angular measurements are used to analyze the patient's malocclusion (**Fig. 1**). The measurement values are compared with the norm, and the amount of deviation for each variable identifies the type of malocclusion. A list of commonly used skeletal, dental, and soft tissue lateral cephalometric variables and the Korean norm are shown in **Table 1**. In patients with facial asymmetry, a posteroanterior cephalogram or computed tomography (CT) is recommended to analyze the asymmetry.

CASE

A 19-year-old female patient presented with the chief complaint of jaw protrusion and facial asymmetry. On a clinical examination, a midface deficiency with chin protrusion was observed (**Fig. 2**). According to the intraoral photographs, an edge-to-edge bite with anterior open bite tendency was observed (**Fig. 3**). Both the left and the right first molars showed a class III relationship, and the lower dental midline was deviated 2.5 mm to the right from the facial midline. In her smile photograph, a flat smile arc was observed.

The lateral cephalometric analysis revealed a class III skeletal pattern with an point A-nasion-point B angle of −2.7°, and Wits appraisal of −7.7 mm. mandibular plane angle (angle between sella-nasion and gonion-gnathion) was 42.7°, indicating a long face. The upper incisors were proclined with a upper incisor inclination (U1-FH) of 132.4°. The lower incisor inclination was 92.4°, measured relative to the mandibular plane (**Fig. 4**, **Table 2**).

According to the cone beam computed tomography (CBCT) images, a maxillary transverse deficiency was observed.

TREATMENT GOAL

The treatment goal was to correct the facial asymmetry and mandibular protrusion and obtain normal occlusion. Maxillary transverse deficiency is often observed in patients with skeletal class III malocclusion. In adult patients, maxillary skeletal

Table 1
Lateral cephalometric variables for analyses of skeletal, dental, and soft tissues

Variable	Definition	Norm
SNA (°)	Angle formed by sella, nasion, and point A	82.4
SNB (°)	Angle formed by sella, nasion, and point B	77
ANB difference (°)	Difference between SNA and SNB	3
A to N-Perp (mm)	Distance from Nasion-perpendicular line to point A	0
Pog to N-Perp (mm)	Distance from Nasion-perpendicular line to pogonion	−5
Wits (mm)	Distance between the points drawn from point A and point B perpendicular to the occlusal plane	−1.3
APDI (°)	Anteroposterior dysplasia indicator	81.4
SN-GoGn (°)	Angle formed by the sella-nasion plane and the mandibular plane	32.5
Occlusal plane (°)	Angle formed by the FH plane and the occlusal plane	10
ODI (°)	Overbite depth indicator	70
U1-FH (°)	Angle formed by the maxillary incisor long axis and the FH plane	116
IMPA (°)	Angle formed by the mandibular incisor long axis and the mandibular plane	95
Upper lip to E-line (mm)	Distance from the outermost point of the upper lip to the E-line (pronasal to soft tissue pogonion)	1.8
Lower lip to E-line (mm)	Distance from the outermost point of the lower lip to the E-line	3.6

Abbreviations: S, sella; A, point A; N, nasion; B, point B; Pog, pogonion; APDI, anteroposterior dysplasia indicator; Go, gonion; Gn, gnathion; ODI, overbite depth indicator; U1, upper incisor; FH, Frankfort horizontal plane; IMPA, incisor to mandibular plane angle; E-line, esthetic line.

expansion can be performed by surgically assisted rapid palatal expansion (SARPE) or miniscrew-assisted rapid palatal expansion (MARPE). In SARPE, corticotomy of the maxilla along the Le Fort I osteotomy line is performed, followed by maxillary expansion using an expansion screw. MARPE uses temporary anchorage devices or miniscrews that are anchored to the midpalatal suture, and then the maxilla is expanded using an expansion screw (**Fig. 5**). Maxillary expansion is an unstable procedure because of the thick keratinized palatal mucosa; therefore, overcorrection and long-term retention are required.

TREATMENT PLAN

Before the surgery, usually presurgical orthodontics is performed. As the teeth are often compensated to the patients' skeletal pattern, a process of decompensation is done to accommodate the postsurgical occlusion. In the case of class III malocclusion, upper and lower incisors often exhibit proclination and retroclination, respectively, to compensate for the skeletal discrepancy (**Fig. 6**). In patients who have severe crowding with upper incisor protrusion, the upper bicuspids could be extracted to relieve crowding and retract the incisors. Lately, the surgery-first approach (SFA) has increased because of advantages, such as the immediate improvement of facial esthetics, patients' psychosocial status, shorter treatment time, and physiologic tooth movement.[5] Despite the advantages of the SFA, care should be taken owing to the unstable occlusion after surgery. There are greater vertical and

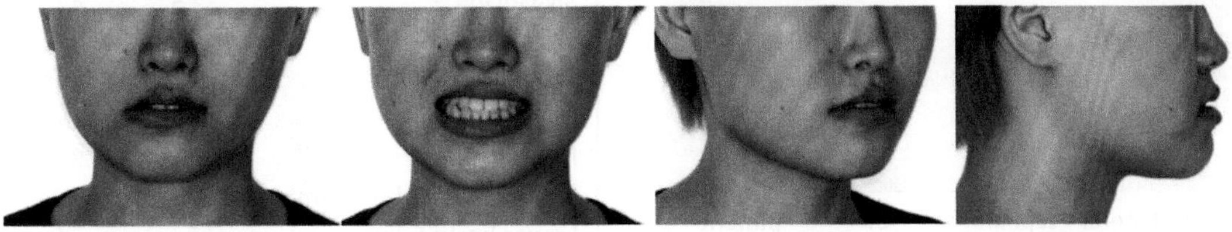

Fig. 2. Facial photograph of the patient.

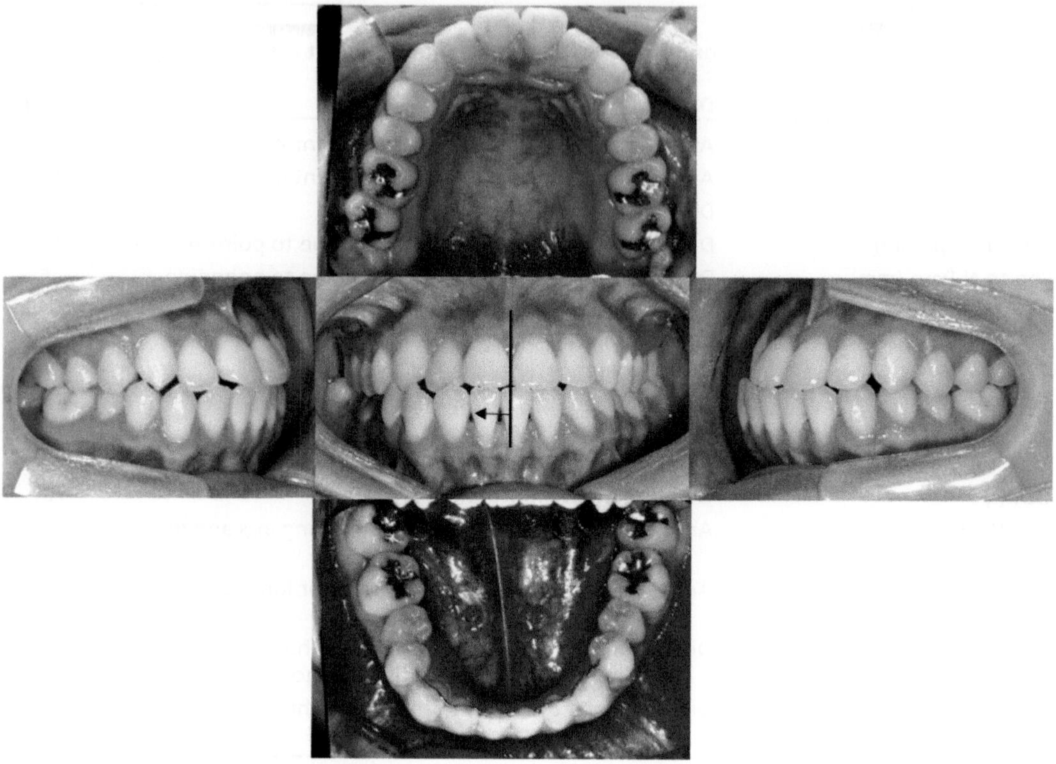

Fig. 3. Intraoral photograph of the patient.

sagittal changes in the occlusion during postsurgical orthodontics, making it less predictable for the final skeletal relationship. In addition, premature contact in the postsurgical occlusion might lead to surgical relapse, and possibly to TMD because of condylar displacement. Therefore, to obtain predictable results in the SFA, accurate diagnosis and treatment planning, accurate laboratory procedures, and much clinical experience are required.

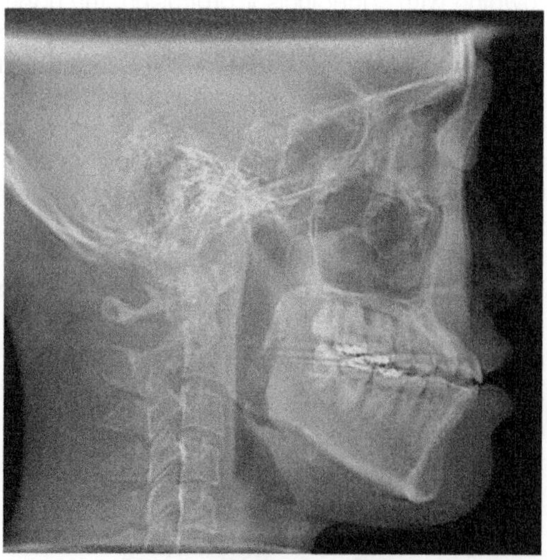

Fig. 4. Lateral cephalogram of the patient at pretreatment.

Table 2
Lateral cephalometric analysis of the patient at pretreatment

Measurements	Norm	Initial
SNA (°)	82.4	78.3
SNB (°)	77	81.1
ANB (°)	3	−2.7
A to N-Perp (mm)	0	0.4
Pog to N-Perp (mm)	−5	4.8
Wits (mm)	−1.3	−7.7
APDI	81.4	90.9
SN-GoGn (°)	32.5	42.7
Occlusal plane (°)	10	3.7
ODI	70	46.5
U1-FH (°)	116	132.4
IMPA (°)	95	92.4
Upper lip to E-line (mm)	1.8	−2.0
Lower lip to E-line (mm)	3.6	2.8

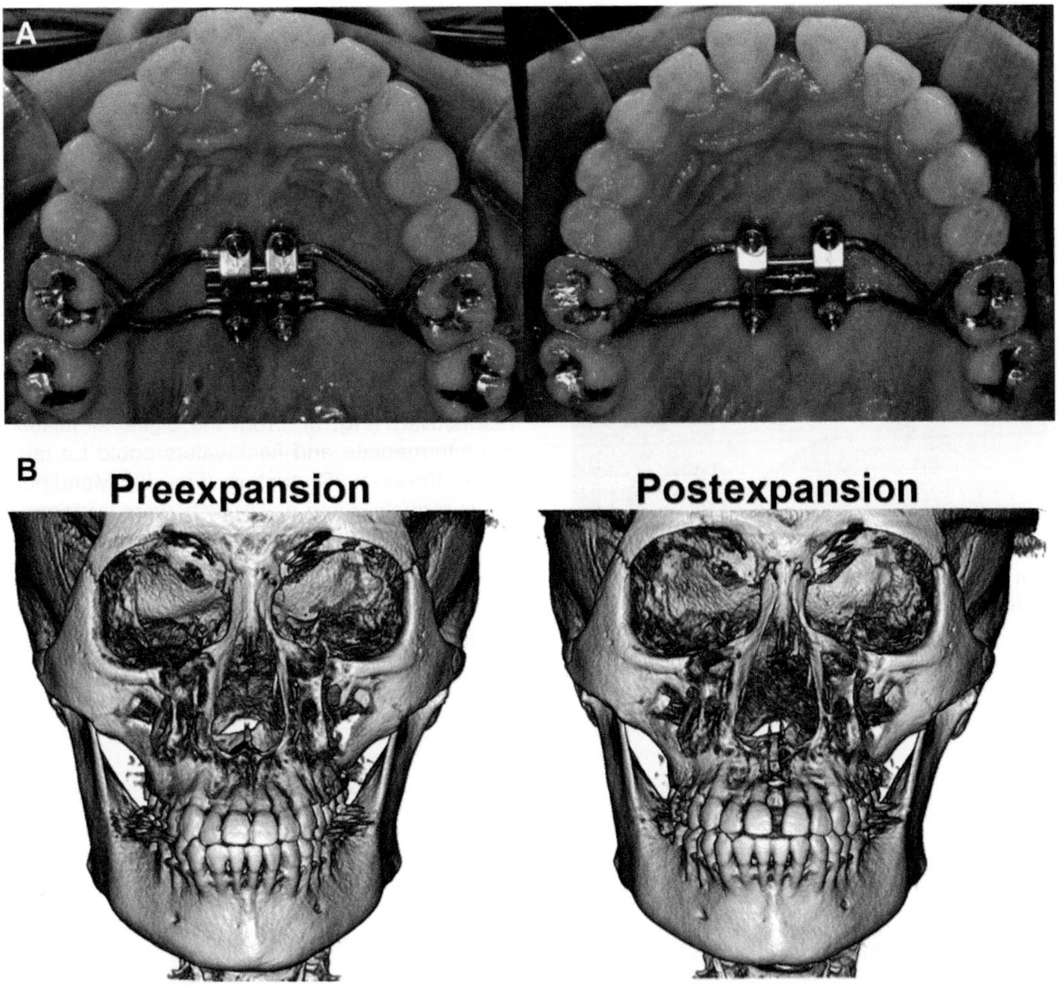

Fig. 5. Maxillary expansion was performed to correct the narrow maxilla. (*A*) MARPE was performed with 4 miniscrews installed in the midpalatal suture. The expansion rate was 1/6 mm per day, and a total of 6 mm was expanded in the maxilla. The appliance was retained for 3 months. (*B*) CBCT of the patient before and after MARPE.

SURGICAL PLANNING

Patients expect an esthetic outcome in addition to the correction of their malocclusion. Therefore, the treatment plan should be based on a careful assessment of the facial soft tissues in addition to analyzing the skeletal and dental anomalies. Arnett and colleagues[6] suggested 7 steps for OGS planning using lateral cephalograms, as follows (**Fig. 7**):

1. Correct the torque of the maxillary incisors (see **Fig. 7**A and B).
   The patient had proclined upper incisors; therefore, the upper incisor torque was corrected.
2. Correct the torque of the mandibular incisors.
   The patient had lower incisor torque within normal ranges; therefore, no changes in the lower incisors were planned.
3. Position the maxillary incisor (Le Fort I).
   The maxilla was moved up and forward (see **Fig. 7**C).
4. Autorotate the mandible to 3 mm of overbite.
   After maxillary repositioning, the mandible was autorotated to occlude with the upper teeth (see **Fig. 7**D).
5. Move the mandible to 3 mm of overjet.
   The mandible was set back to obtain a normal incisor overjet (see **Fig. 7**E).
6. Set the maxillary occlusal plane.
   The patient had a flat occlusal plane; therefore, posterior impaction was performed, resulting in the clockwise rotation of the maxillomandibular complex. This resolves the mandibular protrusion (see **Fig. 7**F).
7. Assess chin projection and height.
   The patient shows normal chin projection with an improved facial profile.

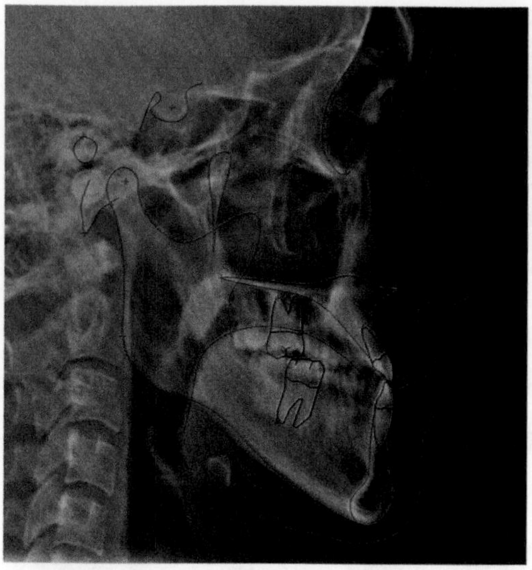

Fig. 6. Proclination of the upper incisors and retroclination of the lower incisors observed in a skeletal class III patient.

In addition, to correct the facial asymmetry, maxillary canting correction was performed; the left maxilla was impacted 2 mm in reference to the upper first molar.

Based on the surgical plan, a virtual surgery was performed using the CBCT data. A 3-dimensional (3D) surface model of the patient was created from the CBCT and intraoral scan data, and the osteotomies in the maxilla and the mandible were performed and repositioned as planned. The canting correction of 2 mm was performed in the maxilla, followed by 5-mm impaction in the posterior nasal spine. The mandible was set back by 7 and 1 mm on the right and left sides, respectively (**Fig. 8**). From the digital simulation, the intermediate and final wafers could be fabricated through 3D printing (**Fig. 9**). Mandibular angle reduction and malarplasty were performed.

POSTOPERATIVE ORTHODONTICS

Postoperative orthodontics usually begins 4 weeks after surgery. The goal of postoperative orthodontics is to stabilize the occlusion according to the

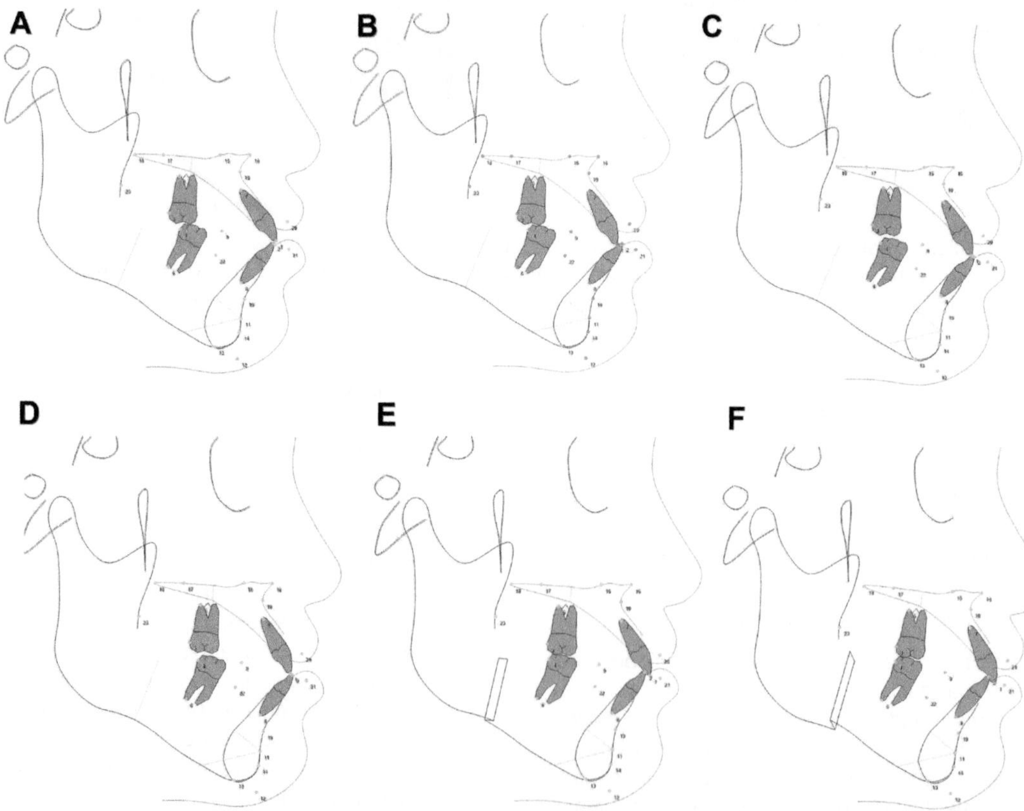

Fig. 7. (*A*) Initial, (*B*) upper incisor torque is corrected. (*C*) Maxilla is moved up and forward. (*D*) Mandible is autorotated. (*E*) Mandible is set back to have normal overjet. (*F*) Clockwise rotation of the maxillomandibular complex is performed to improve the facial profile.

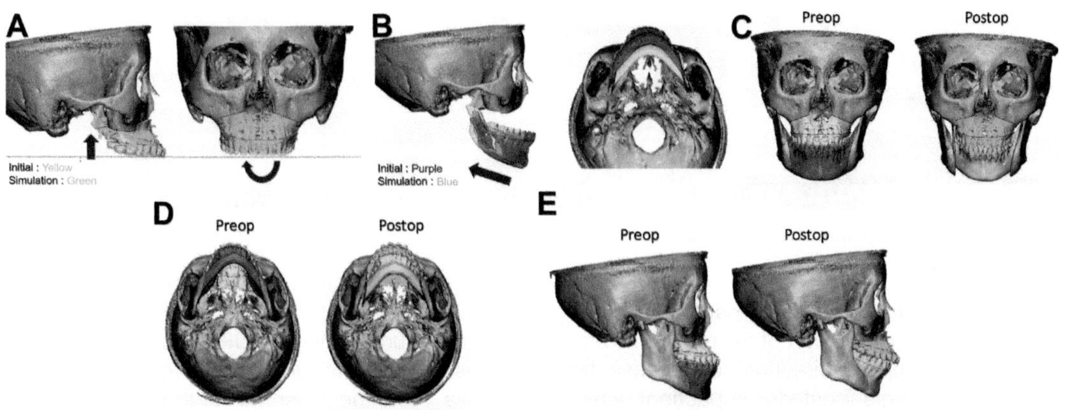

Fig. 8. (*A*) Maxillary canting correction of 2 mm is performed. (*B*) Mandibular setback is performed. (*C–E*) Frontal, submentovertex, and lateral view of before and after simulation surgery.

corrected skeletal relationship. After surgery, the bone remodeling rate is increased, which allows for a rapid alignment of teeth, known as the regional acceleratory phenomenon. The goals of postsurgical orthodontic treatment are as follows[7]: (1) Class I molar relationship—the distal surface of the distal marginal ridge of the upper first molar occludes with the mesial surface of the mesial marginal ridge of the lower second molar; (2) normal crown angulation or mesiodistal tip; (3) normal crown inclination or labiolingual/buccolingual torque; (4) no rotations; (5) tight contact between teeth; and (6) flat curve of Spee.

As a result of surgery, the patient shows facial symmetry in the frontal view, with a normal lateral facial profile (**Fig. 10**). The class I molar and canine key have been achieved with no rotations and interdental spaces (**Fig. 11**). The skeletal and dental changes could be analyzed by superimposing the lateral cephalograms (**Fig. 12**) and CBCT (**Fig. 13**). Dental changes as a result of treatment could also be assessed by using intraoral scan data and superimposing the 2 scans. Tooth alignment and correct inclination are observed (**Fig. 14**).

POPULAR SURGICAL METHODS FOR ORTHOGNATHIC SURGERY IN ASIA

Le Fort I Osteotomy and Maxillary Set Back Surgery

Among the various maxillary osteotomy methods used in OGS, Le Fort I osteotomy is currently the most popular among Asians. Asians tend to have a more protrusive maxilla in the anteroposterior plane than Westerners. Therefore, unlike OGS in

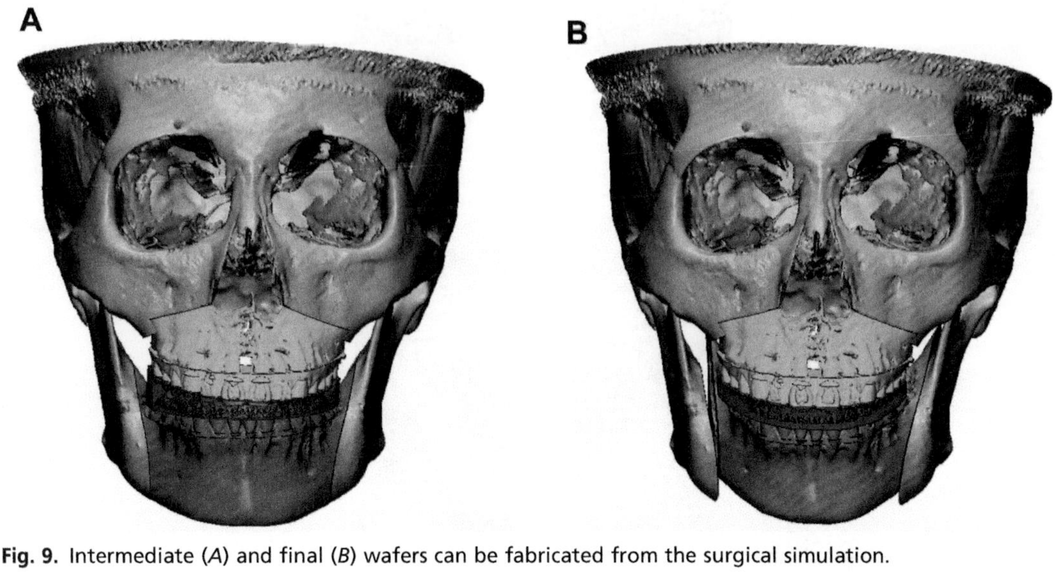

Fig. 9. Intermediate (*A*) and final (*B*) wafers can be fabricated from the surgical simulation.

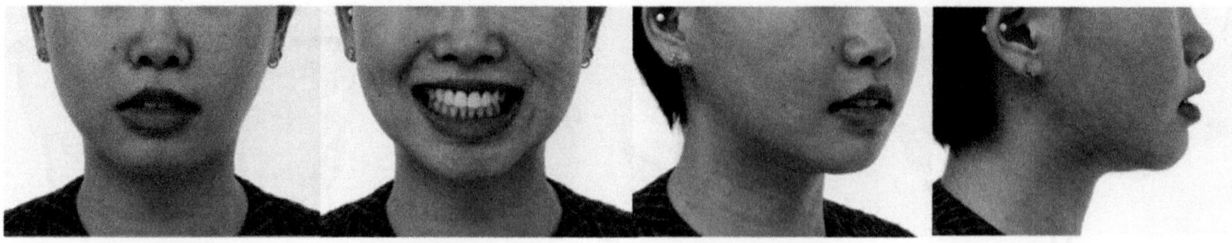

Fig. 10. Facial photograph after treatment.

Westerners, moving the maxilla posteriorly is common. Also, the posterior part of the maxilla is often reposed in the upper direction to increase the occlusal plane angle (posterior impaction), which creates the softer facial impression that Asians prefer (**Fig. 15**). However, the posterior movement of the maxilla requires significant caution because several major blood vessels, such as the pterygoid venous plexus and branches of the maxillary arteries, are located in the area. In addition, it is difficult to access the location of the bleeding point for hemostasis, which might cause fatal and serious bleeding. Hemostasis is often achieved using gauze, Surgicel packing, and electrocautery. The descending palatine artery (DPA) is the key structure when moving the maxilla setback and/or for posterior impaction. It should be carefully dissected or ligated, and the pyramidal bony structure surrounding the DPA should be removed so as to not interrupt proper relocation of the maxilla. Also, the lower part of the pterygoid plate is fractured gently, allowing the backward movement of the maxilla (**Fig. 16**). An excessive setback of the maxilla could cause a narrowing of the nasopharyngeal space after surgery, leading to disorders such as sleep apnea accompanied by severe snoring; hence, care should be taken when establishing a surgical plan. Upward impaction of the maxilla might result in nasal septal deviation and nasal congestion postoperatively; therefore, adequate removal of the nasal septum cartilage and, if necessary, lower nasal turbinectomy are required during surgery. Patients with a postoperatively developed nasal deviation and

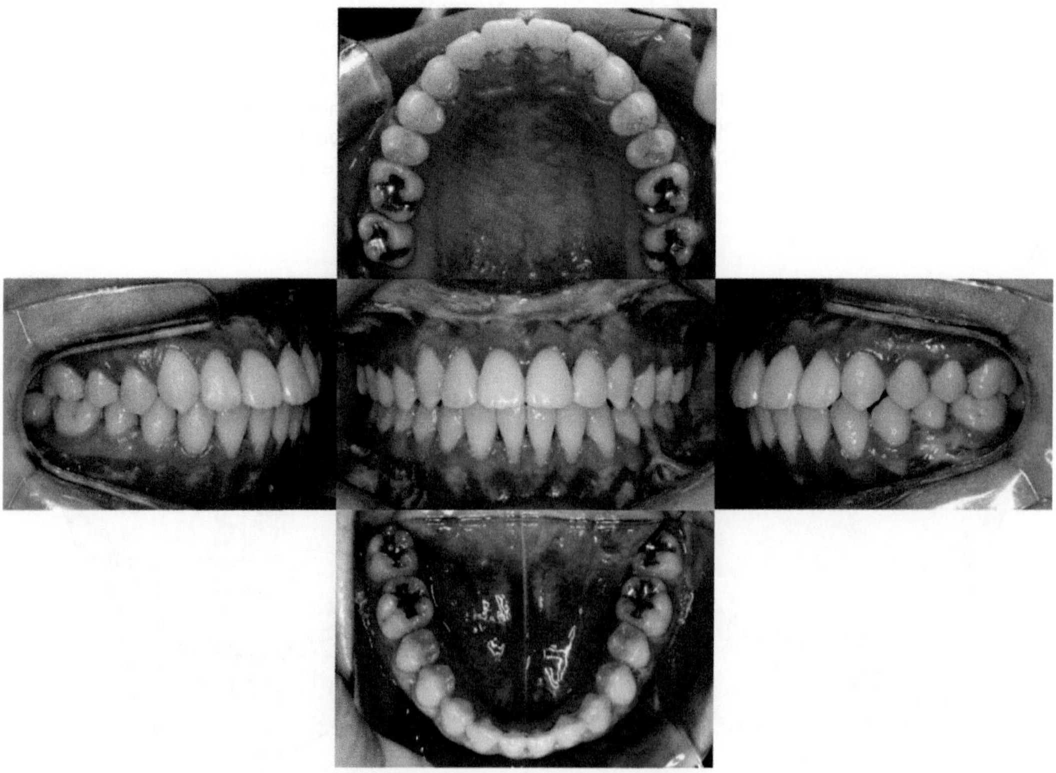

Fig. 11. Intraoral photograph after treatment. Stable occlusion is obtained.

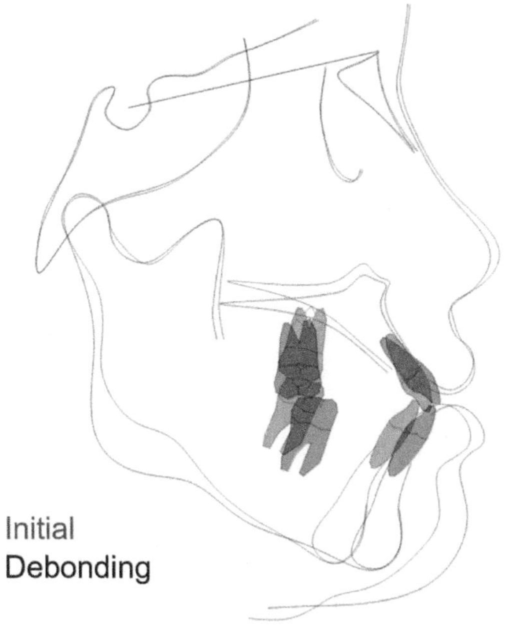

Fig. 12. Lateral superimposition of pretreatment and posttreatment.

other functional nasal problems need to consult an ENT surgeon.

Anterior Segment Osteotomy

Instead of moving the maxilla or the mandible as a whole, a technique in which only a part of the jaw is moved is also widely used. In the past, anterior segment osteotomy (ASO) was the only option to correct deformities of the maxilla.[1] In the case of maxillary protrusion, the most common indication for ASO, extracting the premolar teeth, cutting out the residual bone at the extraction space, and finally, pushing the jawbone segment backward, is simpler and safer than moving the whole maxilla backward (**Fig. 17**). However, this is not indicated in all cases. It is particularly effective in cases whereby the jawbone is long and narrow anteroposteriorly (horseshoe-shaped), as well as when the difference in the width of the maxillary arch between the distal and proximal ends of the extracted premolar teeth is not too large.[8]

Recently, with the development of orthodontic treatments involving a skeletal anchor using screws or miniplates, some cases of skeletal anterior maxillary protrusion that could only be treated through ASO or total setback of the maxilla in the past are now treated effectively with orthodontic treatment. In ASO, the blood supply to the fractured anterior maxillary segment is often limited; therefore, significant care and caution are required during the operation to maintain the blood supply of the premaxilla and to avoid ischemic necrosis of the segment. Maintaining palatal flap continuity between segments of the maxilla is one of the tips for preventing ischemic necrosis of the anterior segment.

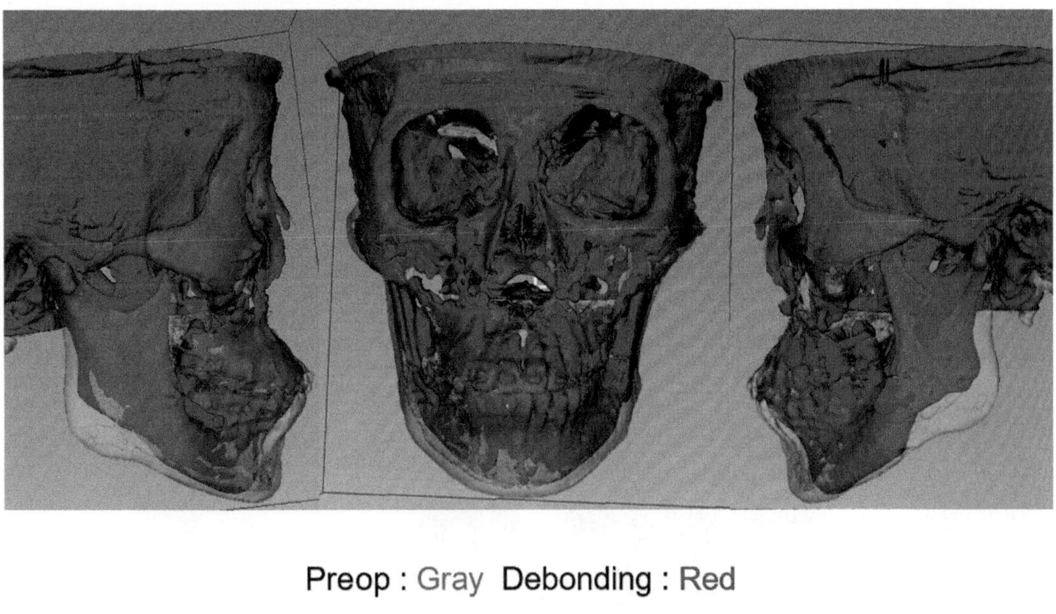

Fig. 13. 3D superimposition of the pretreatment and posttreatment.

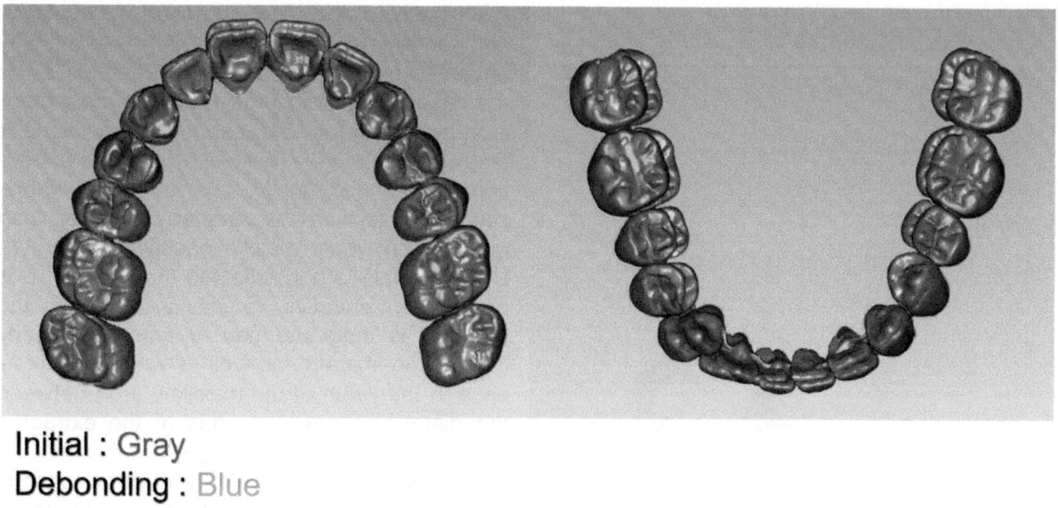

Fig. 14. 3D superimposition of the intraoral scan data before and after treatment.

Bilateral Sagittal Split Osteotomy with Short Lingual Technique versus Intraoral Vertical Ramus Osteotomy

Bilateral sagittal split osteotomy (BSSRO) is the most commonly used mandibular surgery for OGS in Asians. In traditional BSSRO, the posterior portion of the distal segment could push the soft tissue back by the setback amount; therefore, the more the setback, the more the relapse of the mandible after surgery occurs with time. To overcome this problem, the excessive posterior portion of the distal segment should be additionally removed[9] (**Fig. 18**).

Nowadays, a modified BSSRO method called the short lingual technique is popular.[10] This technique prevents the protrusion of the distal segment at the rear from occurring when the mandible is cut with the sagittal plane. This method is also advantageous for the health of the jaw joint, as it can prevent the pathologic rotational pressure of the condyle of the mandible.[11] This modified BSSRO technique could provide more room for the adjustment of the inner surface of the proximal segment

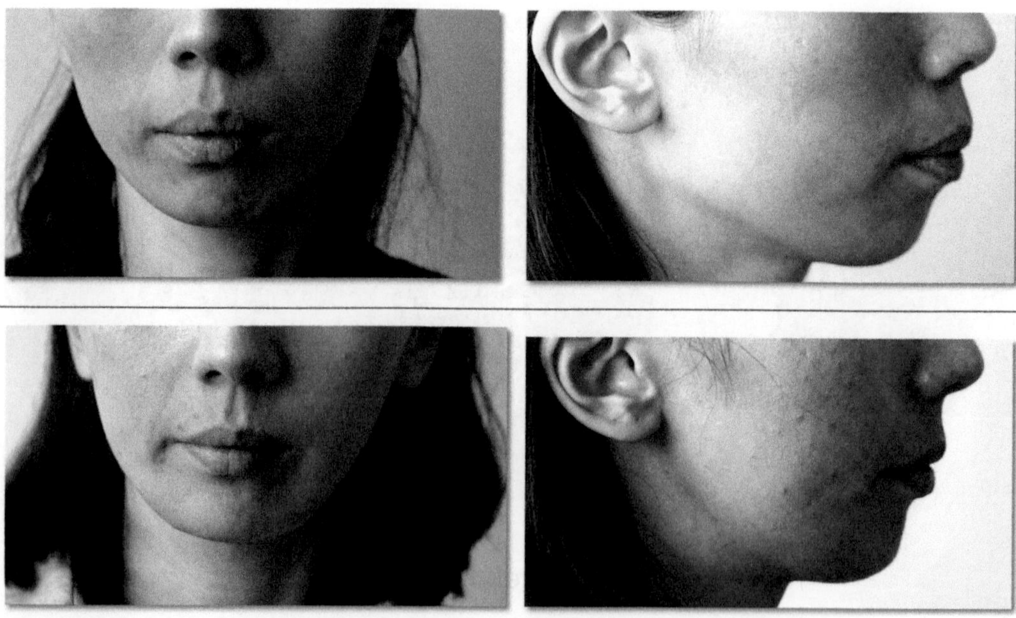

Fig. 15. Maxillary setback and angle reduction (preoperative: upper; postoperative: lower).

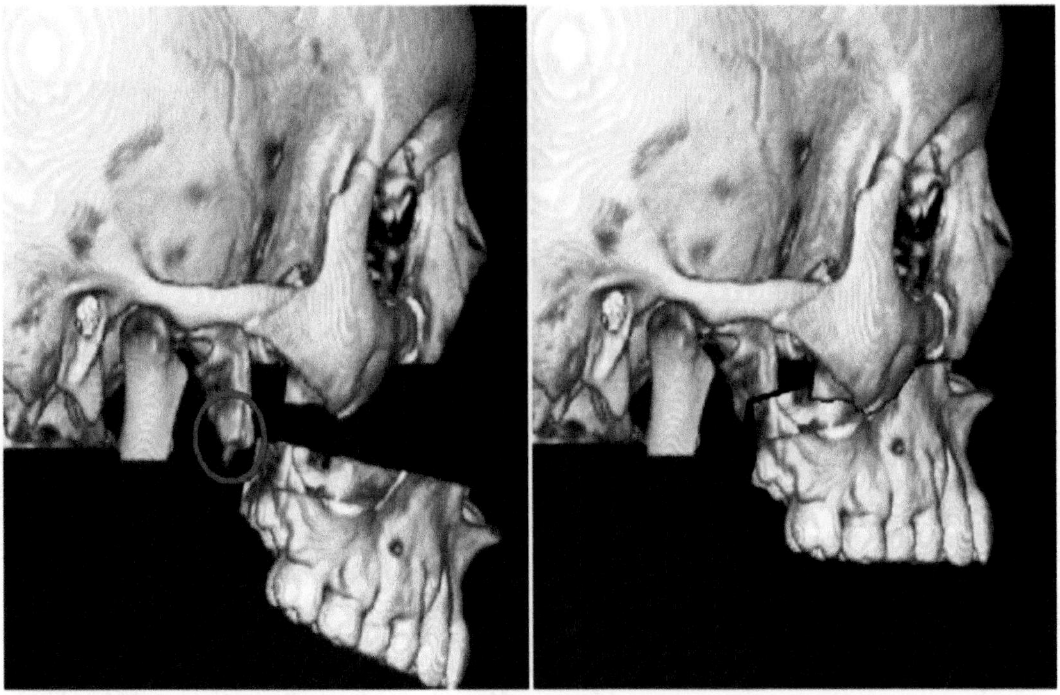

Fig. 16. Inferior resection of the pterygoid process allows maxillary setback. (Reprinted from Schouman T, Baralle MM, Ferri J. Facial morphology changes after total maxillary setback osteotomy. *J Oral Maxillofac Surg*. Jul 2010;68(7):1504-11. https://doi.org/10.1016/j.joms.2009.09.095).

when the split segments are reposed at the planned position. It is another merit that the mandibular angle reduction, which is preferred by Asians, is simultaneously performed with this technique.

In BSSRO, the long screw fixing method using a transbuccal cannula is used rarely these days; instead, a simple monocortical fixation method using various shapes of 4-hole miniplates and mini-screws is common.

Intraoral vertical ramus osteotomy (IVRO) is another popular osteotomy technique of the mandible for OGS (**Fig. 19**). It needs no fixation and lets the proximal segment of the mandible be physiologically reposed and reunited with the distal segment after exercising mandibular opening following surgery. As a result, the proximal segment, including the mandibular condyle, is finally located at a balanced position with the masticatory muscles, which is good for the mandibular condylar health. Therefore, IVRO is known to be helpful for patients undergoing OGS who have temporomandibular joint (TMJ) issues before surgery.[12] However, it has limitations on application, such as mandibular advancement surgery and concomitant mandibular angle reduction surgery. In addition, as the BSSRO short lingual technique could also achieve a beneficial effect for the TMJ and more versatility in terms of application, IVRO is losing its popularity in Korea in recent times.

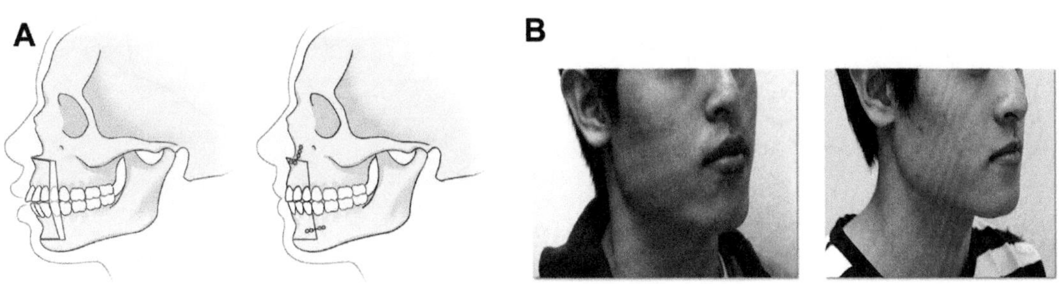

Fig. 17. (*A*) ASO. (*B*) Preoperative (*left*), postoperative (*right*).

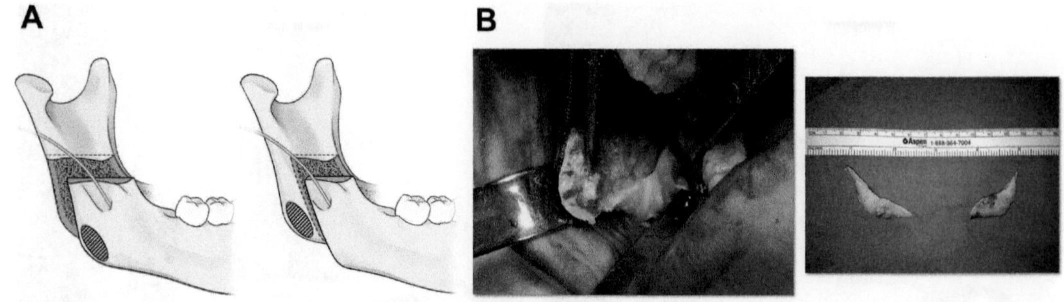

Fig. 18. (*A*) Comparison of classical BSSRO (*left*) and short lingual technique (*right*). Blue mark shows the area of attachment of the medial pterygoid muscle. (*B*) After mandibular splitting via short lingual technique (*left*), mandibular angle reduction can be easily performed (*right*).

TEMPOROMANDIBULAR JOINT CONSIDERATION

The TMJ is the center of mandibular position and movement. Therefore, a change of the mandibular and the maxillary position by OGS significantly affects the function and physiology of the TMJ and masticatory muscles. As most patients with jaw deformity with class II malocclusion or facial asymmetry already have various degrees of TMJ disorders (TMDs),[13] preoperative and postoperative diagnosis and management of TMDs are essential to prevent the postoperative aggravation of TMDs[14] (**Fig. 20**). In addition, the proper positioning of the condylar head of the mandible during the OGS is another key to maintaining condylar health and avoiding a relapse of the mandibular position after surgery.[15] Once TMDs are aggravated after surgery, severe TMJ osteoarthritis and resorption of the condyle could occur, resulting in devastating open bite or deviation of the mandible after surgery.[16]

ADJUVANT JAWBONE SURGERIES DURING ORTHOGNATHIC SURGERY

Mandibular Angle Reduction and Mandibular Border Contouring

As mentioned earlier, Asians, especially women, prefer a soft figure shape with a small mandible. Therefore, when the mandibular width is too large and prominent, mandibular angle reduction and mandibular border contouring surgery can be performed during OGS to make the overall

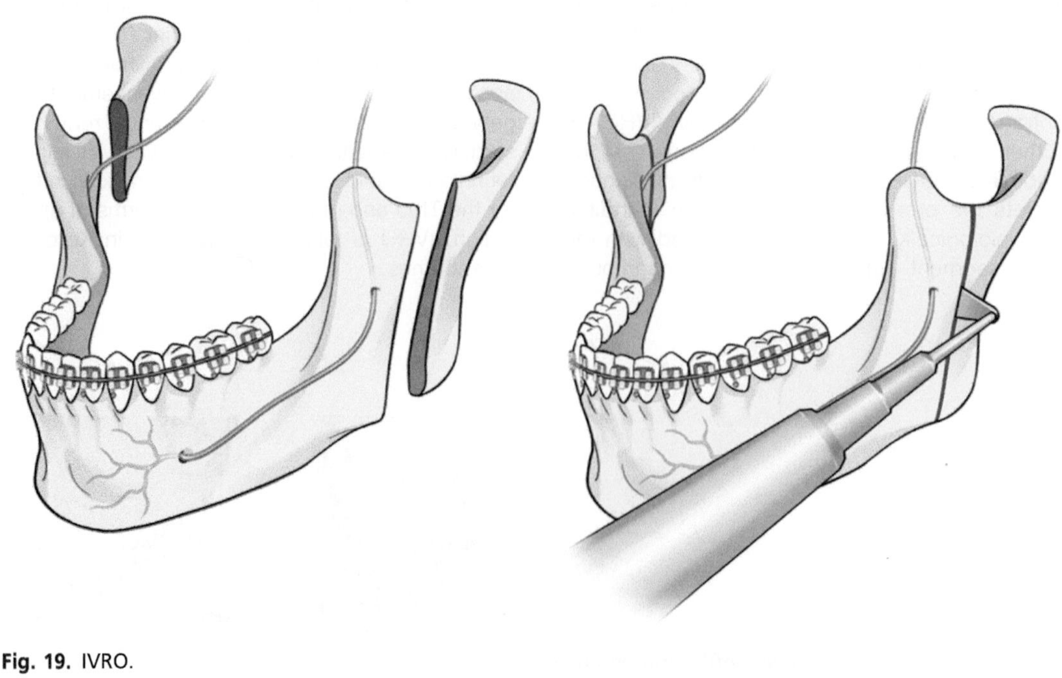

Fig. 19. IVRO.

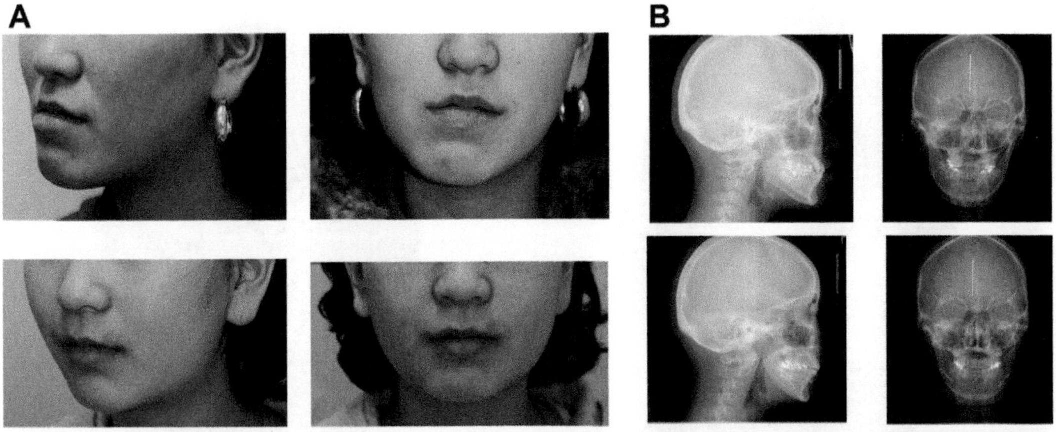

Fig. 20. (*A*) Facial asymmetry patient with temporomandibular disorder. Preoperative (*upper*) and postoperative (*lower*) view. (*B*) Facial asymmetry in a patient with temporomandibular disorder. Preoperative (*upper*) and postoperative (*lower*) radiographic view.

mandibular contour smaller and smoother (**Fig. 21**). Lateral corticotomy of the mandibular body and ramal area is also effective in addition to the resection of the mandibular angle in severe cases.[17] As these can be performed without changing the occlusion, they could be applied to patients regardless of the state of malocclusion.

Malar Reduction

It is known that the cheekbone (malar bone) is relatively prominent in Asians. Various surgical methods for malar reduction have been developed according to the aspect of cheekbone prominence[18] (**Fig. 22**). An intraoral and minimally invasive facial approach with a small incision is common. As the fractured segment could be displaced by the activity of masticatory muscles, such as the masseter muscle, internal fixation using a miniplate and screws should be performed. In addition, as the TMJ is located near the posterior osteotomy or fracture line of the zygomatic arch, additional care should be taken not to affect the jaw joint function. Also, cheek drooping (sagging) is common after surgery; therefore, minimal incisions and dissection are necessary to minimize the side effects.[19,20]

Genioplasty

The shape and position of the chin account for determining a person's impression. After the repositioning of the upper and mandibular bones in 2-jaw surgery, genioplasty is often performed to complete the ideal facial contour (**Fig. 23**). Diverse surgical methods for genioplasty have been

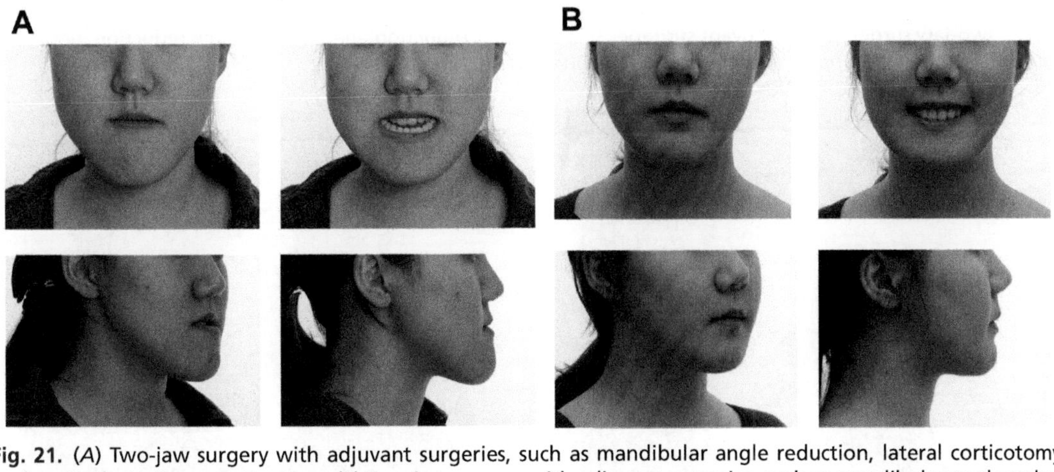

Fig. 21. (*A*) Two-jaw surgery with adjuvant surgeries, such as mandibular angle reduction, lateral corticotomy, and genioplasty. Preoperative view. (*B*) Two-jaw surgery with adjuvant surgeries, such as mandibular angle reduction, lateral corticotomy, and genioplasty. Postoperative view.

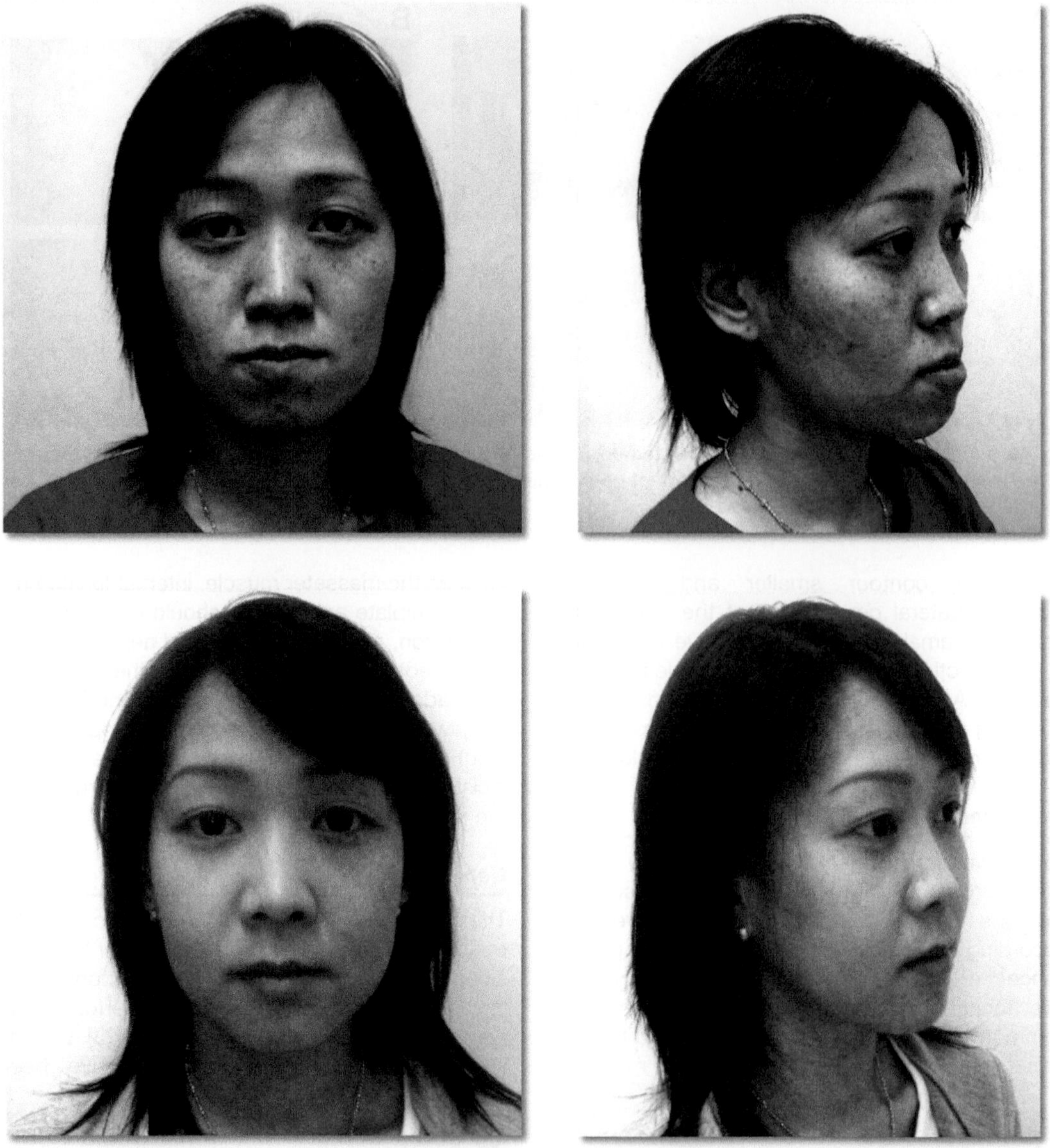

Fig. 22. Two-jaw surgery with adjuvant surgeries such as malar reduction, mandibular angle reduction, and genioplasty. Preoperative (*upper*) and postoperative (*lower*) view.

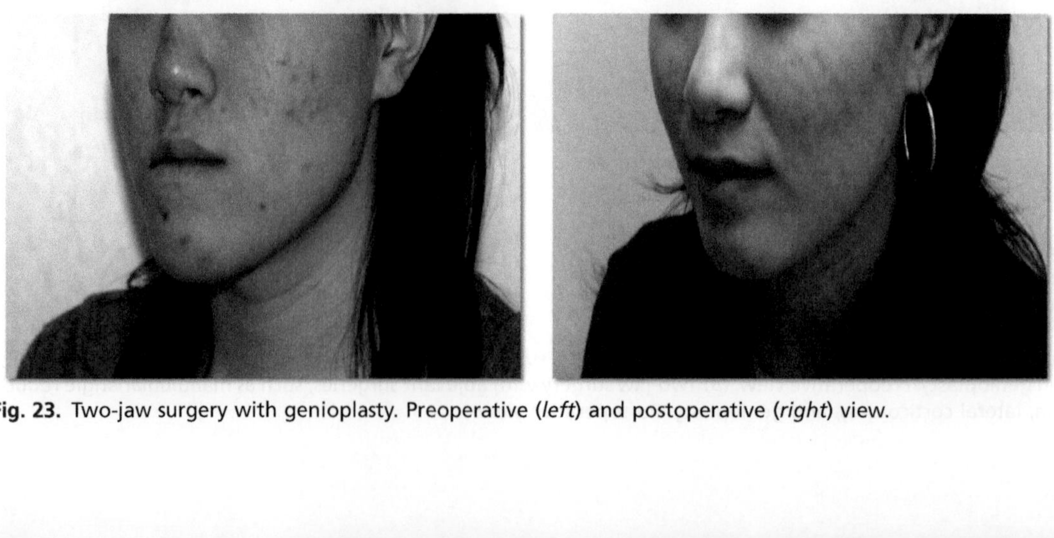

Fig. 23. Two-jaw surgery with genioplasty. Preoperative (*left*) and postoperative (*right*) view.

introduced.[21] Each technique can be applied according to the chin condition and desired chin shape and size. The surgeon and the patient need to fully discuss the esthetics before the operation so that both can be satisfied. The advancement of genioplasty for pulling the geniohyoid muscle forward can be used for the purpose of widening the upper airway of patients with severe snoring or sleep apnea caused by a narrow upper airway.

Although it is a relatively simple operation, in the case of patients with a large incisive nerve, a branch of the inferior alveolar nerve, sensation in the lower anterior gingival area and the inner lower lip may be lost after surgery; therefore, it is necessary to check this through CT before the surgery. In addition, excessive bleeding from the marrow cavity of the chin may occur, causing acute airway obstruction after surgery. Thus, proper hemostasis and postoperative observation are required.

SURGERY-FIRST APPROACH FOR ORTHOGNATHIC SURGERY

In the past, OGS was performed at first without orthodontic treatment because orthodontic treatment for OGS was not fully established. Nowadays, it is the gold standard that the surgical correction for dentofacial deformities is performed when preoperative orthodontic treatment is finished. It is common sense that postoperative stable occlusion is better than an unstable one for the jaw and jaw joint health after surgery. However, recently, contrary to this common sense, some orthodontists and surgeons claim that SFA without preoperative orthodontic treatment is also safe and not harmful to the jaw and jaw joint after surgery.[22–25] They also claim that this approach has more merits, such as early facial esthetic achievement and hastening of the postoperative orthodontic treatment after surgery, reducing the total duration of the treatment. Compared with the past era of surgery-first, it is now quite acceptable because cutting-edge technology, such as 3D CT and simulation software, enables the SFA to be more safe and reliable.[26] Although this approach has become more popular because of its merits, controversy still persists regarding the range of indications, the stability of the jawbone after surgery, and the effect of the jaw joint health.[27] The selection criteria for the SFA are dependent on the expertise and preference of the surgeon and the orthodontist. There is no consensus on the indications and contraindications for the SFA. Early studies on the SFA claimed that it is indicated when there is only little or no transverse discrepancy, no extractions involved, and at least 3 occlusal contact points between the arches. Currently, it is clear that the indication of SFA has become wider with the use of the 3D virtual simulation software.

FUTURE DIRECTIONS

Today, the virtual plan is transferred to the patient using computer-aided designs, computer-aided manufacturing splints, and guide stents, which have completely replaced the plaster casts and analytical model surgery used previously. In addition, osteotomies are stabilized with patient-specific implants to achieve maximal predictability.

Three-Dimensional Virtual Simulation Surgery Software

Substituting 2-dimensional cephaloanalysis, the diagnosis and surgery planning using the recent 3D CT (CBCT) image and simulating software have become more popular in OGS.[28,29] Using a digital articulator, virtual OGS is possible,[26] which enables more precise planning for OGS.

Three-Dimensional Printed Customized Miniplate System and Surgical Guides

After performing simulation surgery with 3D images and a software program, a customized miniplate can be fabricated through the titanium 3D printing system and can be used as a surgical guide during surgery. This system enables more precise surgery as planned before surgery without the process of bending the miniplate by an experienced surgeon during surgery.[30,31]

3D printed customized surgical guides for genioplasty and mandibular angle reduction are now also used.[32]

Navigation System of Major Instruments During Surgery

OGS is performed through areas with poor surgical vision, such as the oral cavity, to prevent facial scars after surgery. Also, the anatomic structure is complex and contains several critical organs, such as major blood vessels and nerves. In addition, these vary from person to person; therefore, the surgical instruments must be placed in the proper place for safe and accurate surgery. The recently developed and increasingly used navigation system could help precise and safe surgery so that the surgical instruments are located in the proper position in real time and minimize the damage to major structures during surgery.[33–36]

Piezoelectric-Powered Osteo-Surgery Devices

Conventionally, bone-cutting or drilling devices are powered by high-pressure nitrogen gas or an electric motor. Currently, piezoelectric-powered bone-cutting devices have become popular. As the maxillofacial area is rich in active blood circulation, it may cause massive bleeding from unwanted damage to critical blood vessels during the surgery. The bone-cutting machine using the piezoelectric power cuts only hard tissues and minimizes damage to soft tissues, such as blood vessels. Therefore, relatively safer bone-cutting is possible, especially in areas where the field of vision is poor and massive bleeding is expected, such as in the posterior part of the maxilla.[37–39]

SUMMARY

The jawbone accounts for two-thirds of the face, and jaw-correction surgery that changes the position of the jawbone significantly alters the facial impression. Thus, well-conducted OGS may provide patients greater esthetic satisfaction. However, OGS also has a significant impact on the jaw's unique functions, such as chewing, swallowing, and pronunciation. Therefore, OGS that does not consider this functional aspect can cause serious problems not only during the surgery but also later, such as TMJ problems or relapse of the corrected jaw position. Furthermore, Asians and Westerners have different anatomies and standards of beauty. Asians, who prefer a soft face shape, often move the maxillary bone to the rear, and additional procedures are often performed on the mandible, which can cause more functional and safety problems when compared with OGS on the Westerners. Therefore, sophisticated surgical planning and operational care should be considered to avoid these side effects. The anatomy of delicate areas should be accurately identified; appropriate surgery should be performed, and adequate hemostasis is also essential. It may be significantly helpful to use the latest variety of virtual surgical software or advanced equipment to this end.

CLINICS CARE POINTS

- Harmonized surgical planning considering functions and esthetic.
- Cooperation of orthodontists and surgeon.
- Special attention around the maxillary posterior part and inferior alveolar nerve.
- Hemostasis and proper fixation of the bony segment during orthognathic surgery for patient safety.
- Proper preoperative and postoperative temporomandibular joint management.
- Application of cutting-edge technologies for precision orthognathic surgery.

DISCLOSURE

There are no conflicts of interest to declare.

ACKNOWLEDGMENTS

The authors gratefully acknowledge the Medical Contents Team of the Asan Medical Center for their excellent illustrations in this article. This study was supported by the National Research Foundation of Korea funded by the Ministry of Science and ICT of South Korea (grant 2019R1C1C1009881).

REFERENCES

1. Bell RB. A history of orthognathic surgery in North America. J Oral Maxillofac Surg 2018;76(12):2466–81.
2. Pachêco-Pereira C, Abreu LG, Dick BD, et al. Patient satisfaction after orthodontic treatment combined with orthognathic surgery: a systematic review. Angle Orthod 2016;86(3):495–508.
3. Lee LH, Jun JH, Danganan M, et al. Orthognathic surgery for the Asian patient and the influence of the surgeon's background on treatment. Int J Oral Maxillofac Surg 2011;40(5):458–63.
4. Lee ST, Choi NR, Song JM, et al. Three-dimensional morphometric analysis of mandibule in coronal plane after bimaxillary rotational surgery. Maxillofac Plast Reconstr Surg 2016;38(1):49.
5. Peiró-Guijarro MA, Guijarro-Martínez R, Hernández-Alfaro F. Surgery first in orthognathic surgery: a systematic review of the literature. Am J Orthod Dentofacial Orthop 2016;149(4):448–62.
6. Arnett GW, Jelic JS, Kim J, et al. Soft tissue cephalometric analysis: diagnosis and treatment planning of dentofacial deformity. Am J Orthod Dentofacial Orthop 1999;116(3):239–53.
7. Andrews LF. The six keys to normal occlusion. Am J Orthod 1972;62(3):296–309.
8. Bloomquist DS. Anterior segmental mandibular osteotomies for the correction of facial-skeletal deformities. Oral Maxillofac Surg Clin North Am 2007;19(3):369–79, vi.
9. Kim MJ, Kim SG, Park YW. Positional stability following intentional posterior ostectomy of the distal

segment in bilateral sagittal split ramus osteotomy for correction of mandibular prognathism. J Craniomaxillofac Surg 2002;30(1):35–40.
10. Wolford LM, Bennett MA, Rafferty CG. Modification of the mandibular ramus sagittal split osteotomy. Oral Surg Oral Med Oral Pathol 1987;64(2): 146–55.
11. Yang HJ, Lee WJ, Yi WJ, et al. Interferences between mandibular proximal and distal segments in orthognathic surgery for patients with asymmetric mandibular prognathism depending on different osteotomy techniques. Oral Surg Oral Med Oral Pathol Oral Radiol Endod 2010;110(1): 18–24.
12. Huh JW, Kim SY, Lee YB, et al. Three-dimensional changes of proximal segments in facial asymmetry patients after bilateral vertical ramus osteotomy. Int J Oral Maxillofac Surg 2020;49(8):1036–41.
13. Al-Ahmad HT, Al-Bitar ZB. The effect of temporomandibular disorders on condition-specific quality of life in patients with dentofacial deformities. Oral Surg Oral Med Oral Pathol Oral Radiol 2014; 117(3):293–301.
14. Toll DE, Popović N, Drinkuth N. The use of MRI diagnostics in orthognathic surgery: prevalence of TMJ pathologies in Angle class I, II, III patients. J Orofac Orthop 2010;71(1):68–80.
15. Bénateau H, Chatellier A, Leprovost N, et al. [Condylar positioning during mandibular orthognatic surgery]. Rev Stomatol Chir Maxillofac Chir Orale 2014;115(4):245–9.
16. Hori M, Okaue M, Hasegawa M, et al. Worsening of pre-existing TMJ dysfunction following sagittal split osteotomy: a study of three cases. J Oral Sci 1999; 41(3):133–9.
17. Song G, Zong X, Guo X, et al. Single-stage mandibular curved ostectomy on affected side combined with bilateral outer cortex grinding for correction of facial asymmetry: indications and outcomes. Aesthet Plast Surg 2019;43(3):733–41.
18. Kang M. Three-dimensional approach to zygoma reduction: review of 221 patients over 7 years. Ann Plast Surg 2016;76(1):51–6.
19. Shim HS, Seo BF, Rha EY, et al. Endotine midface for soft tissue suspension in zygoma fracture. J Craniofac Surg 2015;26(6):e496–500.
20. Hong SE, Liu SY, Kim JT, et al. Intraoral zygoma reduction using L-shaped osteotomy. J Craniofac Surg 2014;25(3):758–61.
21. Park S, Noh JH. Importance of the chin in lower facial contour: narrowing genioplasty to achieve a feminine and slim lower face. Plast Reconstr Surg 2008;122(1):261–8.
22. Bardet I, Goudot P, Kerbrat JB, et al. [Surgery first: prediction for skeletal objectives through structural analysis. Comparison of Sassouni and Delaire analysis]. Orthod Fr 2019;90(1):37–54.
23. Yamauchi K, Takahashi T, Yamaguchi Y, et al. Effect of "surgery first" orthognathic approach on temporomandibular symptoms and function: a comparison with "orthodontic first" approach. Oral Surg Oral Med Oral Pathol Oral Radiol 2019;127(5):387–92.
24. Sugawara J, Aymach Z, Nagasaka DH, et al. "Surgery first" orthognathics to correct a skeletal class II malocclusion with an impinging bite. J Clin Orthod 2010;44(7):429–38.
25. Villegas C, Uribe F, Sugawara J, et al. Expedited correction of significant dentofacial asymmetry using a "surgery first" approach. J Clin Orthod 2010; 44(2):97–103 [quiz 105].
26. Biao Y, Jung JA, Kook MS, et al. Application of the digital articulator in surgery-first approach. J Craniofac Surg 2021. https://doi.org/10.1097/SCS.0000000000007477.
27. Jung S, Choi Y, Park JH, et al. Positional changes in the mandibular proximal segment after intraoral vertical ramus osteotomy: Surgery-first approach versus conventional approach. Korean J Orthod 2020;50(5):324–35.
28. Ferraz FWDS, Iwaki-Filho L, Souza-Pinto GN, et al. A comparative study of the accuracy between two computer-aided surgical simulation methods in virtual surgical planning. J Craniomaxillofac Surg 2021;49(2):84–92.
29. Oh HJ, Moon JH, Ha H, et al. Virtually-planned orthognathic surgery achieves an accurate condylar position. J Oral Maxillofac Surg 2021. https://doi.org/10.1016/j.joms.2020.12.048.
30. Figueiredo CE, Paranhos LR, da Silva RP, et al. Accuracy of orthognathic surgery with customized titanium plates-systematic review. J Stomatol Oral Maxillofac Surg 2021;122(1):88–97.
31. Mascarenhas W, Makhoul N. Efficient in-house 3D printing of an orthognathic splint for single-jaw cases. Int J Oral Maxillofac Surg 2021. https://doi.org/10.1016/j.ijom.2020.12.016.
32. Oth O, Mestrallet P, Glineur R. Clinical study on the minimally invasive-guided genioplasty using piezosurgery and 3D printed surgical guide. Ann Maxillofac Surg 2020;10(1):91–5.
33. Chen C, Sun N, Jiang C, et al. Randomized controlled clinical trial to assess the utility of computer-aided intraoperative navigation in bimaxillary orthognathic surgery. J Craniofac Surg 2021. https://doi.org/10.1097/SCS.0000000000007512.
34. Koyachi M, Sugahara K, Odaka K, et al. Accuracy of Le Fort I osteotomy with combined computer-aided design/computer-aided manufacturing technology and mixed reality. Int J Oral Maxillofac Surg 2020. https://doi.org/10.1016/j.ijom.2020.09.026.
35. DeLong MR, Gandolfi BM, Barr ML, et al. Intraoperative image-guided navigation in craniofacial surgery: review and grading of the current literature. J Craniofac Surg 2019;30(2):465–72.

36. Lartizien R, Zaccaria I, Noyelles L, et al. Improvement in accuracy of maxillary repositioning of Le Fort I osteotomy with Orthopilot™ Navigation System: evaluation of 30 patients. Br J Oral Maxillofac Surg 2020;58(9):1116–22.
37. Bilge S, Kaba YN, Demirbas AE, et al. Evaluation of the pterygomaxillary separation pattern in Le Fort I osteotomy using different cutting instruments. J Oral Maxillofac Surg 2020;78(10):1820–31.
38. Cascino F, Aboh IV, Giovannoni ME, et al. Orthognathic surgery: a randomized study comparing piezosurgery and saw techniques. Ann Ital Chir 2020;9.
39. Schouman T, Baralle MM, Ferri J. Facial morphology changes after total maxillary setback osteotomy. J Oral Maxillofac Surg 2010;68(7):1504–11.

Special Considerations in Facial Reconstruction in the Non-White Patient

Jenica Su-ern Yong, MBBS[a], Stephen S. Park, MD[b,*]

KEYWORDS

• Facial reconstruction • Non-White • Ethnic differences in reconstruction

KEY POINTS

- Ethnic distinctives should be identified before consideration of reconstructive options.
- Non-White skin is different in terms of anatomy and physiology from White skin.
- For nasal reconstruction, the subunit principle is often modified from the White model.
- The skin soft tissue envelope (SSTE) is usually thicker and more inelastic compared with White patients. Wider undermining may be required to achieve tension-free closure.
- Nonanatomic cartilage grafting of the nose is used extensively but primarily to prevent alar notching rather than lateral wall collapse.

INTRODUCTION

Facial cutaneous defects with subsequent reconstructions form a large part of a typical facial plastic surgical practice. Facial defects are usually a result of either resection of a tumor or trauma. Although the incidence of skin malignancies is higher in the White population, they also occur in other ethnic groups and present an equally challenging repair. Hispanic, Asian, and African American individuals account for 4% to 5%, 2% to 4%, and 1% to 2% of skin cancer cases, respectively.[1] Because of the scarcity of skin cancers in non-Whites, there is less experience and literature on this topic.

It is imperative to realize that there are nuances when performing facial reconstruction in the non-White group of patients. As globalization occurs, the idea of beauty takes on a broader and more universal view.[2] Despite this, there are ethnic distinctives that should be respected.

DISCUSSION

Ethnic Differences

Before delving into the differences in reconstruction, the basic structural and physiologic difference in skin should be examined.

Skin structure

Contrary to common belief, there are no racial differences in the number of melanocytes.[3] Differences in skin color are attributed to variations in melanosomes, which are the melanin-containing organelles in melanocytes and keratinocytes.[4] The skin's response to UV irradiation is dependent on the epidermal content of melanin and distribution of melanosomes. Because of the increased melanin in Asians, Hispanics, and African Americans, the classic signs of photodamage often manifest later in life. However, this increase in melanin also predispose other darker-skinned ethnic groups to postinflammatory hyperpigmentation (PIH). This

No financial disclosures relevant to this research.
Conflict of interest: None.
[a] Department of Otolaryngology–Head and Neck Surgery, KK Women's and Children's Hospital, 100 Bukit Timah Road, Singapore 229899, Singapore; [b] Department of Otolaryngology–Head and Neck Surgery, University of Virginia, PO Box 800713, Charlottesville, VA 22908, USA
* Corresponding author.
E-mail address: ssp8a@virginia.edu

Facial Plast Surg Clin N Am 29 (2021) 567–573
https://doi.org/10.1016/j.fsc.2021.06.007
1064-7406/21/

may have a significant role when considering the normal course of healing with darker-skinned individuals, especially as it pertains to incision planning, scar revision, dermabrasion, and cosmetic facial surgery.

Skin phototype

The system of categorizing skin phototype was developed by Fitzpatrick.[5] This differentiates the skin type based on color and response to sunlight and UV radiation. This classification allows clear and consistent communication when classifying patients across different ethnic groups. It also helps alert the physician to be aware that patients with higher Fitzpatrick skin types are more prone to developing PIH.

Skin healing

During the healing phase, PIH results from overproduction of melanin or an irregular dispersion of pigment after cutaneous inflammation.[6] The intensity of the PIH may correlate with high skin phenotypes.[7]

The incidence of keloids is variable and patients with darker skin tend to have a higher prevalence compared with lighter-skin individuals.[8] It is the most common skin disease among ethnic Chinese in Asia and the fifth most common disease among Africans in the United Kingdom.[9,10]

Facial proportion

When performing reconstruction, aesthetics and form should be a substantial consideration. There is some ethnic deviation of what is considered to be attractive. Asian women tend to prefer a small and less angular face, whereas Whites tend to accept a more defined mandible and protruding cheeks.[11] In a study looking at facial anthropometric differences among workers in the United States, they found that African Americans have larger features than Whites with larger faces. Hispanics also have faces larger than Whites but have shorter nasal protrusion.[12] Comparing North American Whites and Asians, there were significantly smaller mouth widths, greater intercanthal widths, shorter palpebral fissures and wider noses among the Asian population.[13] These ethnic distinctions are real and should be considered before embarking on facial reconstruction. It is important to recognize that only rarely does a person of one ethnicity actually desire to look like another race.

Aging

A dynamic process, such as aging, can affect races differently for several reasons, including variations in fibroelastic fibers, sebaceous glands, skin thickness, and environmental exposures. A comparison between Chinese and European populations has shown that Chinese women are affected by wrinkles later than French women. As expected, both races have pigmented lesions as they get older; however, when Chinese women acquire these lesions they tend to have a greater number than French women.[14] The knowledge of the differences in aging can play a role in surgical planning.

Cultural significance/sensitivities

In many Asian countries, elderly individuals often prefer a less extensive approach to repair of their cutaneous defects as compared with other ethnicities.[15] The ultimate choice of reconstruction option obviously lies with the patient but the surgeon–patient interaction can have a significant impact and influence decision making. There are cultural beliefs and social values toward facial proportions that may affect the patient's choice of reconstruction. The shape of the nose, mouth, lips, and forehead are said to influence one's life and wealth. This could have a role in selecting the appropriate reconstruction option, especially if the surgery involves narrowing the nose and lips. A thick fleshy nose is believed to indicate wealth and prosperity, whereas thicker lips are said to reflect such positive traits as enthusiasm and kindness. Surgeons should have an honest, open discussion with patients about procedures that can potentially change the shapes of their nose and lips.

Treatment of Nasal Defects

Nasal anatomy

Studies have shown that African Americans have shorter, wider, and shallower noses.[12] Ethnic variations of nasal morphology have been categorized to three general forms:

- Leptorrhine ("tall and thin") nose, which is associated with White or Indo-European descent.
- Platyrrhine ("broad and flat") nose associated with African descent. It is characterized with thick skin, low radix, bulbous and lower projected tip, short dorsum, and flared nostrils.
- Mesorrhine ("intermediate") nose that is associated with Asian or Latino nose. It is characterized by a low radix, rounded and less projected tip, variable anterior dorsal projection, and rounded nostrils.

These ethnic variations are only meant as a guide and categorizing all non-White noses to be just "ethnic" is overly simplistic.

Skin thickness plays a major role when planning for reconstruction. This is most apparent in the nose, where skin thickness differs depending on the location. The nasal skin is thinner in the upper portion and becomes tighter and more adherent in the lower portion. Patients with thinner skin soft tissue envelope (SSTE) often have a higher risk of postoperative atrophy and possible discoloration from vascular congestion, whereas patients with thicker SSTE are more likely to have increased postoperative edema. The edema may impact scar healing and camouflage and refinement of the nasal tip and fullness to the supratip.[16]

Asians and African Americans tend to have thicker and less extensible skin with more abundant subcutaneous soft tissue than noses of Whites.[17] Eggerstedt and colleagues[18] have demonstrated that African American patients have significantly thicker SSTE at the supratip than all other races. Asian Americans also demonstrate thicker SSTE at the supratip than occidental patients.[18]

Nasal subunits

Generally, in the White population, reconstruction using the subunit principle has yielded good results. These subunits were not as appropriate for Asian patients. The soft tissue triangle is not distinct; the distinction between other subunits is not as sharp as with Whites. This is mainly caused by the thick skin and weaker underlying cartilages.[19] When considering the resultant scars for a nasal reconstruction, these ethnic differences must be considered at the forefront. Generally speaking, the softer and more rounded nature of the non-White nose leads to less defined aesthetic units and thus they have a more minor role in flap selection and design.

Functional difference

The internal nasal valve is defined as the area between the caudal border of the upper lateral cartilages and the dorsal cartilaginous septum. In White noses, this angle is said to be 10° to 15°. In African American and Asian noses, this angle of more obtuse, making them less susceptible to internal nasal valve collapse and nasal obstruction. Knowledge about the internal nasal valve is crucial in the White and non-White population because there are maneuvers that could potentially cause narrowing and collapse.

Management of specific nasal defect

Primary closure is considered if the nasal defect is small and there is minimal distortion of the nose. In non-White noses, where the skin is less extensible, this technique may not be used as much.

Skin grafting is an easy technique and useful in closure of various defects. However, for most defects of the nose, it is not an ideal choice because of the difficulty in matching texture and color. This is especially true in non-White noses where the SSTE is thicker.

Local flaps tend to be the reconstructive option of choice for many nasal defects. Local flaps are often robust and provide good texture and color match. Because of the thicker and less extensible nature of the SSTE in non-White patients, wider undermining is usually required to achieve the stretch required for tensionless defect closure. Additionally, the Asian nose tends to be smaller in size and local flaps are more limited in versatility. Many tables and algorithms found in the medical literature reference the White nose in terms of overall size. This is misleading.

Case study 1

Fig. 1 shows a middle-aged Korean man with basal cell carcinoma. After Mohs surgery, he had a small nasal defect at the nasal tip. The nasal tip skin is more sebaceous especially in Asian subjects. Bilateral advancement flap was designed for closure of the defect, with standing cutaneous defects immediately above and below the defect. The resultant scar is in the midline with minimal distortion of alar rims.

Case study 2

Fig. 2 shows an elderly Chinese man with basal cell carcinoma and 8-mm defect of the nasal tip after excision. While planning for reconstruction, note the SSTE of the nasal tip is thick and sebaceous. In planning the East-West flap, the inferior standing cutaneous deformity was moved to the midline infratip lobule segment. Wide undermining is generally required because of the relative inelasticity of the sebaceous skin.

Similar to White nasal defects, nonanatomic cartilage grafting is used extensively. However, according to Jin and colleagues, nasal grafting is often used to prevent alar notching rather than for functional purposes and lateral wall collapse.[15]

Choice of local flaps used depends on mainly the site, size, and depth of the defect. For many alar defects, the flap of choice is an interpolated melolabial flap. For larger defects, forehead flap should be considered.

In the design of forehead flaps, there are subtle modifications as suggested by Hsiao and colleagues[20] for reconstruction of Asian noses. The Asian SSTE is generally thicker with more fibrofatty tissue at the nasal tip. For this reason, flap thinning is less imperative and performed in a more conservative manner. They found that framework reinforcement was necessary in patients because of the unpredictable flap contracture. Therefore, it was recommended to thin the flap conservatively

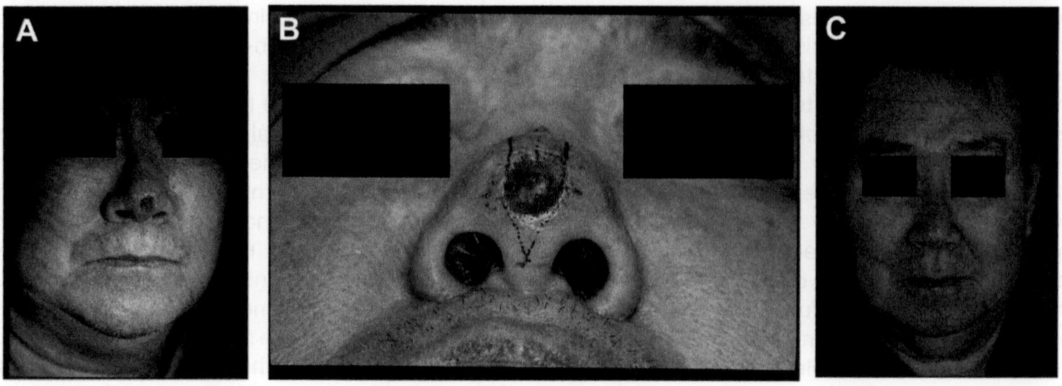

Fig. 1. (*A*) Middle-aged Korean man with small nasal defect at the nasal tip. (*B*) Bilateral advancement flap designed for closure of the defect. (*C*) Final result about 3 weeks after surgery.

to match the skin thickness and to strengthen and overbuild the structural framework to counter the contractile forces of a healing forehead flap.[20]

Case study 3

Fig. 3 shows a middle-aged African American man with extensive basal cell carcinoma involving the nasal tip, dorsum, and the alar. After Mohs excision, the patient had a large, full-thickness nasal defect involving the nasal dorsum, nasal tip, left nasal sidewall, and left nasal alar. He underwent multiple staged reconstruction with forehead flap as skin coverage, full-thickness skin graft for nasal lining, costal cartilage for framework support, and composite concha grafts for support and lining. Left cheek advancement flap was also performed. Costal cartilage was used to reconstruct the dorsal strut. Composite concha graft was harvested from the right ear and used to reconstruct the lining and the left alar rim.

Case study 4

Fig. 4 shows a middle-aged Chinese man with right nasal basal cell carcinoma involving the nasal tip, the right nasal alar, with a resultant large nasal defect after excision involving the nasal tip and alar. Forehead flap was planned for skin coverage and concha cartilage nonanatomic grafting to support the nasal alar. Cartilage graft was mainly used to prevent alar notching. During the harvest of forehead flap, it is important to match the skin thickness of the surrounding skin.

Treatment of Periorbital Defects

Periorbital anatomy

It is well known that there are many differences between the Asian and White eyelid. There is generally more prominent subcutaneous, suborbicularis, and pretarsal fat tissue in the Asian upper eyelid. This pretarsal fat is considered to be a spacer that prevents levator aponeurosis from extending to the subdermal tissue in single eyelid crease people.[21] In Asians, the preaponeurotic fat is much lower than that in Whites.[22] Epicanthi are folds of skin in the medial canthal area and Asians tend to have this fold of skin that hides the caruncle.

Globe protrusion and interpupillary distance in African American patients tend to be greater compared with White patients.[23,24]

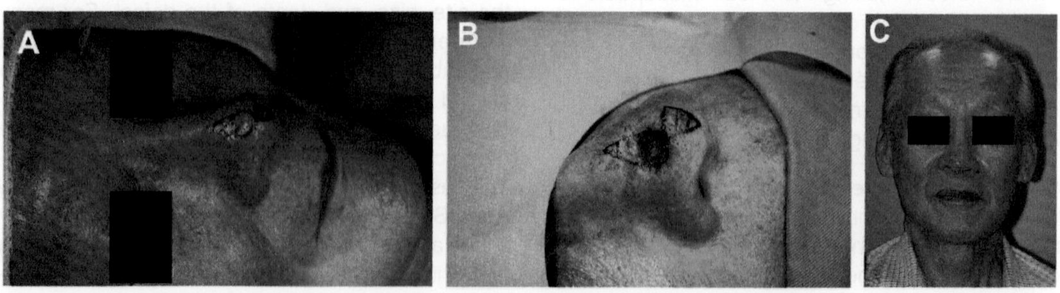

Fig. 2. Elderly Chinese man with basal cell carcinoma and 8-mm defect of the nasal tip, reconstructed with East-West flap. (*A*) Planning for excision of the basal cell carcinoma. (*B*) Planning the East-West flap with wide undermining required because of the relative inelasticity of the sebaceous skin. (*C*) Final result about 2 weeks after the surgery.

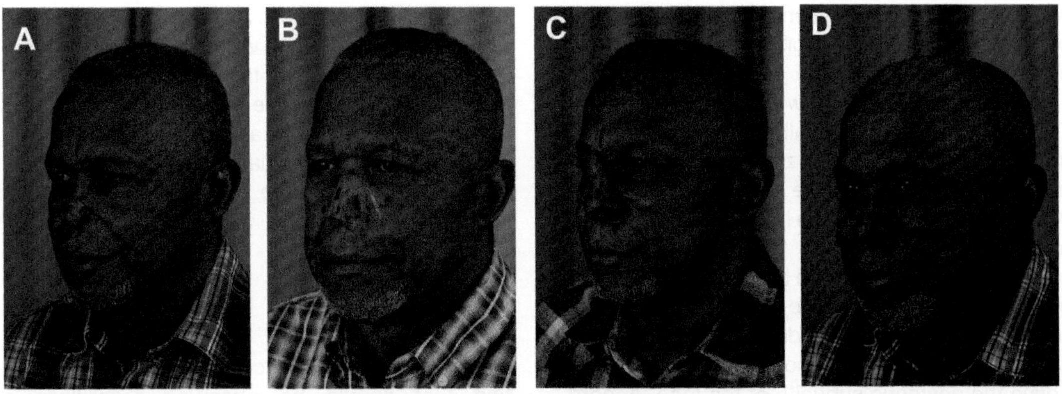

Fig. 3. (*A*) Middle-aged African American man with extensive basal cell carcinoma involving the nasal tip, dorsum, and the alar. (*B*) Large nasal defect after Mohs excision. (*C*) Staged reconstruction with forehead flap, full-thickness skin graft, composite concha cartilage graft for alar form and lining, and costal cartilage for framework support. (*D*) Final result about 6 months after surgery.

Whites also have more prominent supraorbital bones, whereas Asians have low supraorbital bones.[25]

Management of specific periorbital defects

Local skin flaps are the preferred reconstructive option of choice in anterior lamellar defects. Skin grafts usually do not have appropriate color and texture match. The color mismatch maybe more apparent in other ethnic groups because of the PIH. Common flap designs are rhombic flaps and V-Y and Y-V advancement flaps. For superior eyelid defects, the absence of supratarsal creases in the Asian population can lead to increased difficulty in hiding the resultant scar.

Generally, second intent healing is not acceptable in upper eyelid defects. The exception is the medial canthal region where defects less than 1 cm can heal well with second intent. However, in the Asian population with prominent epicanthal folds, the scarring is difficult to predict and this may result in asymmetry, which can be jarringly obvious, especially if the epicanthal fold is disrupted unilaterally. Medial canthal symmetry in the Asian patient is especially challenging to correct and requires a more elaborate and thoughtful repair from the onset.

Treatment of Cheek Defects

Cheek anatomy

The surface anatomy and contour of the face depends on the underlying bony structures and on the overlying soft tissues. The facial skeleton,

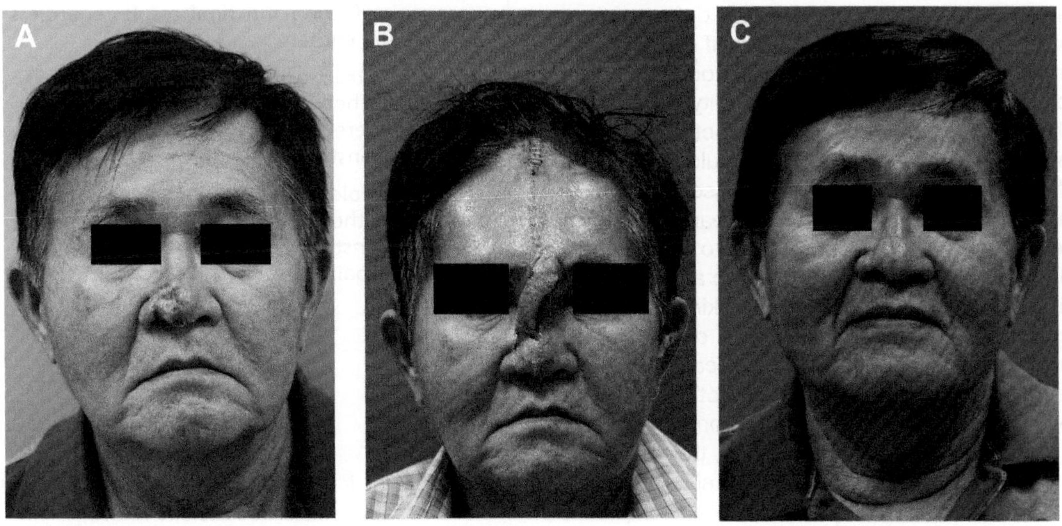

Fig. 4. (*A*) Middle-aged Chinese man with right nasal basal cell carcinoma involving the nasal tip, the right nasal alar, with a resultant large nasal defect after excision. (*B*) Forehead flap planned for skin coverage and concha cartilage nonanatomic grafting to prevent alar notching. (*C*) Postoperative result about 3 months after surgery.

which forms the foundation of the face, is obviously different depending on the ethnicities. There are also differing physical characteristics of the skin and the soft tissue between the ethnic groups. The Asian skeleton generally has a wide and flat midface, with prominent zygomas, small nasal bones, and wide mandible angles.[26] The African American skeleton tends to have a bimaxillary protrusion, orbital proptosis, with increased facial convexity. The Latino and Hispanic face generally has increased bizygomatic distance, bimaxillary protrusion, with more receded chin.[27]

Different authors have sought to describe and define the aesthetic subunits of the face. According to Gonzalez-Ulloa and coworkers,[28] the cheek is divided into three aesthetic subunits: zone I includes the suborbital region, zone II involves the preauricular region, and zone III encompasses the bucomandibular region. Bradley and Murakami[29] have divided the cheek into medial, lateral (mandibular), zygomatic, and buccal divisions. It is generally agreed that the primary goal during reconstruction is to restore skin color and texture, which are more obvious than contour and subunit outline variations.

Reconstruction of specific defects

Generally, the same principles apply in White and non-White patients. Reconstruction should be tailored accordingly in each patient, taking note of their defect size and their location. Immobile landmarks should be respected and care must be taken to avoid any shift or distortion. Resultant scars are always considered but different across ethnicities.

Direct closure in general should be considered as the first line for closure of cheek defects if there is no distortion of adjacent tissue. If direct closure is not possible, the next option is a local flap. When planning for cheek flaps, the mobility and laxity of the skin surrounding the defect should be assessed. The resultant scars should ideally lie at the border of aesthetic units, the nasofacial sulcus, alar-facial sulcus, melolabial crease, or along relaxed skin tension lines (RSTL) to best camouflage them. This may be difficult to achieve in patients with taut and wrinkle-free skin. In Kim and coworkers'[30] study on cheek defects, they avoided the use of bilobed flaps because of unsatisfactory scarring in Asians. They opted instead for either V-Y advancement flap or rhombic flap.

For cheek defects adjacent to the nasal ala, lateral nasal wall, and inferior orbital rims, usually large cervicofacial flaps or rotational flaps are required. In younger patients or patients with better orbicularis oculi tone, the scar is camouflaged in the subciliary line. However, care has to be taken to avoid ectropion and inferior lid retraction, especially in individuals with lax lower lids.[31]

With larger defects, the cervicofacial flap remains the reconstructive option of choice. With a large flap and visible scar, the concept of healing in the non-White population becomes pertinent. Meticulous tension-free skin closure with good wound care form the foundation to achieving good results.

SUMMARY

There are a few key principles in facial reconstruction that should be observed regardless of ethnicity. The principles of restoring facial harmony and symmetry should be foremost in any reconstructive surgeon's mind. With different ethnicities, however, there are nuances to consider that include facial anatomy, skin physiology, and cultural norms and expectations. Integrating these variables improves outcomes and patient satisfaction.

CLINICS CARE POINTS

- Ethnic distinctions are part of the consideration of reconstructive planning.
- Different ethnic groups have different skin anatomy and physiology and that should be taken into consideration. Variations in aesthetic units can lead to different flap selection and design.
- Healing differs among the different ethnic groups, affecting the final result regardless of method chosen.
- For reconstruction of nasal defects, the SSTE difference between the ethnic groups has to be considered before choosing an appropriate reconstructive option.
- The principles of symmetry and harmony remain as the central pilar when performing facial reconstruction with the goal of allowing the repair to appear as inconspicuous as possible.

REFERENCES

1. Gloster HM Jr, Neal K. Skin cancer in skin of color. J Am Acad Dermatol 2006;55(5):741–60.
2. Sands NB, Adamson PA. Global facial beauty: approaching a unified aesthetic ideal. Facial Plast Surg 2014;30(2):93–100.

3. Staricco RJ, Pinkus H. Quantitative and qualitative data on the pigment cells of adult human epidermis. J Invest Dermatol 1957;28(1):33–45.
4. Goldschmidt H, Raymond JZ. Quantitative analysis of skin color from melanin content of superficial skin cells. J Forensic Sci 1972;17(1):124–31.
5. Fitzpatrick TB. The validity and practicality of sun reactive skin type I through VI. Arch Dermatol 1988;124:869–71.
6. Grimes PE. Managment of hyperpigmentation in darker racial ethnic groups. Semin Cutan Med Surg 2009;28:77–85.
7. Davis EC, Callender VD. Postinflammatory hyperpigmentation: a review of the epidemiology, clinical features, and treatment options in skin of color. J Clin Aesthet Dermatol 2010;3(7):20–31.
8. LeFlore IC. Misconceptions regarding elective plastic surgery in the black patient. J Natl Med Assoc 1980;72:947–8.
9. Child FJ, Fuller LC, Higgins EM, et al. A study of the spectrum of skin disease occurring in a black population in south-east London. Br J Dermatol 1999;141: 512–7.
10. Alhady SM, Sivanantharajah K. Keloids in various races: a review of 175 cases. Plast Reconstr Surg 1969;44:564–6.
11. Gao Y, Niddam J, Noel W, et al. Comparison of aesthetic facial criteria between caucasian and East Asian female populations: an esthetic surgeon's perspective. Asian J Surg 2018;41(1):4–11.
12. Zhuang Z, Landsittel D, Benson S, et al. Facial anthropometric differences among gender, ethnicity, and age groups. Ann Occup Hyg 2010;54(4): 391–402.
13. Le TT, Farkas LG, Ngim RC, et al. Proportionality in Asian and North American caucasian faces using neoclassical facial canons as criteria. Aesthet Plast Surg 2002;26:64–9.
14. Nouveau S, Yang Z, Mac-Mary S, et al. Skin ageing: a comparison between Chinese and European populations. A pilot study. J Dermatol Sci 2005;40(3): 187–93.
15. Jin HR, Jeong WJ. Reconstruction of nasal cutaneous defects in Asians. Auris Nasus Larynx 2009; 36(5):560–6.
16. Ozucer B, Yildirim YS, Veyseller B, et al. Effect of postrhinoplasty taping on postoperative edema and nasal draping: a randomized clinical trial. JAMA Facial Plast Surg 2016;18(3):157–63.
17. Lessard ML, Daniel RK. Surgical anatomy of septorhinoplasty. Arch Otolaryngol 1985;111(1):25–9.
18. Eggerstedt M, Rhee J, Buranosky M, et al. Nasal skin and soft tissue thickness variation among differing races and ethnicities: an objective radiographic analysis. Facial Plast Sugr Anesthet Med 2020;22(3):188–94.
19. Yotsuyanagi T, Yamashita K, Urushidate S, et al. Nasal reconstruction based on aesthetic subunits in Orientals. Plast Reconstr Surg 2000;106(1):36–44.
20. Hsiao YC, Chang CS, Zelken J. Aesthetic refinements in forehead flap reconstruction of the Asian nose. Plast Surg (Oakv) 2017;25(2):71–7.
21. Jeong S, Lemke BN, Dortzbach RK, et al. The Asian upper eyelid: an anatomical study with comparison to the caucasian eyelid. Arch Ophthalmol 1999; 117(7):907–12.
22. Kiranantawat K, Suhk JH, Nguyen AH. The Asian eyelid: relevant anatomy. Semin Plast Surg 2015; 29(3):158–64.
23. Pivnick EK, Rivas ML, Tolley EA, et al. Interpupillary distance in a normal black population. Clin Genet 1999;55:182–91.
24. Barretto RL, Mathog RH. Orbital measurement in black and white populations. Laryngoscope 1999; 109:1051–4.
25. Watanabe K. Measurement method of upper blepharoplasty for Oriental. Aesthet Plast Surg 1993;17: 1e8.
26. Kim SJ, Kim SJ, Park JS, et al. Analysis of age-related changes in Asian facial skeletons using 3D vector mathematics on picture archiving and communication system computed tomography. Yonsei Med J 2015;56(5):1395–400.
27. Vashi NA, de Castro Maymone MB, Kundu RV. Aging differences in ethnic skin. J Clin Aesthet Dermatol 2016;9(1):31–8.
28. Gonzalez-Ulloa M, Castillo A, Stevens E, et al. Preliminary study of the total restoration of the facial skin. Plast Reconstr Surg (1946) 1954;13:151–61.
29. Bradley DT, Murakami CS. Reconstruction of the cheek. In: Baker SR, editor. Local flaps in facial reconstruction. Philadelphia: Mosby Elsevier; 2007. p. 521–56.
30. Kim JH, Jeong HS, Lee BH, et al. Reconstructive modalities according to aesthetic consideration of subunits of the cheek after wide excision of skin cancer. Arch Aesthet Plast Surg 2016;22(1):28–34.
31. Hanks JE, Moyer JS, Brenner MJ. Reconstruction of cheek defects secondary to Mohs microsurgery or wide local excision. Facial Plast Surg Clin North Am 2017;25(3):443–61.

Approach for Rhinoplasty in African Descendants

Lucas G. Patrocinio, MD, PhD[a,b,*], Tomas G. Patrocinio, MD, PhD[b], Jose A. Patrocinio, MD, PhD[a,b]

KEYWORDS

• Rhinoplasty • African-American • African descendants • Grafts • Thick skin • Isotretinoin • Triamcinolone

KEY POINTS

- The main objectives of rhinoplasty in African descendant patients are to improve the definition and projection of the nasal tip, augment the dorsum, and reduce the alar base.
- Open rhinoplasty with costal cartilage graft is the preferred technique for rhinoplasty in African descendants.
- Lateral crural tensioning with septal extension graft associated with en bloc dorsal augmentation is the workhorse in rhinoplasty of African descendants.
- The use of isotretinoin in pre- and postoperative periods may lead to better outcomes in tip definition.
- Postoperative injections of triamcinolone can help reduce supra-tip edema and tip definition.

INTRODUCTION

The study of anthropometry in Negroid (originally named Ethiopian) faces and noses has been well documented for decades.[1–6] More recently, an increase in the number of patients of African descent searching for aesthetic procedures has brought a lot of new scientific information to the field.[7–13]

Based on a survey,[14] the American Society of Plastic Surgeons (ASPS) estimates that 18 million cosmetic procedures were performed in United States during 2019. Segmenting, 30% of those procedures were performed on non-Caucasian patients. In 2005, non-Caucasian patients accounted for 22% of all cosmetic procedures.[15] In 2019, 9% of the patients were black or African American, representing approximately 1.7 million cosmetic procedures.[13] In 2004, this population comprised 5% of cosmetic procedures.[15,16] From 1999 to 2001, there was a reported 340% increase in African American patients requesting cosmetic procedures.[17]

The same survey from the ASPS estimates that more than 200,000 rhinoplasties were performed in 2019, whereas 7% of those were performed on patients of African descent, which translates to approximately 14,000 rhinoplasties.[14] This article discusses new advances in surgical techniques and clinical care for rhinoplasty in African descendants.

ANATOMY AND CLINICAL FEATURES

The African descendant's nose presents specific anatomic characteristics that are relevant to rhinoplasty.

Skin and Subcutaneous Features

The skin on the nose of the African descendants is thicker, sebaceous, and inelastic, especially at the tip, which is bulbous, flattened, and ill-defined. It is necessary to remember, at the time of grafting, that over the upper nasal third the nasal skin and subcutaneous fat is fairly thick and becomes relatively thin over the middle third.

In the subcutaneous tissue, mainly in the nasal tip, there is a greater amount of fibrofatty tissue

[a] Department of Otolaryngology, Medical School, Federal University of Uberlandia, Rua Arthur Bernardes, 555, Uberlandia, Minas Gerais 38400-368, Brazil; [b] Private Practice, OTOFACE, Uberlandia Medical Center, Rua Arthur Bernardes, 555, Uberlandia, Minas Gerais 38400-368, Brazil
* Corresponding author.
E-mail address: lucaspatrocinio@clinicaotoface.com.br

Facial Plast Surg Clin N Am 29 (2021) 575–588
https://doi.org/10.1016/j.fsc.2021.06.008

(about 2–4 mm), one of the factors that compete for not defining the tip.[18]

This traditional description may not reflect the whole diversity of skin thickness encountered among patients of African descent. Categorizing the African nasal skin envelope as mild, intermediate, or severely thick is more helpful in anticipating its response to rhinoplasty.[8]

Nasal Tip

Lower lateral cartilages (LLCs), skin, and subcutaneous tissue form the nasal tip. The LLCs are not thinner and weaker than those of Caucasians, as was thought initially.[18,19] The large amount of fibrofatty tissue between the domes, the obtuse angle (>90°) between the medial and lateral crura, the acute lateral crural cartilage angle of inclination relative to the maxilla, 3 short columella, and the hypodeveloped nasal spine cause the lack of projection and definition of the nasal tip, creating an aspect of a flat and bulbous tip.

In African descendants, the projection of the tip of the nose is generally smaller than in Caucasians (0.67 times the ideal nasal length), approximately 0.5 times the ideal nasal length. The rotation may vary, but, in general, there is an under-rotated tip (African American vs Caucasian is 86–91 vs 99 in women and 83 vs 98–100 in men, respectively).[4–6]

Nasal Pyramid

The nasal bones in African descendant patients are shorter and have an obtuse angle between each other, resulting in a flatter and broader appearance of the dorsum, both in the upper and the middle thirds.[20]

The nasofrontal angle is usually at the height or caudal to the pupil line and varies from equal to more obtuse than in Caucasians, because the radix is deeper set and wider (25–27 mm compared with 15–16 mm in Caucasians).[4–6]

Alar Base

In the African descendants, the columella is short and wide, contributing to the ovoid shape and horizontal oriented nostril. The columella to tip lobule relationship is usually 1.4 to 1.5:1, which is shorter than the classic 2:1 ratio.[5,6,21,22] The nasolabial angle is acute because of the more cephalic position of the nasal septum and the underdevelopment of nasal spine.

The pyriform aperture shape more ovoid and with a shorter vertical height compared with Caucasians, contributing to an extremely wide alar base.[4,20] Compared with the traditional ratio of a 1:1 relationship between intercanthal distance and nasal base width, the relationship is 1:1.25 and 1:3 in African American women and men.[5,6]

Further, a more horizontal orientation of the LLCs leads the ala to flare beyond the alar base attachment in African descendants by more than 2 mm.[18] The lateral wall of the nostril can be bulky.

GOALS

Among patients of African descent, the final ideal result should be a balanced-looking nose that blends in with the patient's face, preserving the ethnic features. The objective is to have a nose as close possible of the standard of beauty, maintaining its ethnic characteristics and creating better harmony and nasofacial balance.[11] Therefore, the objectives of rhinoplasty in African descendants are to improve the definition and projection of the nasal tip, augment the dorsum, and reduce the alar base.

To operate on the nose of African descendants, one must first have a careful conversation with the patient, realistically defining the changes proposals, keeping the nose as close as possible to the standard of beauty, without losing its ethnic characteristics.[23,24]

PREOPERATIVE CLINICAL TREATMENT

The medical treatment of the skin-soft tissue envelope with isotretinoin is recommended.[25] There are few studies; however, evidence suggests that the use of oral isotretinoin in patients with thick skin accelerates improvement in cosmetic results during the early months after surgery,[26] and the patients were more satisfied with their operation outcomes and experienced fewer skin problems.[27] On the other hand, it seems that isotretinoin does not significantly affect the final cosmetic result in 1 year.[26]

Patients usually receive a drug regimen a dose ranging from 0.25 mg/kg to 0.5 mg/kg for a period of 4 to 6 months. The authors' protocol starts 30 to 60 days before surgery and is suspended 7 days before surgery. Then, 15 days after surgery it is resumed and kept for approximately 6 months (**Fig. 1**). All patients should be monitored with hepatic function tests.

SURGICAL TECHINIQUE

Anesthesia

All procedures are performed under general anesthesia with remifentanil and propofol (topical anesthesia with cotton soaked in 2% tetracaine with adrenaline 1: 1,000, which remains in the nasal cavity for 10 minutes; local anesthesia with

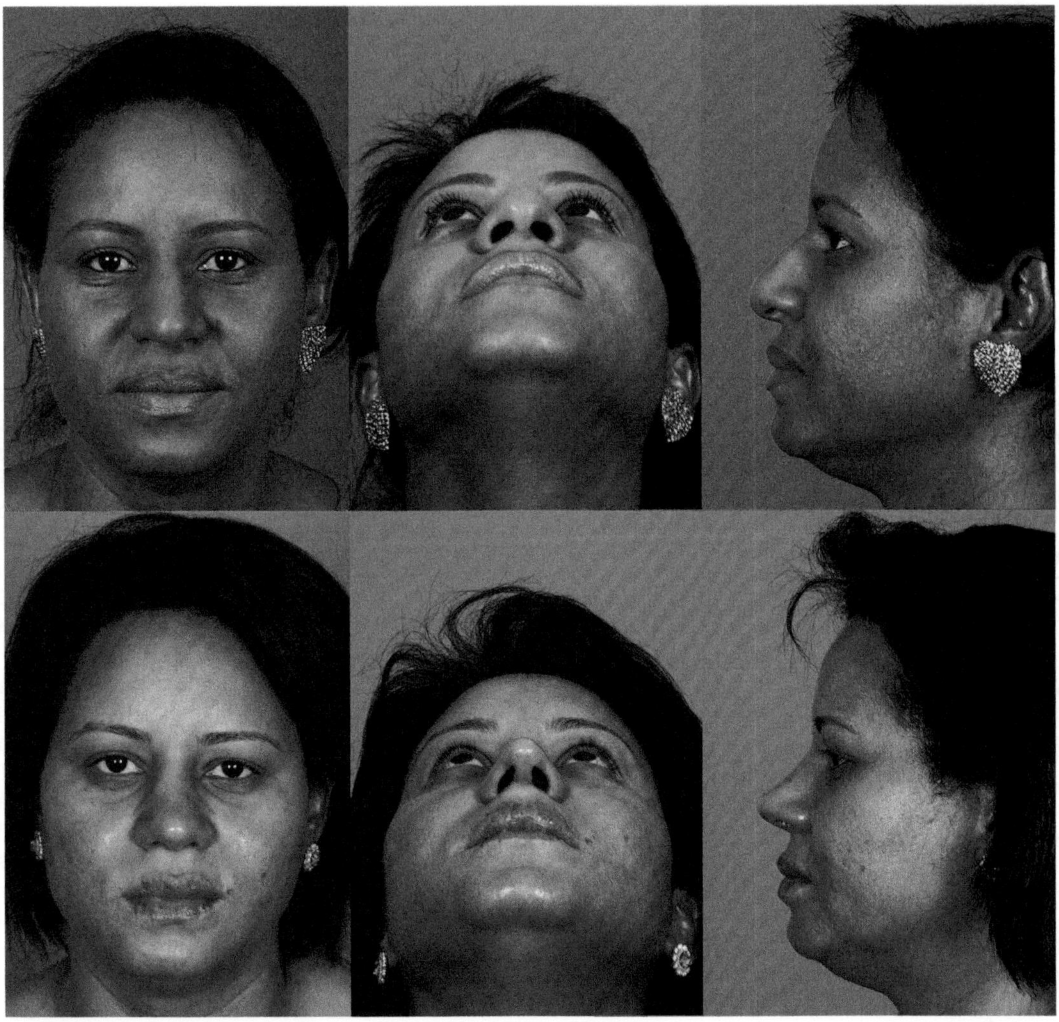

Fig. 1. Pre and postoperative photographs of a patient submitted to rhinoplasty and oral isotretinoin for 6 months after surgery.

extravascular infiltration of 5 mL of 1% ropivacaine with adrenaline 1: 100,000).

Obtaining Autologous Grafts

The grafts can be obtained from septal cartilage, conchal cartilage, or costal cartilage. However, in most rhinoplasties in African descendants, the septal cartilage is weak; thus it is strongly recommended to harvest costal cartilage.[28] Implants should be avoided.

The nasal septum cartilage is obtained through routine septoplasty with elevation of the mucosa, releasing the cartilage septum from its junction with the perpendicular plate of the ethmoid (PPE) and incising it dorsally and caudally, preserving 1.5 cm anteriorly and 1.5 cm dorsally. It can be used as a septal extension graft (SEG), a tip graft, alar contour grafts, and dorsum augmentation. The PPE can also be harvested and used as a splint to the septum or to the SEG. As previously stated, there are few cases in which the septal cartilage is enough for rhinoplasty in African descendants.

The conchal cartilage, because of its flabbiness, can be used as camouflage or dorsum augmentation, but cannot be used as structural grafts, so it is almost never used.

Costal cartilage is the preferred material for grafts in rhinoplasty of African descendants. A piece with 5.0 to 7.0 cm can be obtained with a 1.5 to 2.0 cm incision. Rectus abdominis fascia can also be harvested through the same incision.[29] Using the oblique split technique to carve the grafts avoids cartilage wrapping.[30]

Incision/Dissection

Open rhinoplasty is the preferred approach.[31] Despite the skin being thick and oily, the transcolumellar scar is inconspicuous.[32] Bilateral marginal incisions are joined with an inverted V incision in the middle of the columella. Dissection of the lower lateral cartilages is performed in the supraperichondrial plane. The subperichondrial plane may be tricky, because the weakness of the LLC may jeopardize tip sutures. Care should be taken exposing the Pitanguy ligament in the midline; it should be transected carefully and preserved for reconstruction as a final step of the surgery.[33] The bony dorsum is dissected in a subperichondrial/subperiosteal plane, creating a pocket limited to the area in which reduction or augmentation is planned.

Osteotomies

The nasal bone of African descendants usually has a broad base, requiring lateral osteotomies with a 3 mm chisel, with upward perforation at the nasomaxillary angle, with fracture in the medial direction for narrowing the nose.[31] In cases with the nasal dorsum excessively low and in which a large augmentation will be necessary, the osteotomy might be unnecessary. Other osteotomies are reserved for crooked noses.

Nasal Tip

The maneuvers performed on the tip of the African descendant's nose aim to improve projection and definition of the nasal tip, to set rotation desired by the patient, and balance it with the height of the dorsum.[34] The algorithm of treatment of tip is defatting, SEG, LCT, tongue in groove, tip graft, and alar rim graft.

The defatting is an important step to help control skin thickness (**Fig. 2**). Selective debulking allows one to maintain the highlights in the center of the tip and to help keep the shadows in the supra tip and scroll areas, giving a better refined tip.[8,10] The Pitanguy ligament should be totally dissected, transected at the supra tip area, and preserved for reinsertion at the end of the procedure. Carrying the dissection further posteriorly to the anterior nasal spine between the medial crura creates a soft tissue flap that can be used at end of the operation to cover all the grafts of the tip.[35]

The SEG is the most important graft in modern rhinoplasty, especially in African descendants in whom there is total absence of nasal tip support a very thick skin. Without adequate tip support is unlikely to achieve long-term tip definition and projection.[36] The SEG is fixed to the caudal septal to increase septal length and height. The position of the graft will set the tip rotation and projection; therefore, it should be carved carefully and may receive minor adjustments after its fixation. The stabilization of the SEG with additional cartilage or bone splints is mandatory. In end-to-end fixation, bilateral extended spreader grafts and bilateral splints in the posterior septal angle must be used to avoid tilting (**Fig. 3**). In lateral-to-lateral fixation, a contralateral splint should be used to set the midline. The authors advocate the use of lateral-to-lateral fixation, but with the use of bilateral costal cartilage SEG to have the maximum support possible to counteract skin thickness and scar contracture (**Fig. 4**). The graft is carved to span the whole height of the caudal septum and to set the tip position 10 to 12 mm above the final dorsum height. The 2 SEGs are fixated to the caudal septum with several 5-0 polydioxanone mattress sutures. After desired projection and rotation are achieved, the tip of the SEG should be trimmed to achieve better tip refinement and projection.

The LCT[37] is the workhorse in thick skin with a wide and amorphous nasal tip, which is the case of African descendant rhinoplasty. The LCT is a modification of the lateral crural steal.[38] LCT stretches and flattens the lateral crura with a noticeable reduction in crural convexity and bulbosity, increasing tension and strength, thus achieving tip definition and better support of nasal valve and preventing alar retraction. Transdomal oblique 5-0 polydioxanone mattress sutures are used to set the new domes in a position that creates a flat lateral crus.[39] Paradomal trimming is used to adjust the domes to 5 to 6 mm width. Complete separation of the scroll ligament is necessary for adjustment of the lateral crura in the correct resting angle.

The tongue in groove is initiated with the interdomal suture to the SEG. A 5-0 polydioxanone 5-0 mattress suture is used, starting from the right side, transfixing the SEG 2 mm bellow the margin, then transfixing the center of the dome 1 mm below the margin, returning 2 mm cephalic to this point; then, transfixing again the SEG, 2 mm posterior and cephalic to the first point, and then transfixing the right dome the same way as the other one. The knot is tied carefully so the 2 domes are positioned symmetrically and the lateral crus everted, with the caudal margin higher than the cephalic one. The next suture is an intercrural 5-0 polydioxanone mattress suture, 6 to 8 mm bellow the domes, with the knot medially (**Fig. 5**). If further increase in columella projection is needed, a small strut can be interpolated to this suture to correct retractions and set better infratip angle.

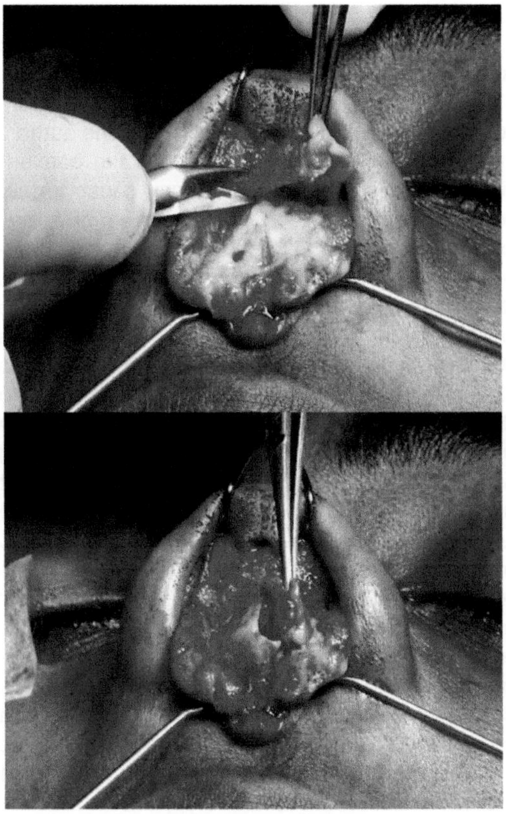

Fig. 2. Photographs showing selective deffating of the nasal tip.

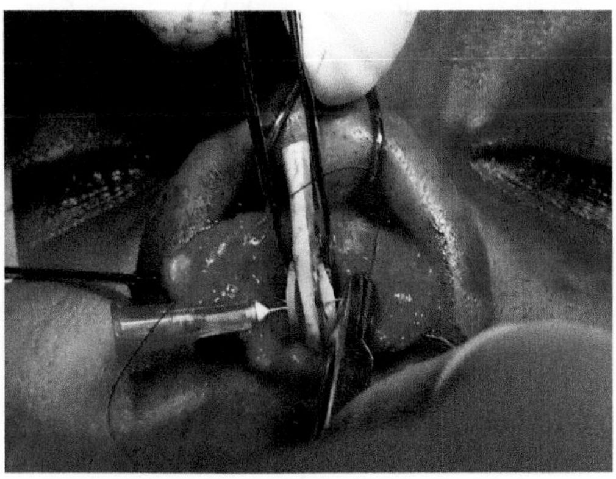

Fig. 3. Photograph showing suturing of costal cartilage, end-to-end, septal extension graft, stabilized with bilateral splints.

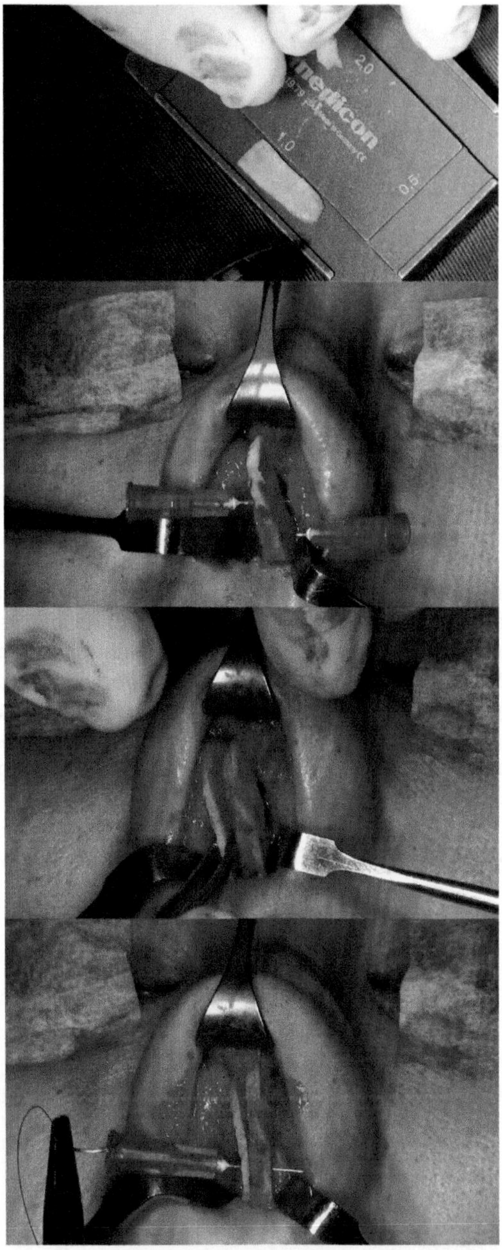

Fig. 4. Photographs showing suturing of costal cartilage, lateral-to-lateral, bilateral septal extension grafts.

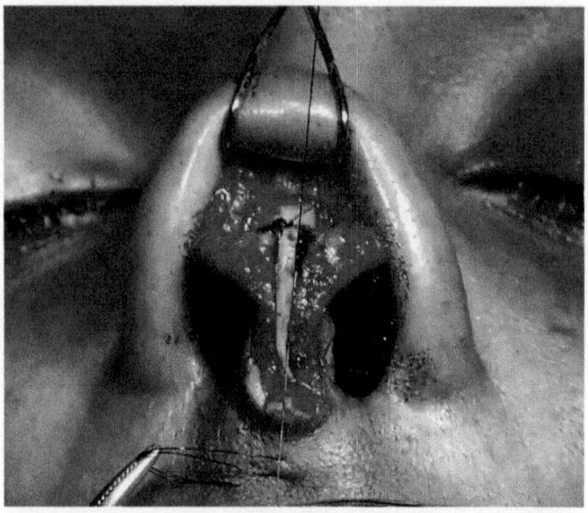

Fig. 5. Photograph showing lateral crural tensioning and tongue-in-groove of the lower lateral cartilages.

Tip grafts are a good option to further increase tip definition and camouflage. Small pieces of lateral crus trimming or of the costal cartilage are used to camouflage the SEG and might give 1 to 2 mm more of tip projection if desired.[34] Shield graft with a buttress graft can also be used, but generally it is not necessary if costal cartilage is used and there is enough graft to carve 2 strong SEGs, with correct length and width.

Alar margins are weak in noses of African descendants. Usually there is an important concavity around the alar ridge.[40] Thus, lateral crus spanning sutures and alar contour grafts should be added to achieve better aesthetic and function to the tip. The first step is to apply the lateral crura suture to set the best resting angle possible. The authors prefer the pulley suture rather than the conventional spanning suture, which may cause further rotation of the tip and some degree of lateral crus cephalization. In the pulley technique, the suture is passed in the shape of a loop that embraces the lateral crus from the contralateral side of the nasal septum or the SEG. The needle transfixes the SEG or the dorsal septum and upper laterals (2–3 mm from the anterior border) contralateral to the crus that will be rotated. Then, the needle transfixes the lateral crus, from outside in, creating a loop that will act as a pulley to rotate the short axis. The entry point is in the upper face of the lateral crus, approximately 3 mm from the cephalic margin and 3 mm lateral to the dome. Next, the needle transfixes back the SEG or the dorsal septum and upper laterals back to the contralateral side, 2 mm bellow the first entry. The anteroposterior and cephalocaudal position of the suture may be modified, depending on each case. Finally, the knot is tightened on the same side as the first entry, observing the rotation of the short axis of the lateral crus, until it reaches the desired position (**Fig. 6**). Each crus is sutured separately, because the desired tension of the

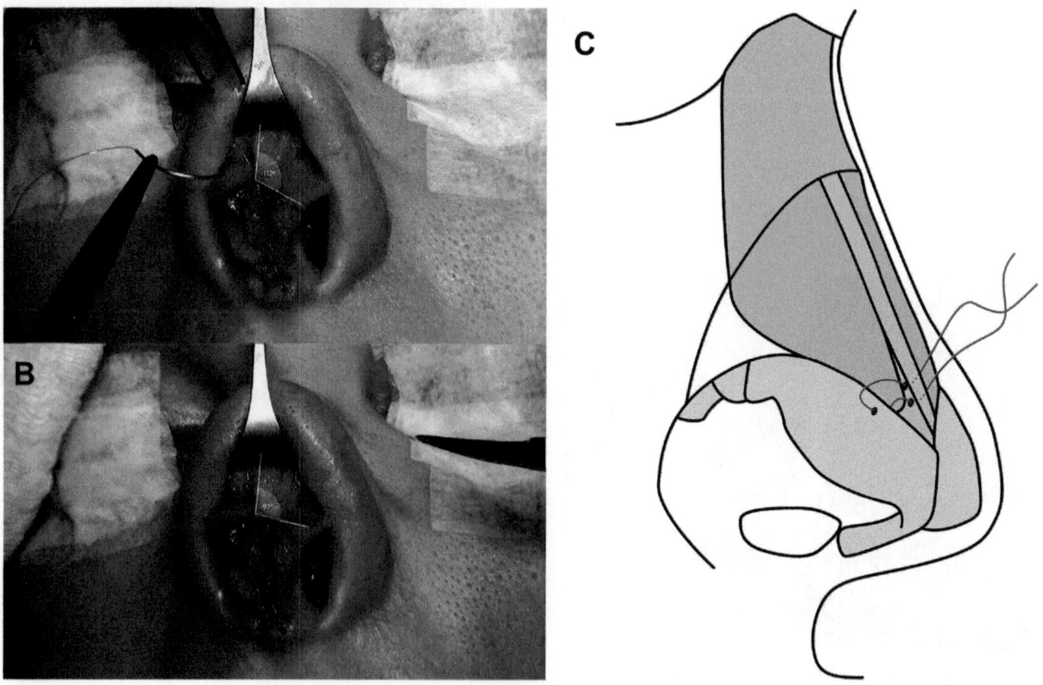

Fig. 6. Photographs (*A,B*) and drawing (*C*) showing the pulley suture and its effect in enhancing the resting angle.

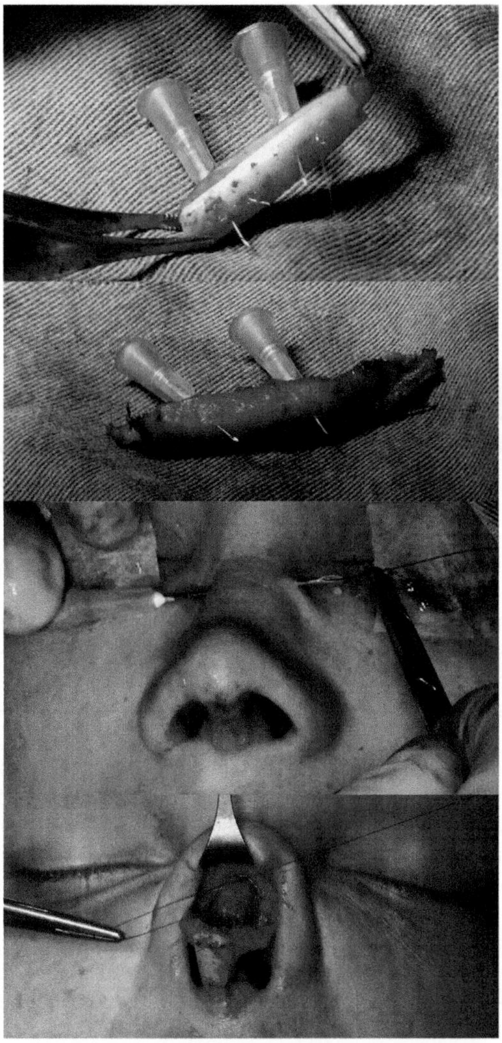

Fig. 7. Photographs showing en bloc costal cartilage wrapped in rectus abdominis fascia sutured in the dorsum with transcutaneous transosseous suture.

suture may differ for each side. If further reinforcement of the caudal margin of the lateral crus is needed, alar rim grafts (articulate or floating) or lateral crus caudal extension grafts can also be added.[40] The authors prefer lateral crus caudal extension grafts, because they are limited to the region of the alar ridge and no further flaring of the nostrils or alar base widening occur. It is a 4 to 6 mm graft suture in a pocket underneath the lateral crus, just spanning the region of the alar ridge and creating a smooth lobule-ala transition.

Nasal Dorsum

Most rhinoplasties in African descendants require some degree of dorsum augmentation. Diced or en bloc cartilage can be used to achieve the desired dorsum projection. Diced cartilage (with or without fascia) is better indicated in small augmentations. In the other hand, large augmentation requires en bloc costal cartilage augmentation.

For diced carriage augmentation, the graft should be diced in minuscule pieces to avoid visibility.[41] Precise pocket also is important to avoid displacement. The use of fascia to wrap the diced cartilage may be helpful to precisely fit the graft, and it also can be sutured to the dorsum to avoid displacement.[42]

En bloc augmentation is more predictable; however, several steps should be followed to avoid wrapping. The oblique split[30] is important, so lower ribs are helpful because of the thickness. Several layers of cartilage can be sutured together achieve the desired projection. If there is irregular dorsum augmentation, small pieces should be sutured to the whole graft in the region needed. When the graft reaches the correct size, all margins should be beveled, and the graft should be wrapped 360° with fascia to avoid viability of the edges and to increase adhesion to the nasal bones. One or 2 transosseous cerclage 4-0 polydioxanone sutures should be used to further stabilize and fix the graft to the dorsum (**Fig. 7**).[43] Another 1 or 2 sutures should be added in the cartilaginous dorsum to achieve the same goals.

Resuturing of the Ligaments

Repositioning and resuturing the Pitanguy ligament and the vertical scroll ligament are helpful to avoid dead space and redraping of the skin, leading to better outcomes in tip definition.

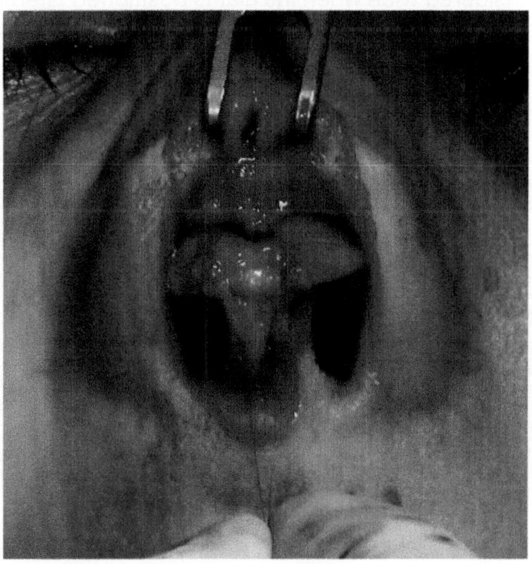

Fig. 8. Photograph showing resuture of the Pitanguy ligament.

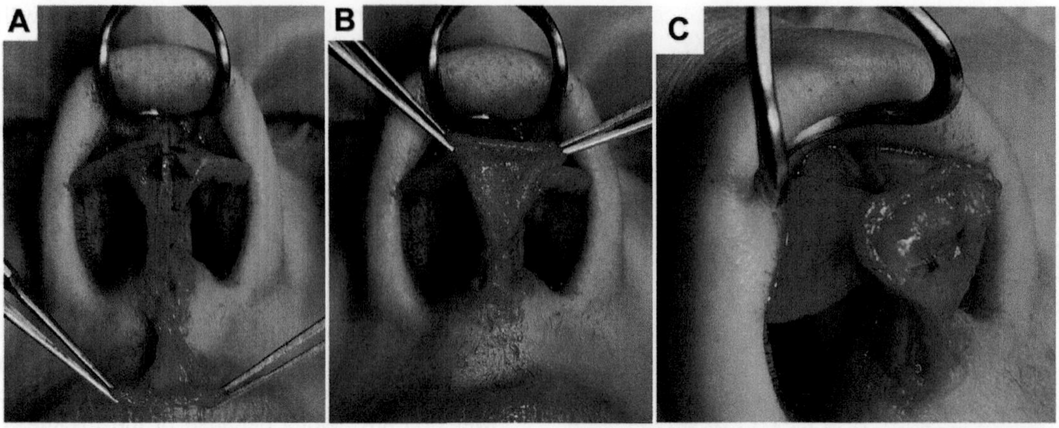

Fig. 9. Photographs showing the carving (*A*), reposition (*B*) and suturing (*C*) of the Protection of Augmented Tip (PAT) flap to camouflage the tip.

The deep Pitanguy ligament is reinserted using 4-0 polydiaxonone sutures between the medial crura and the vestibule mucosa reaching the preserved ligament and them returning to the contralateral medial.[44] This suture increases supratip break and prevents pollybeak deformity (**Fig. 8**). The vertical scroll ligaments are resutured in the same fashion, but the suture is passed through the inner lining of the scroll region. Care should be taken with the knot pressure not to damage the vascularization to the skin. The flap created at the beginning of the surgery (PAT flap) can be redraped to the tip to cover all the grafts (**Fig. 9**).[35]

Alar Base

Wide alar base is the most common reason for rhinoplasty in African descendants. The alar base is considered wide when the alar is positioned lateral to the intercaruncular point. Surgery of the nasal base is performed at the end of the procedure. The alar resection is used to correct the wide nasal base and the alar flare, and then for nostril reshaping. The design for soft tissue excision for alar base reduction is selected based on whether nostril reduction and alar flare modification are simultaneously planned.[31]

In patients with large nostrils with adequate flare, only sill excision is needed. In patients with mild to moderate alar flare, correction can be achieved with tip projection, soft tissue excision, and alar rim grafts. For patients with an excess of alar base, alar flare and large nostrils, a combination of alar and sill resection allows correction. According to the defect, the skin incisions are designed on the medial and lateral vestibular sill and alar skin, being careful not to injure the deep musculature and, then, sutured with 3 to 4 separate 6-0 polypropylene mattress sutures. Residual asymmetry can persist even after a careful attempt to correct, and patients should be educated on that topic.

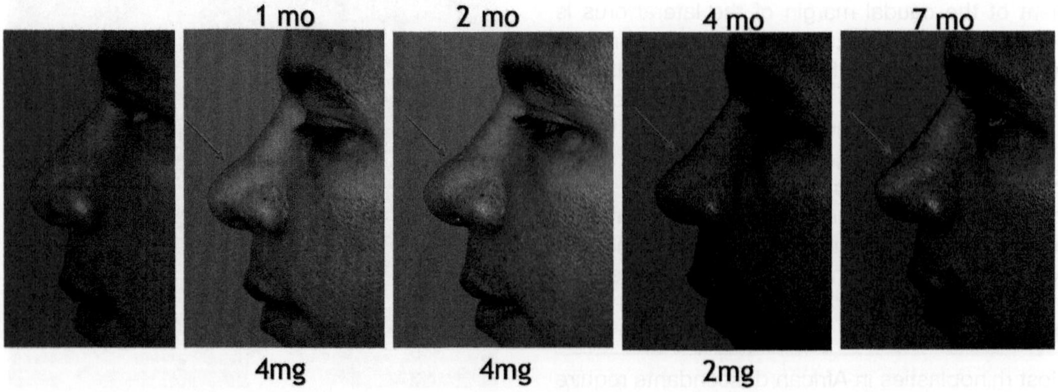

Fig. 10. Pre and postoperative photographs of a patient submitted to rhinoplasty and serial infiltration of triamcinolone showing improvement of the supratip break 7 months after surgery.

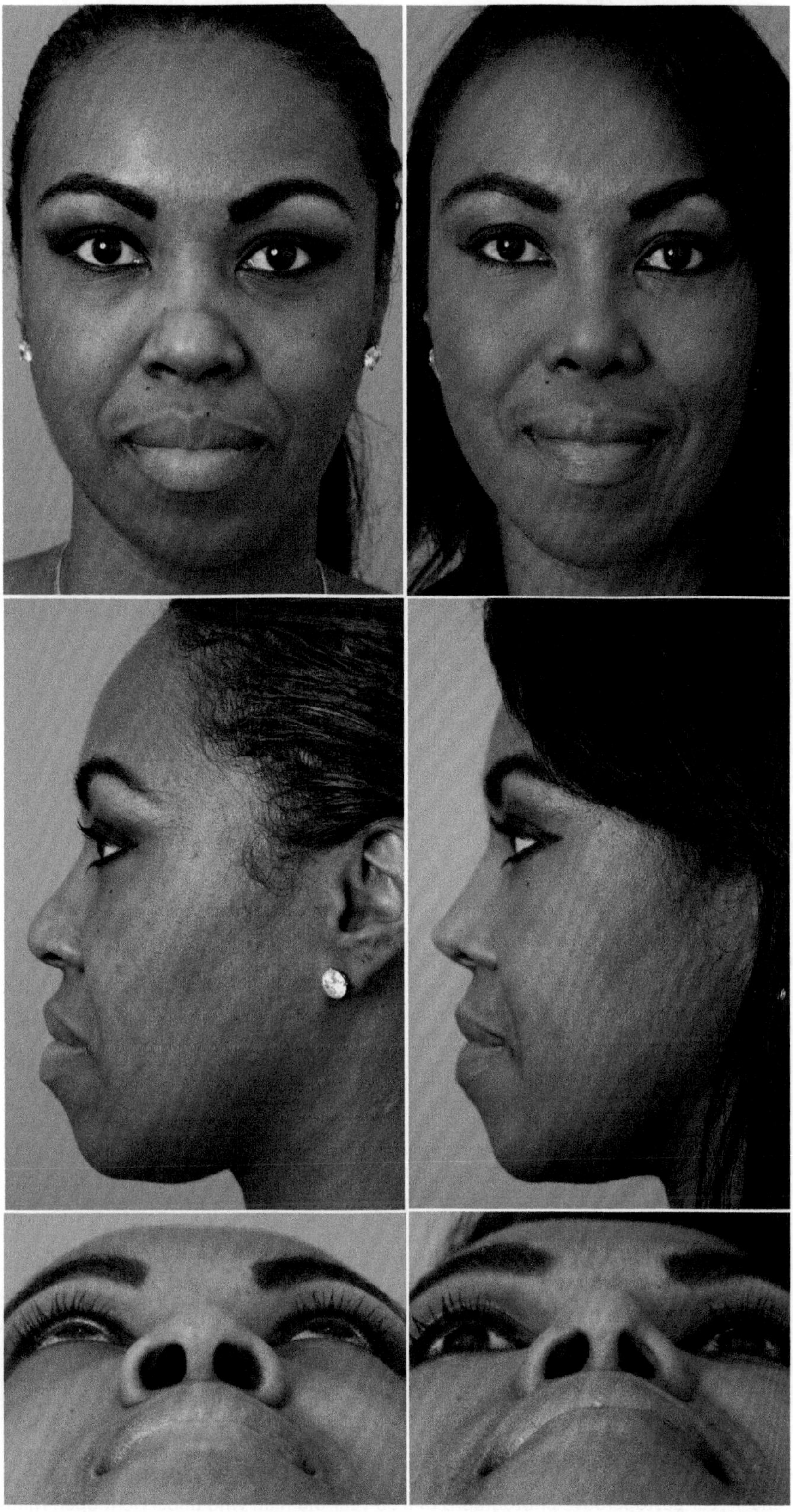

Fig. 11. Pre- and 2-year postoperative photographs of a 35-year-old woman who underwent open rhinoplasty with lateral crural tensioning, achieving better tip rotation, projection, and definition, better balance of the profile, and reduction of the alar base and flare.

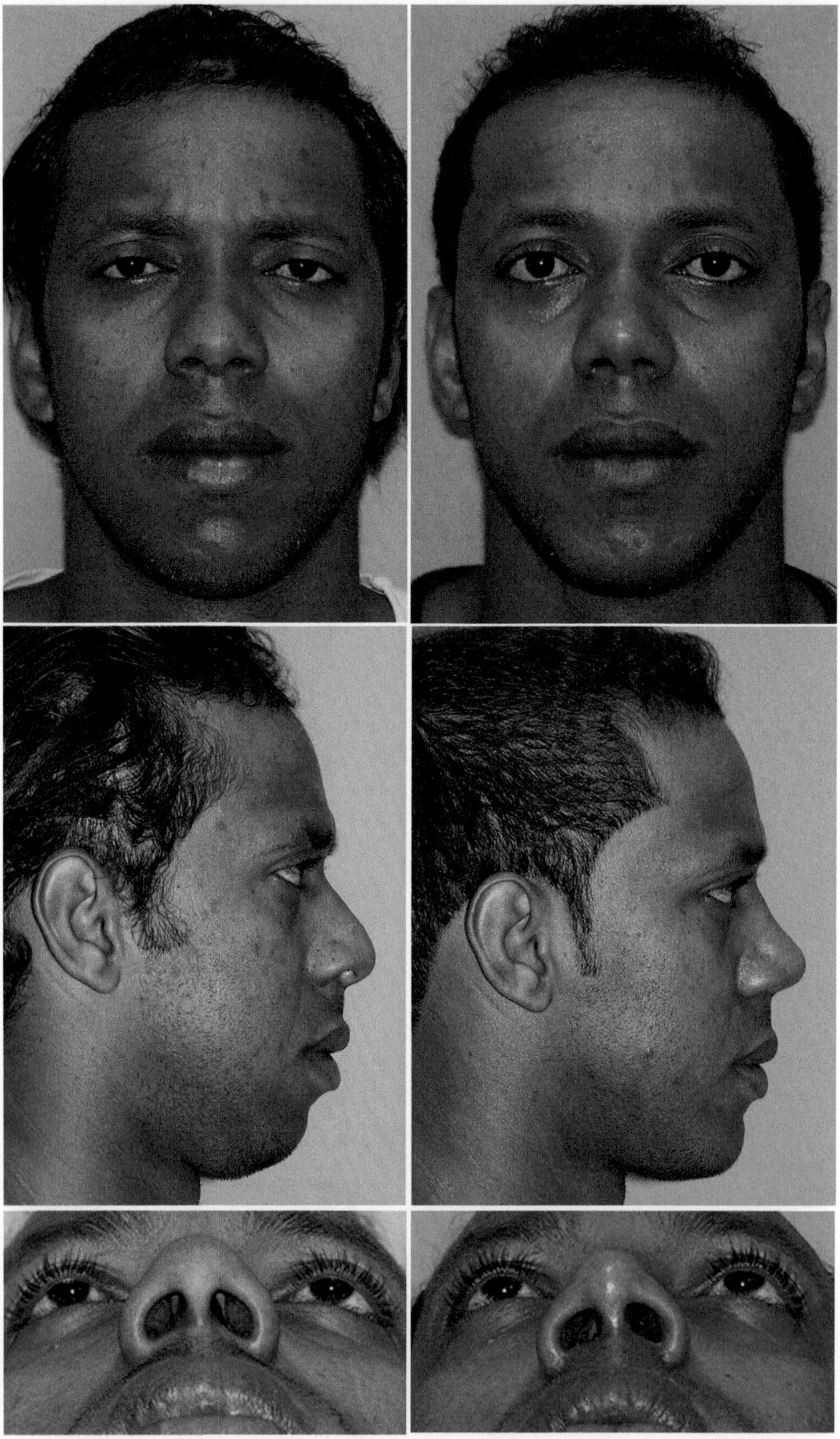

Fig. 12. Pre- and 1-year postoperative photographs of a 38-year-old man who underwent open rhinoplasty with lateral crural tensioning, pulley suture, and articulated alar rim grafts to both lateral crura, achieving better tip rotation, projection, and definition, associated with en bloc dorsal augmentation and sliding genioplasty to balance the profile and enhance refinement of the bridge.

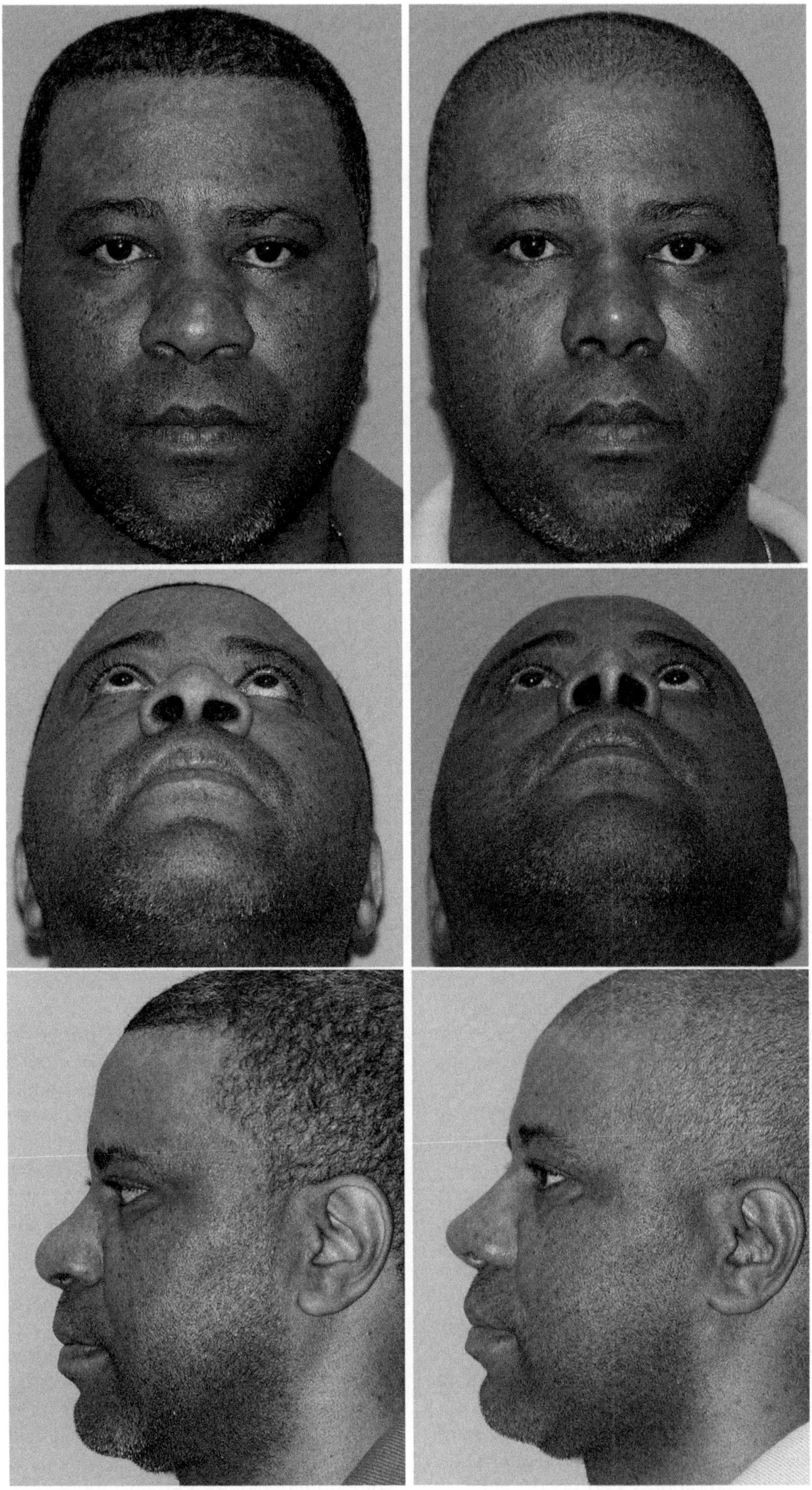

Fig. 13. Pre and 1-year postoperative photographs of a 41-year-old man who underwent open rhinoplasty, achieving better tip rotation, projection, and definition, better balance of the profile, and reduction of the alar base and flare.

The alar volume can also be reduced. The skin is excised in a triangular shape. The base is posterior, and the medial incision is hidden inside the nostril so that there is no visible scar. Some 6-0 polypropylene separated sutures are used to close the incision.

POSTOPERATIVE CARE

Postoperative care is usually extended in rhinoplasty of African descendants because of the thickness of the skin and the prolonged edema. Patients should be aware that final results can be reached only after 2 to 3 years.

External splinting remains for 7 days. Taping is used for another month during the night. Physical activity is forbidden for 30 days. Sun screen should be reinforced for at least 1 year because of the initial bruising and for the incision healing.

Subcutaneous injections of corticosteroids (triamcinolone) postoperatively can help reduce the edema in the supratip area.[45] The dose of 0.2. to 0.4 mL of 10 mg/mL is used 2 weeks after surgery and repeated subsequently every 4 weeks depending on the response obtained (**Fig. 10**).

COMPLICATIONS

The most common complications are the same for all rhinoplasty, including hematoma, epistaxis, edema, synechia, infection, dorsum irregularities, asymmetries, nasal obstruction, altered sense of smell, and septal perforation.

Specifically in rhinoplasty of African descendants, other complications can occur. The most common are related to the incisions, such as hyper- or hypopigmentation and hypertrophic scars. Dermabrasion might be applied to help reduce these effects.[46] Because of the thickness of the skin, the edema can last up to 3 years and delay the final outcome of the nasal tip. This fact should be advised to the patient before surgery, so that it does not create anxieties and false expectations regarding the tip definition. Therefore, reviews, when necessary, should be postponed until at least 1 or 2 years after surgery.

Although much less common with the technique described previously, loss of tip projection because of the skin weight or SEG dislocation can also occur and lead to patient dissatisfaction.

Regarding the costal cartilage harvesting, complications such as keloid formation, unsightly scar, infection, and pneumothorax can occur, and the patient should be educated about this.

CLINICS CARE POINTS

- Noses of African descendants present thick skin and subcutaneous tissue; wide nasal bones with under projected dorsum; under-projected, bulbous and amorphous tip, under developed; and retroprojected anterior nasal spine, weak septum cartilage, and wide alar base with horizontal nostrils.
- The main objectives of rhinoplasty in African descendants are to improve the definition and projection of the nasal tip, augment the dorsum, and reduce the alar base.
- Open rhinoplasty with costal cartilage graft is the preferred technique for rhinoplasty in African descendants.
- Lateral crural tensioning with septal extension graft associated with en bloc dorsal augmentation is the workhorse in rhinoplasty of African descendants.
- The use of isotretinoin in pre and postoperative periods may lead to better outcomes in tip definition.
- Postoperative injections of triamcinolone can help reduce supratip edema and improve tip definition.
- Complications related the skin (conspicuous scars and later tip edema) must be disclosed and discussed with the patient.

SUMMARY

The modern approach to facial plastic surgery has at its central core, the precept of embracing individuality.[47] Technical skill is not the most important obstacle to be overcome to achieve favorable aesthetic results in patients of different races. Techniques can be taught and learned. Surgical success ultimately depends on the ability of the surgeon to accurately identify the anatomic variables and reconcile these anatomic realities with the patient's aesthetic expectations and his or her sense of ethnic identity (**Figs. 11–13**).

Rhinoplasty is a challenging surgery. On African descendants, it becomes an even greater challenge because of ethnic peculiarities. The surgery involves augmenting the dorsum, increasing tip projection, improving nasal tip definition, and reducing the alar base, using various grafts and suturing techniques, certainly more complex than in Caucasian rhinoplasty.

Objectively, harmony and facial balance should be maintained, with a straight and narrow dorsum, a projected and well-defined tip, and normal interalar distance. Finally, resections should be minimal.

DISCLOSURE

None of the authors have any commercial or financial conflicts of interest to disclose.

REFERENCES

1. Zingaro EA, Falces E. Aesthetic anatomy of the non-Caucasian nose. Clin Plast Surg 1987;14(4):749–65.
2. Baker HL. Anatomical and profile analysis of the female black American nose. J Natl Med Assoc 1989; 81(11):1169–75.
3. Ofodile FA, Bokhari FJ, Ellis C. The black American nose. Ann Plast Surg 1993;31(3):209–18.
4. Ofodile FA, Bokhari F. The African-American nose: part II. Ann Plast Surg 1995;34(2):123–9.
5. Porter JP. The average African American male face: an anthropometric analysis. Arch Facial Plast Surg 2004;6(2):78–81.
6. Porter JP, Olson KL. Analysis of the African American female nose. Plast Reconstr Surg 2003; 111(2):620–6.
7. Eggerstedt M, Rhee J, Buranosky M, et al. Nasal skin and soft tissue thickness variation among differing races and ethnicities: an objective radiographic analysis. Facial Plast Surg Aesthet Med 2020;22(3):188–94.
8. Boahene KDO. The African rhinoplasty. Facial Plast Surg 2020;36(1):46–52.
9. O'Connor K, Brissett AE. The changing face of america. Otolaryngol Clin North Am 2020;53(2):299–308.
10. Boahene KDO. Management of the nasal tip, nasal base, and soft tissue envelope in patients of African Descent. Otolaryngol Clin North Am 2020;53(2): 309–17.
11. Patel PN, Most SP. Concepts of facial aesthetics when considering ethnic rhinoplasty. Otolaryngol Clin North Am 2020;53(2):195–208.
12. Villanueva NL, Afrooz PN, Carboy JA, et al. Nasal analysis: considerations for ethnic variation. Plast Reconstr Surg 2019;143(6):1179e–88e.
13. Saad A, Hewett S, Nolte M, et al. Ethnic rhinoplasty in female patients: the neoclassical canons revisited. Aesthet Plast Surg 2018;42(2):565–76.
14. American Society of Plastic Surgeons. Plastic surgery statistics report 2019. Available at: https://www.plasticsurgery.org/documents/News/Statistics/2019/plastic-surgery-statistics-full-report-2019.pdf. Accessed February 1, 2021.
15. American Society of Plastic Surgeons. Plastic surgery statistics report 2005. Available at: https://www.plasticsurgery.org/documents/News/Statistics/2005/cosmetic-procedures-ethnicity-2005.pdf. Accessed February 1, 2021.
16. Wimalawansa S, McKnight A, Bullocks JM. Socioeconomic impact of ethnic cosmetic surgery: trends and potential financial impact the African American, Asian American, Latin American, and Middle Eastern communities have on cosmetic surgery. Semin Plast Surg 2009;23(3):159–62.
17. Sturm-O'Brien AK, Brissett AE. Ethnic trends in facial plastic surgery. Facial Plast Surg 2010;26(2):69–74.
18. Rohrich RJ, Muzaffar AR. Rhinoplasty in the African-American patient. Plast Reconstr Surg 2003;111(3): 1322–39.
19. Ofodile FA, James EA. Anatomy of alar cartilages in blacks. Plast Reconstr Surg 1997;100(3):699–703.
20. Ofodile FA. Nasal bones and pyriform apertures in blacks. Ann Plast Surg 1994;32(1):21–6.
21. Boyette JR, Stucker FJ. African American rhinoplasty. Facial Plast Surg Clin North Am 2014;22(3): 379–93.
22. Stucker FJ, Lian T, Sanders K. African American rhinoplasty. Facial Plast Surg Clin North Am 2005; 13(1):65–72.
23. Kridel RW, Rowe-Jones J. Ethnicity in facial plastic surgery. Facial Plast Surg 2010;26(2):61–2.
24. Weeks DM, Thomas JR. Beauty in a multicultral world. Facial Plast Surg Clin North Am 2014;22(3): 337–41.
25. Cobo R, Vitery L. Isotretinoin use in thick-skinned rhinoplasty patients. Facial Plast Surg 2016;32(6): 656–61.
26. Sazgar AA, Majlesi A, Shooshtari S, et al. Oral isotretinoin in the treatment of postoperative edema in thick-skinned rhinoplasty: a randomized placebo-controlled clinical trial. Aesthet Plast Surg 2019; 43(1):189–95.
27. Yahyavi S, Jahandideh H, Izadi M, et al. Analysis of the effects of isotretinoin on rhinoplasty patients. Aesthet Surg J 2020;40(12):NP657–65.
28. Toriumi DM, Swartout B. Asian Rhinoplasty. Facial Plast Surg Clin North Am 2007;15(3):293–307.
29. As'adi K, Salehi SH, Shoar S. Rib diced cartilage-fascia grafting in dorsal nasal reconstruction: a randomized clinical trial of wrapping with rectus muscle fascia vs deep temporal fascia. Aesthet Surg J 2014;34(6):NP21–31.
30. Taştan E, Yücel ÖT, Aydin E, et al. The oblique split method: a novel technique for carving costal cartilage grafts. JAMA Facial Plast Surg 2013;15(3): 198–203.
31. Patrocinio LG, Patrocinio JA. Open rhinoplasty for African-American noses. Br J Oral Maxillofac Surg 2007;45(7):561–6.
32. Ofodile F, Bokhari FJ. Columella incision in open rhinoplasty in blacks. Plast Reconstr Surg 1992;89(5): 991–2.

33. Abdelwahab M, Patel PN. Conventional resection versus preservation of the nasal dorsum and ligaments: an anatomic perspective and review of the literature. Facial Plast Surg Clin North Am 2021; 29(1):15–28.
34. Patrocinio LG, Patrocinio TG, Maniglia JV, et al. Graduated approach to refinement of the nasal lobule. Arch Facial Plast Surg 2009;11(4):221–9.
35. Patrocinio TG, Patrocinio LG, Patrocinio JA. The Protection of Augmented Tip (PAT) flap technique for tip camouflage. JAMA Facial Plast Surg 2018;20(4): 326–7.
36. Davis RE, Hrisomalos EN. surgical management of the thick-skinned nose. Facial Plast Surg 2018; 34(1):22–8.
37. Davis RE. Lateral crural tensioning for refinement of the wide and underprojected nasal tip: rethinking the lateral crural steal. Facial Plast Surg Clin North Am 2015;23:23–53.
38. Patrocinio LG, Patrocinio TG, Barreto DM, et al. Evaluation of lateral crural steal in nasal tip surgery. JAMA Facial Plast Surg 2014;16(6):400–4.
39. Toriumi DM. Nasal tip contouring: anatomic basis for management. Facial Plast Surg Aesthet Med 2020; 22(1):10–24.
40. Kao WTK, Davis RE. Postsurgical alar retraction: etiology and treatment. Facial Plast Surg Clin North Am 2019;27(4):491–504.
41. Hoehne J, Gubisch W, Kreutzer C, et al. Refining the nasal dorsum with free diced cartilage. Facial Plast Surg 2016;32(4):345–50.
42. Daniel RK. Rhinoplasty: dorsal grafts and the designer dorsum. Clin Plast Surg 2010;37(2): 293–300.
43. Haack S, Hacker S, Mann S, et al. Bony fixation of the nasal framework. Facial Plast Surg 2019;35(1): 23–30.
44. Hoehne J, Brandstetter M, Gubisch W, et al. How to reduce the probability of a pollybeak deformity in primary rhinoplasty: a single-center experience. Plast Reconstr Surg 2019;143(6):1620–4.
45. Hanasono MM, Kridel RW, Pastorek NJ, et al. Correction of the soft tissue pollybeak using triamcinolone injection. Arch Facial Plast Surg 2002; 4(1):26–30.
46. Kridel RW, Castellano RD. A simplified approach to alar base reduction: a review of 124 patients over 20 years. Arch Facial Plast Surg 2005;7(2):81–93.
47. Cobo R, Montes JJ, Patrocinio LG, et al. Rhinoplasty across Latin America: case discussions. Facial Plast Surg 2013;29(3):193–205.

Cosmetic Augmentation Rhinoplasty for East Asians

Man-Koon SUH, MD

KEYWORDS

• Rhinoplasty • Nasal tip plasty • Asian rhinoplasty • Short nose correction

KEY POINTS

- Implants for dorsal augmentation should be placed under the periosteum and the caudal end of the implant should be placed at the supratip area.
- Three-dimensional printed nasal implants can exactly fit the patient's nasal dorsal contour, decreasing the chance of deviation and malpositioning.
- Vertically oriented folded dermal graft and block costal cartilage are the choices of autogenous material for major dorsal augmentation.
- Derotation graft allows supple and movable nasal tip while enabling enough tip lengthening, even if the septal extension graft is the most commonly performed procedure for short nose correction.

NASAL DORSAL AUGMENTATION

Low nasal dorsum is one of the main characteristics of Asian noses. Thus, nasal dorsal augmentation is one of the most frequently performed rhinoplasty procedures in Asian countries.[1]

Materials used for dorsal augmentation are divided into implants and autogenous tissues.

There is no doubt that the autogenous tissues are superior to the implants in the aspect of complications. However, autogenous tissues have disadvantages of lesser satisfaction aesthetically, donor site morbidity, and tissue resorption. Thus, implant is still the preferred material for dorsal augmentation in Asia.

NASAL DORSAL AUGMENTATION USING IMPLANTS

Because of the thick skin envelope of Asian noses, as opposed to that of Westerners' noses, implant showing through the skin or skin thinning and redness after dorsal augmentation with implant is considerably less likely than in white patients.

A high-quality implant carved accurately to match dorsal contour, if placed in the appropriate surgical plane under the correct surgical technique, can minimize the chance of adverse effects and bring esthetically beautiful results for Asians who have thicker skin.

The most commonly used alloplastic implant for Asian dorsal augmentation is silicone implants, followed by expanded polytetrafluoroethylene (e-PTFE) implants.[2,3]

OPERATIVE TECHNIQUES

Marking for Implant Placement

The cephalic starting point of the implant is determined individually, but implants are usually placed between the double eyelid line and the upper pupillary line[4] (**Fig. 1**).

The face may look longer and older after nasal dorsal augmentation in the long face, so it is necessary to set the starting point of the implant to a caudal position and to lower the implant height.

Implant use is limited to dorsal augmentation. Tip projection should be done with a variety of

The author has no disclosures.
JW Plastic Surgery Center, Seoul, Korea
E-mail address: smankoon@hanmail.net

Facial Plast Surg Clin N Am 29 (2021) 589–609
https://doi.org/10.1016/j.fsc.2021.06.010

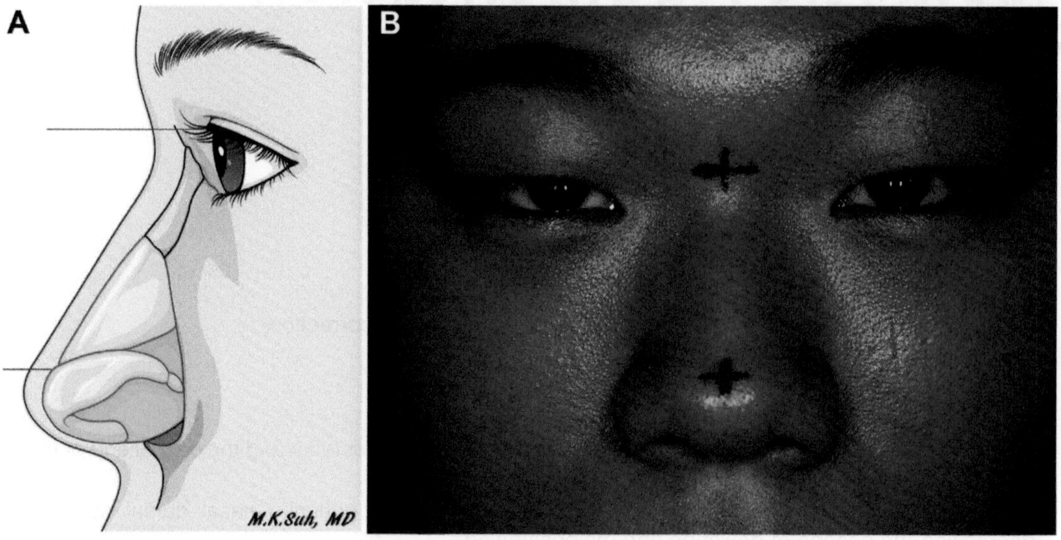

Fig. 1. Cephalic starting and caudal ending points of dorsal implants (*A, B*).

tip plasty techniques, including suture techniques and cartilage grafts. It is safe to use the implant only from the nose to supratip area (**Fig. 2**). Long or L-shaped implants should not be used.

Carving an Implant

The procedure for an implant carving is as follows (**Fig. 3**):

1. Among various types of implants with various heights, widths, and curvatures, the operator chooses the most appropriate implant that fits the dorsal contour and the desired height/shape of the patient.
2. Implant is placed on the nasal dorsum, the cephalic part of the implant being placed on the point marked on the radix, and then the caudal ending point of the implant is marked.
3. The marked distal end of the implant is cut, and then the thick distal end is thinly carved.
4. The bottom of the implant is carved and trimmed to match the contour of the dorsum.

Dissection

A dissection to form a straight and symmetric pocket is the most significant part of dorsal augmentation.

Dissection is performed above the perichondrium in the lower lateral and upper lateral cartilages (supraperichondrial plane) and under the periosteum in the nasal bone area (subperiosteal plane). Implant should be placed under the periosteum to avoid movable implant and to decrease visibility of the implant through the skin. Metzenbaum scissors are used for the dissections over

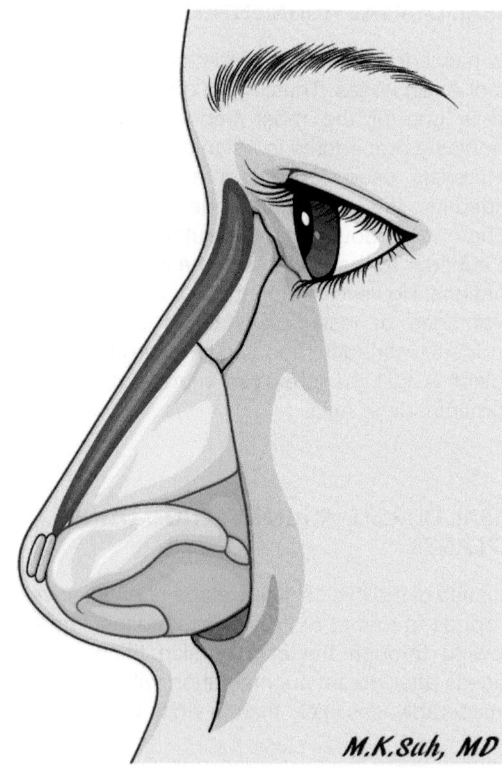

Fig. 2. Dorsal and tip augmentation in Asian rhinoplasty. Short I-shaped implant for dorsal augmentation and cartilage graft for the tip projection. This technique is recommended for augmentation rhinoplasty.

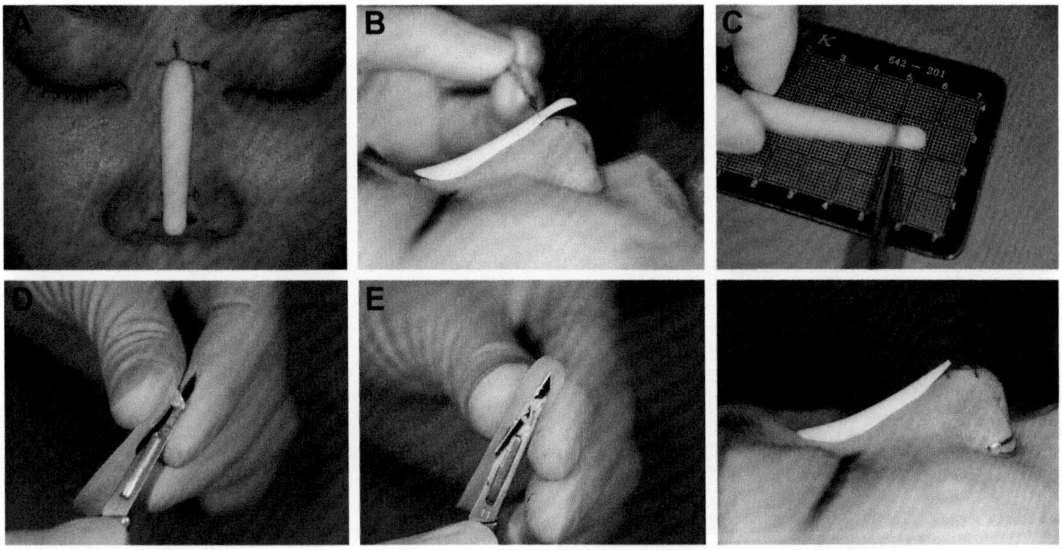

Fig. 3. Silicone implant carving. (*A*) Placing an implant on the nasal dorsum. (*B, C*) Caudal end of the implant is marked and cut. (*D, E*) Thinning of the cephalic tip of implant and carving of the implant undersurface to match the dorsal contour. (*F*) Final shape of the implant.

the lower and upper lateral cartilages. It is important to make sure a maximum amount of the soft tissue is included in the skin envelope (**Fig. 4**).

A Joseph knife is used to make incision on the periosteum transversely about 1 mm above the inferior margin of the nasal bone. Then, a Joseph elevator is used to elevate the periosteum.

Dissection and pocket formation are performed through the bilateral incision to ensure a symmetric pocket. Regarding pocket size, this author recommends a slightly larger pocket size than the width of the implant.

After pocket formation, irrigating the pocket with a povidone-iodine solution mixed with an antibiotic is helpful for the prevention of infection.

Implant Insertion

Implant is placed in the center of the pocket without deviation to one side. There is no need to fix the caudal end of an implant. However, when the operator is not sure of the straight symmetric implant positioning, then suturing the caudal end of implant to the septal angle may be helpful.

Fig. 5 shows an example of dorsal augmentation using implants in a male patient.

AUGMENTATION RHINOPLASTY WITH THREE-DIMENSIONAL PRINTING TECHNOLOGY

Recently, three-dimensional (3D) printing technology has gained traction in the medical fields. With the rapid growth of 3D printing technology, the paradigm shifted to patient-specific treatment, giving surgeons the opportunity to plan and apply more precise and visible surgery by designing patient-specific medical devices.[5]

Before 3D printing technology, surgeons had to create the shape of the implant they wanted to use, and they had to further process (carve) the ready-made products to suit the patient's nasal dorsum at the intraoperation step.

However, 3D printing technology allows surgeons to produce the implant desired by the surgeon at the preoperation step, without the need for carving at the operation step. Implant contour reflecting the asymmetry and irregularity of the nasal bone and upper lateral cartilages can be produced through this technique. It can also reflect the other surgical plans, such as osteotomy, cartilage graft, and lower lateral cartilage realignment (**Fig. 6**). Patients can participate in the determination of the desired height and profile line before surgery through the simulation program.

Design and Manufacturing Process

Patient-specific nasal implants for augmentation rhinoplasty are manufactured in the following 5 steps (**Fig. 7**):

1. Medical images of the nose are acquired through computed tomography or MRI.
   a. It must be possible to obtain 3D information of human tissue from medical images.
2. Segment a specific part from the medical image and infer the side where the implant is inserted.

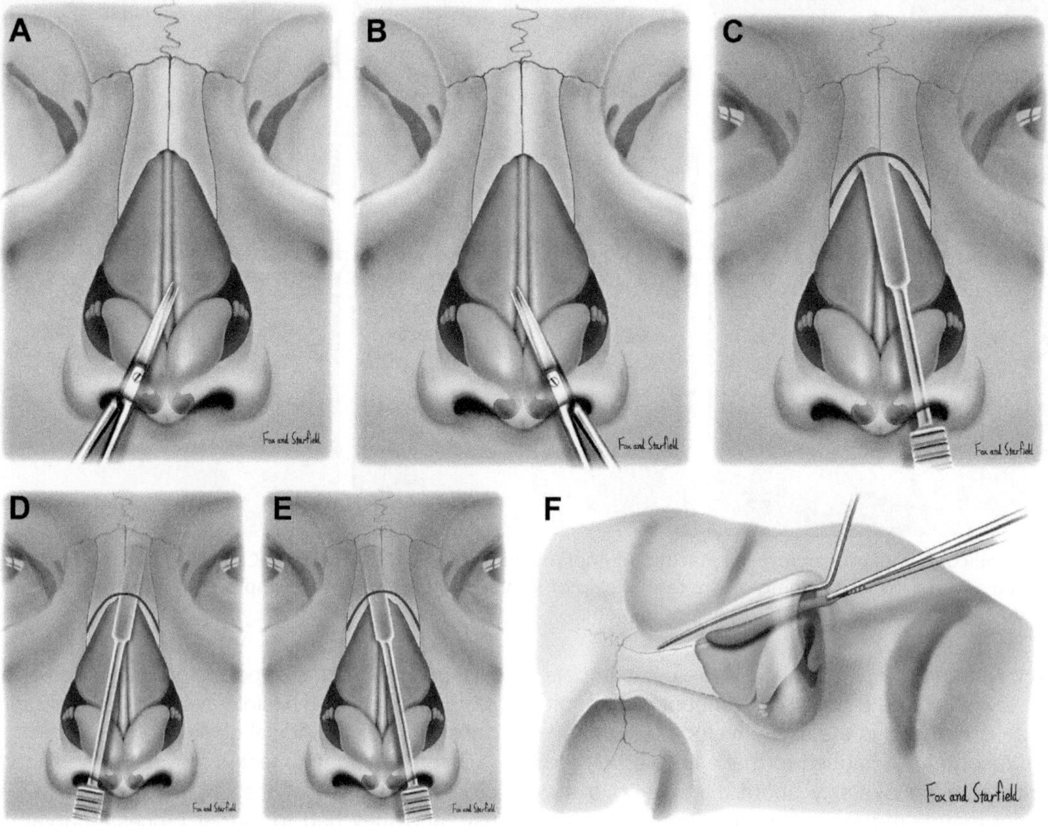

Fig. 4. Dissection and pocket formation. (*A, B*) Dissection over the upper lateral cartilages. (*C–E*) Periosteal elevation. (*F*) Implant insertion.

   a. Divide the skin, the bone in the region (including the nasal bone and the orbital bone), and the nasal cavity.
   b. It can be segmented using snake algorithm and U-net deep learning algorithm.
   c. Because most medical images are not of adequate quality to segment nasal cartilages, they are inferred through medical statistical analysis and deep learning.
3. Computation of the implant volume required for predicted outcome after surgery.
   a. Predicted outcome after surgery usually refers to two-dimensional information in which the outline of the expected shape is drawn on a picture taken from the side or the back.
   b. Using virtual plastic surgery technology, 3D information on the predicted outcome can be obtained, which means more accurate information on the predicted outcome.
4. Design an implant that reflects the surgical plan and the doctor's request form.
   a. For example, when glabellar-radix augmentation is required, a long implant capable of glabellar augmentation can be designed.
   b. The width or angle of nasofrontal slope of the implant can be designed as desired by the doctor.
5. The implant is fabricated using a 3D printer.

Three-way communication between patient, doctor, and manufacturer is required in patient-specific nasal implant fabrication.

1. In cosmetic surgery, it is important to express what the patient wants.
2. The manufacture of patient-specific nasal implants is the result of both the patient's desire and the doctor's surgical plan (**Table 1**).

Fig. 8 shows preoperative and postoperative results of nasal dorsal augmentation using 3D printed nasal implant.

Advantages and Disadvantages of Three-dimensional Printed Nasal Implant

Advantages of 3D printed patient-specific nasal implant are as follows: first, implants that exactly fit the patient's nasal dorsal contour can be manufactured (**Fig. 9**). The implant is manufactured to

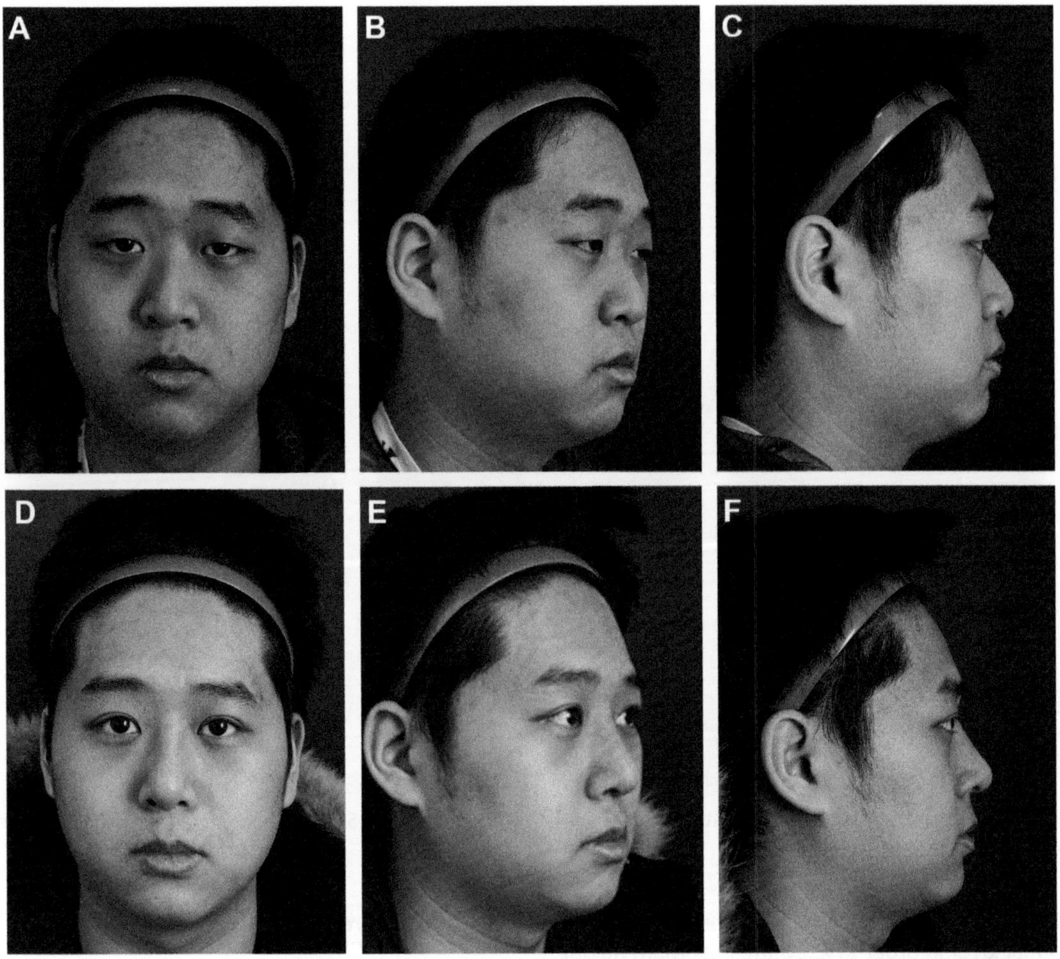

Fig. 5. Dorsal augmentation using silicone implant (6.0 mm in height) and tip projection using columellar strut graft with septal cartilage and septal cartilage onlay graft. (*A–C*) Before operation, (*D–F*) after operation.

match the contour irregularity of nasal bone and upper lateral cartilages, and also reflects the nasal dorsal asymmetry. Therefore, implant carving is unnecessary or significantly reduced compared with ready-made implants. In the intraoperation process, the time and effort required to carve an implant can be significantly reduced.

Because the shape of the implant is consistent with the patient's nasal dorsal irregular contour and asymmetry, it is expected that the possibility of implant deviation and migration can be reduced. Because the dead space between the implant and the underlying nasal framework is minimized, it is speculated that the chance of thick formation of posterior capsule and resulting capsule contracture is also minimized.

Second, patients can participate in simulation surgery and making the desired implant through a virtual plastic surgery application.

Nevertheless, the disadvantage of this technique is that it takes several days for the implant to be manufactured before surgery.

NASAL DORSAL AUGMENTATION USING AUTOGENOUS TISSUES

Autogenous tissues are appropriate for dorsal augmentation in patients with extremely thin dorsal skin, and in secondary operation for implant-related complication, such as dorsal skin redness and thinning, or capsular contracture.

DORSAL AUGMENTATION WITH VERTICALLY ORIENTED FOLDED DERMAL GRAFT

Resorption of generally performed dermofat graft occurs in both the dermal layer and the fat layer, but more resorption takes place in the fat layer. Therefore, it is important to minimize the thickness

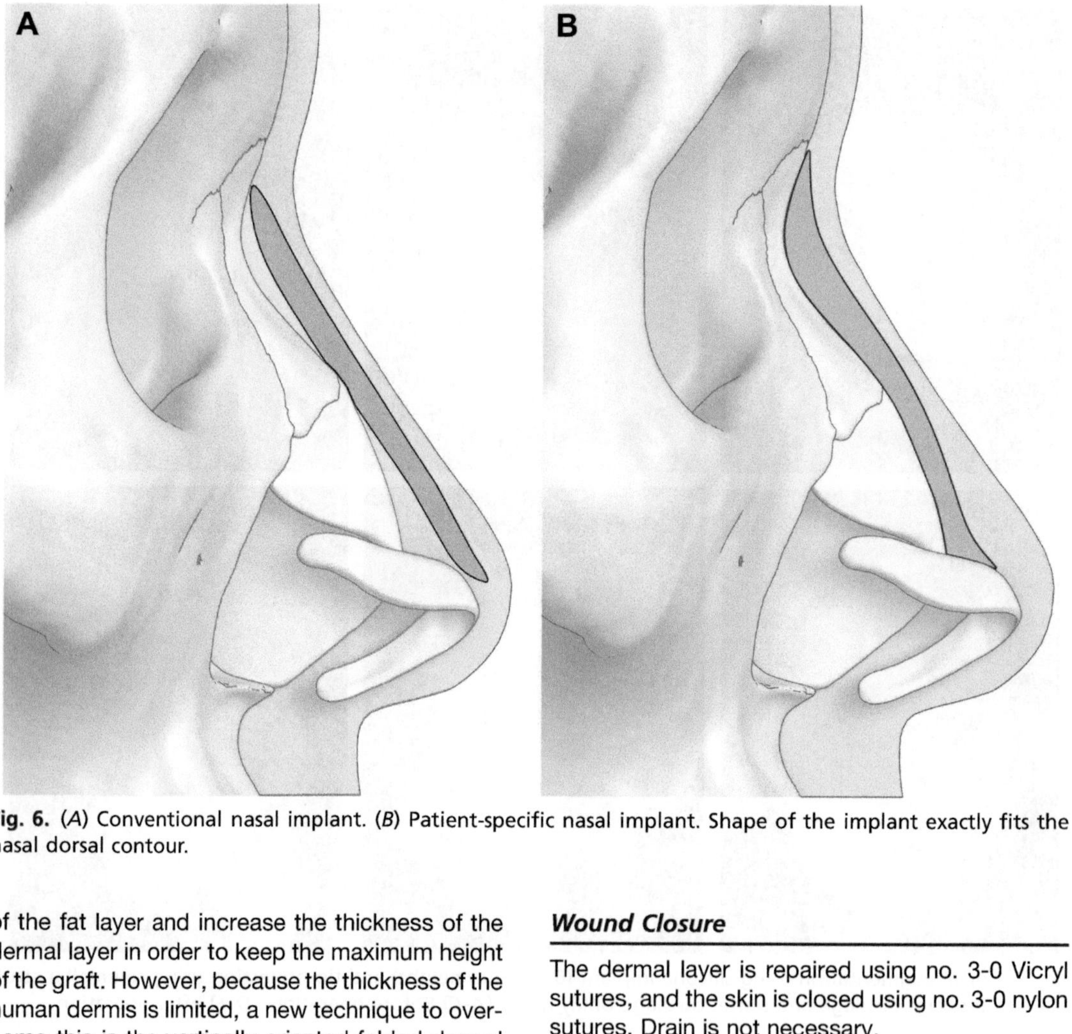

Fig. 6. (*A*) Conventional nasal implant. (*B*) Patient-specific nasal implant. Shape of the implant exactly fits the nasal dorsal contour.

of the fat layer and increase the thickness of the dermal layer in order to keep the maximum height of the graft. However, because the thickness of the human dermis is limited, a new technique to overcome this is the vertically oriented folded dermal graft technique.

This technique contains minimal fat in the graft, and is mainly a technique of dorsal augmentation using dermal components.[6]

Graft Design

As shown in **Fig. 10**, the graft is designed on the sacrococcygeal area. The caudal margin of graft is located 2 cm superior to the coccyx. The cephalic portion of the graft needs to be wider for greater augmentation of the radix area.

Harvest of the Graft

As shown in **Fig. 10**, harvest of the graft begins with half-thickness incision through dermis followed by deepithelization. Thereafter, full-thickness dermal incision is performed. The graft is elevated and a minimal amount of the fat is incorporated into the graft.

Wound Closure

The dermal layer is repaired using no. 3-0 Vicryl sutures, and the skin is closed using no. 3-0 nylon sutures. Drain is not necessary.

Fabrication of the Harvested Graft

The graft fabrication is a procedure to fold and compact the graft horizontally, and to erect the graft vertically by multiple sutures to the graft, such that it becomes more compact horizontally and provides maximal height.

The harvested dermal graft is fixated to a thick paper plate with a pin on each end (**Fig. 11**). A straight line is drawn along the central axis of the graft. The graft is folded along the central line by placing 5 6-0 nylon sutures through the offset lines. The folded edges are brought together using 5-0 nylon sutures. Then, the graft is made more compact by multiple outer vertical or horizontal sutures (5-0 nylon). If bulging of the graft's base occurs because of these sutures, the base should be trimmed to make it flat. Next, the outer circular sutures are placed using 5-0 nylon. At this point, the graft should stand vertically on its base, as shown

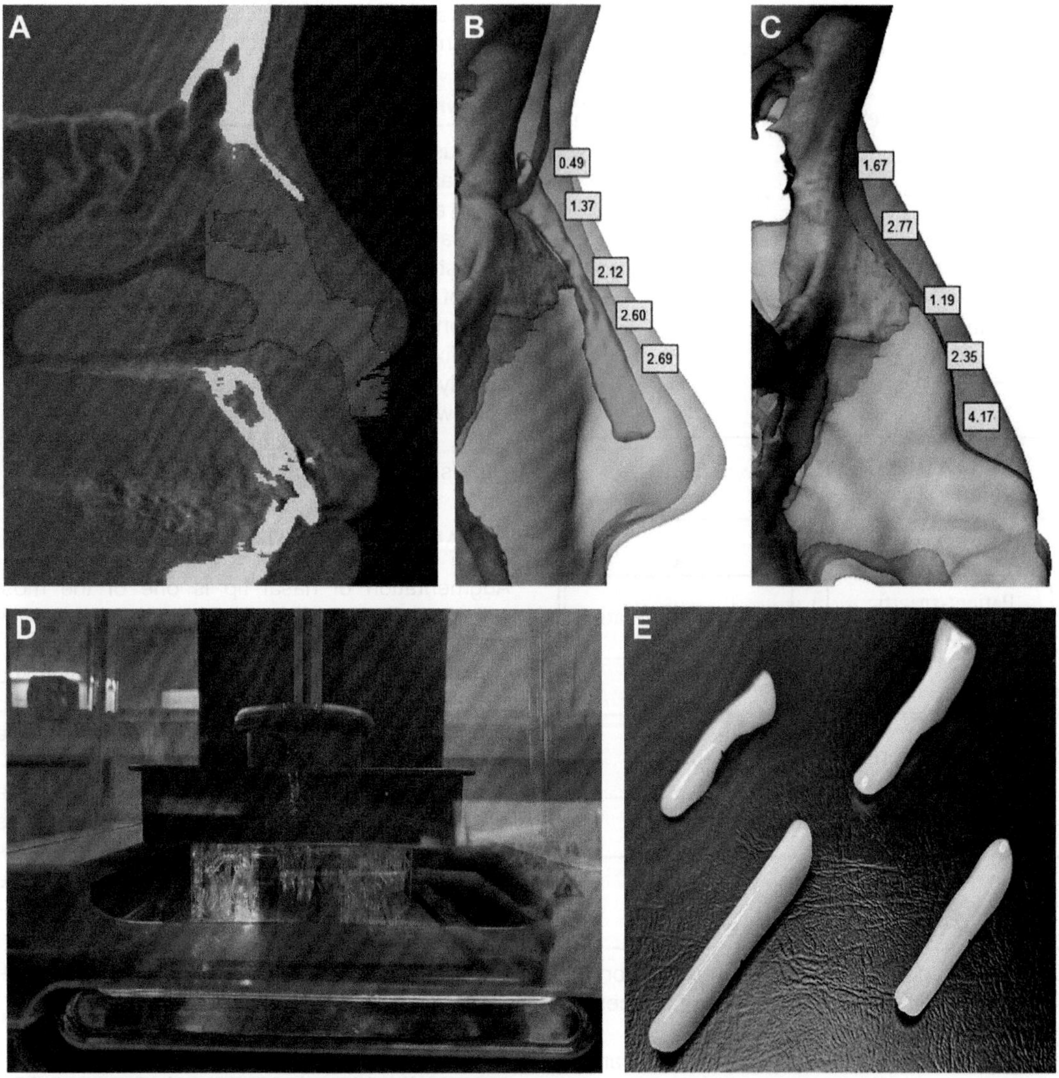

Fig. 7. Manufacturing process of patient-specific nasal implant. (*A*) Segmentation of specific area. (*B*) Computation volume change. (*C*) Implant design. (*D, E*) Implant fabrication.

in **Fig. 11**F. The vertically oriented folded dermal graft augments the dorsal height not by the thickness but by the folded height of the graft. This concept is totally different from conventional dermofat graft. Because of this, the graft base should be flat enough not to fall to the side when placed on the dorsum.

The final height of the fabricated graft is around 10 to 12 mm.

Placing the Graft on the Dorsum

The cephalic end of the graft is fixated using a pull-out suture. The caudal end is fixed to the septal angle or to the dome of lower lateral cartilages.

Although the resorption rate of horizontally oriented folded dermal graft is known to be 40% after 1 year,[7] the resorption rate for the vertically oriented folded dermal graft has not been reported yet (**Fig. 12**).

DORSAL AUGMENTATION WITH SOLID COSTAL CARTILAGE

Costal cartilage is the choice of autogenous material for major dorsal augmentation because it is abundant in graft volume and has a very low absorption rate compared with dermofat graft.

Cartilage approximately 5 to 6 cm long is required for dorsal augmentation. Sixth and seventh costal cartilage is preferred for this purpose.[8]

Table 1
Flow chart of patient-specific rhinoplasty

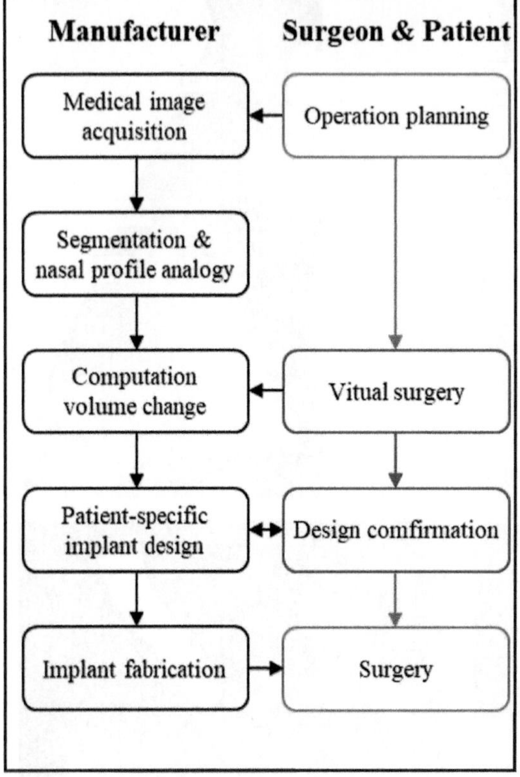

Carving of the Costal Cartilage

Costal cartilage carving is the most important, difficult, and time-consuming step of successful dorsal augmentation.

The typical solid block costal cartilage carving technique is performed according to the balanced intrinsic stress by using the core portion of the cartilage (**Fig. 13**). Graft must be accurately carved to fit the radix and dorsal contours. A carved costal cartilage will have undergone the maximum amount of warping after an hour. The carved graft should therefore be placed in a saline solution for an hour, after which the graft is further trimmed before insertion.

Multilayered costal cartilage graft technique

Multilayered costal cartilage graft technique,[9] developed to minimize graft warping, can be an effective alternative technique to solid costal cartilage graft for dorsal augmentation.

The harvested costal cartilage is sliced into thin pieces and soaked in a saline-filled container for at least 30 minutes to allow sufficient warping. Using a 5-0 polydioxanone (PDS) suture, a few slices of cartilage are stacked to the desired height. Stacked multi-layer cartilage blocks are trimmed into shape with a 15-blade scalpel (**Fig. 14**).

Placement of the Graft

Because the solid costal cartilage graft is slippery, it is easy to deviate after it is placed on the nasal bone and upper lateral cartilage. To avoid this, there are a few key points to keep in mind: the subperiosteal pocket should not be wide. The caudal part of the graft is fixed to the cephalic and caudal portion of the upper lateral cartilage. Kirschner-wire fixation through the graft at the radix is not usually required, but can be used in some situations when graft deviation cannot be avoided.

Fig. 15 shows an example of dorsal augmentation using a solid block costal cartilage graft.

NASAL TIP AUGMENTATION

Augmentation of nasal tip is one of the most commonly performed tip plasty in Asian noses with low and short nasal tips.

Asian nasal tips are characterized by small and weak lower lateral cartilages, which makes tip augmentation of Asians difficult. Moreover, the nasal tip is not a static part but a dynamic and mobile structure. Ideally, a nasal tip should be mobile and have sufficient tip projection. However, this is not always possible. The more tip projection is performed, the more rigid tip is obtained, and the emphasis on the mobile tip may result in insufficient projection or drooping in the long term. It is rhinoplasty surgeons' job to strive to make the nasal tip movable and sufficiently projected.

Correction of Low Tip

Tip projection in Asian noses is accomplished through 1 or a combination of the following surgical techniques (**Fig. 16**):

1. Cartilage onlay/shield graft on the dome of lower lateral cartilages
2. Medialization of lateral crura (lateral crural steal)[10]
3. Suspension of lower lateral cartilages: columellar strut graft, septal extension graft

TIP ONLAY/SHIELD GRAFT

Cartilage onlay/shield graft is the most commonly performed and the preferred tip projection technique in Asians. Auricular cartilage is the preferred donor source, although septal cartilage can also be used. Both cavum concha and cymba concha can be used, but, for simple onlay/shield graft, cavum concha with thicker cartilage is preferred.

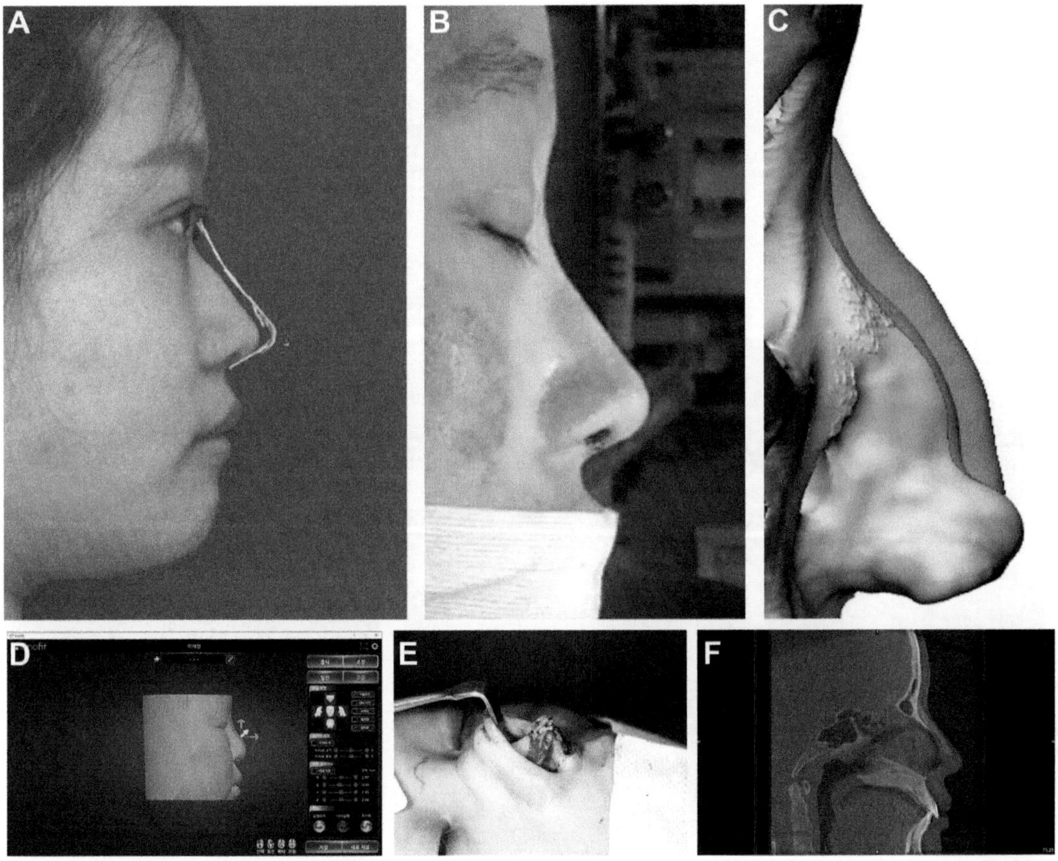

Fig. 8. Applied case of patient-specific nasal implant (INNOFIT, Anymedi Inc, Seoul, Korea). (*A*) Before operation. The line drawn with a pencil is the height and line the patient wants. (*B*) After operation. (*C*) 3D model of patient-specific implant and nasal profile. (*D*) Virtual surgery with the simulation program (Anymedi Inc). (*E*) After tip plasty, the 3D implant (INNOFIT) is placed on the dorsum and fits the nasal contour perfectly. (*F*) On computed tomography, the implant is precisely matched to the nasal dorsal contour.

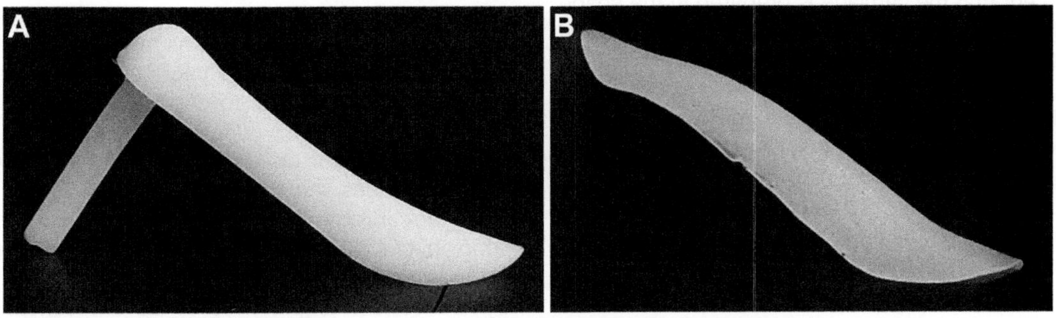

Fig. 9. (*A*) Conventional ready-made implant and (*B*) patient-specific 3D printed implant (INNOFIT).

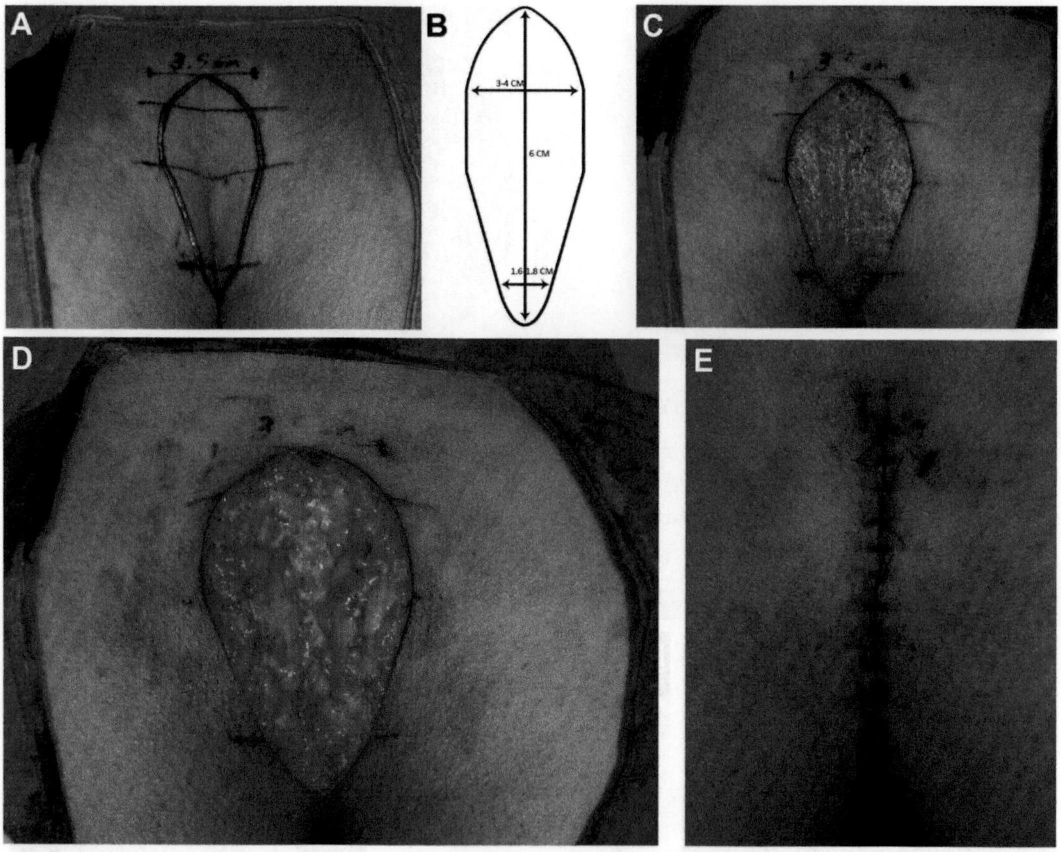

Fig. 10. Design and harvest of the vertically oriented folded dermal graft. (*A*) The graft is located at the midline of the sacrococcygeal area, and the caudal margin of the graft is located 2 cm above the coccyx. The length of the graft is 6 cm, whereas the width of the cephalic area is ~3 to 4 cm and that of the caudal area is ~1.6 to 1.8 cm. (*B*) Half-thickness incision into dermal layer. (*C*) The epidermis has been peeled off from the dermal layer. (*D*) A full-thickness dermal incision is made and dermal layer has been harvested. (*E*) Skin closure.

To avoid visibility of the graft through the tip skin, graft margin should be tapered thin to have a beveled edge or slightly crushed using cartilage crusher, and the graft should be fixed to the underlying dome meticulously.

Shield graft can advance the infratip lobule caudally as well as projecting the tip. The operative technique is the same as the onlay graft technique, except that the cartilage is prepared in the shape of a shield and that it is located from the caudal part of dome to the middle crura.

Although the cartilage onlay/shield graft is a simple and very effective surgical method for tip projection in firm and stable lower lateral cartilages, if this is performed on lower lateral cartilages with weak and short medial crura, tip drooping may occur with time as the medial crura is compressed or twisted[11] (**Fig. 17**). Short and retruded columella is a sign of weak and unstable medial crura.

Considering these 2 points, it is required to perform columellar strut graft and cartilage onlay graft together to form stable tip projection and a harmonious infratip lobule ratio in most Asians with weak medial crura.

COLUMELLAR STRUT GRAFT

The mechanisms by which this graft can increase the nasal tip can be explained as follows:

First, it straightens twisted medial crura, which is congenital or secondary to cartilage onlay graft (**Fig. 18**).

Secondly, it lifts up and suspends the lower lateral cartilages anteriorly.

Septal cartilage is most commonly used as a donor but, if the septal cartilage is too small or not available, auricular cartilage can be used. Cymba concha is preferred to cavum concha, and, because cartilage has curvature, cartilage is

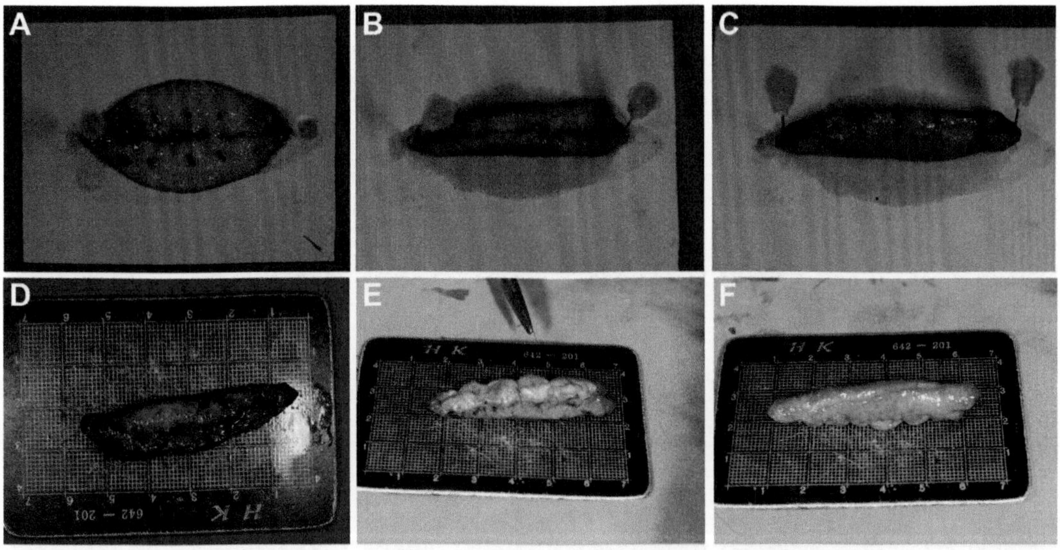

Fig. 11. Fabrication of a graft. (*A*) Marking for 5 inner sutures. (*B*) To fold the graft, 5 inner sutures were placed using a no. 6-0 nylon suture. (*C*) Four base sutures were placed using a no. 5-0 nylon suture. (*D*) After multiple outer horizontal sutures using a no. 5-0 nylon suture, the bulging graft base was trimmed. (*E*) The outer circular sutures were placed. (*F*) The graft is erected in a vertical orientation after all the sutures have been placed.

folded along the midline and sutured to itself to make a straight graft (**Fig. 19**).

Because the length of the graft is not usually enough for the fixed type to reach the anterior nasal spine, the columellar strut graft is performed as a floating type. Pockets between medial crura for floating type should not be too deep. By preserving the soft tissue between the posterior end of the graft and the anterior nasal spine (ANS), the spring effect of the soft tissue to the graft must be preserved (**Fig. 20**). While graft is being gently pushed posteriorly, the domes are pulled anteriorly. Then, 3 fixation sutures are applied using no. 5-0 PDS.

Additional tip projection can be achieved by medialization of lateral crura. Medialization of lateral crura (lateral crural steal) is the conversion of the lateral crura into the middle crura with suture techniques to increase the tip height.

When the tip projection is performed by columellar strut graft, tip is rotated cephalically. Measures to prevent this unwanted rotation include spanning suture of lateral crura, derotation suture (tip extension suture),[12] or derotation graft.[13,14]

CORRECTION OF SHORT NOSE

Short nose with upturned nasal tip and visible nostrils requires 1 of 2 surgical methods: septal extension graft and derotation graft.

SEPTAL EXTENSION GRAFT

Septal extension graft[15] is the most commonly performed procedure for low tip and short nose correction in Asian countries. The first and the most important step of this technique is the repositioning of the lower lateral cartilages caudally. For caudal repositioning, lower lateral cartilage should be released from surrounding structures.

Release of Lower Lateral Cartilages

The lower lateral cartilages are released from the scroll area and hinge complex. The scroll area is the connection between the upper and lower lateral cartilages. Release of the scroll area is the most important step in the release of lower lateral cartilages. The fibrous connective tissue between 2 cartilages is sufficiently released, leaving mucosa intact (**Fig. 21**). The hinge complex should also be sufficiently dissected and released, cutting accessory ligament in some cases.

Release of the Skin and Soft Tissue Envelope

The second key factor for successful short nose correction is sufficient stretching of skin and soft tissue envelope. The skin and soft tissue are released through wide dissection. The extent of skin/soft tissue dissection varies depending on how short the nose is and how tense the skin is. For a very short nose with tight skin, the dissection

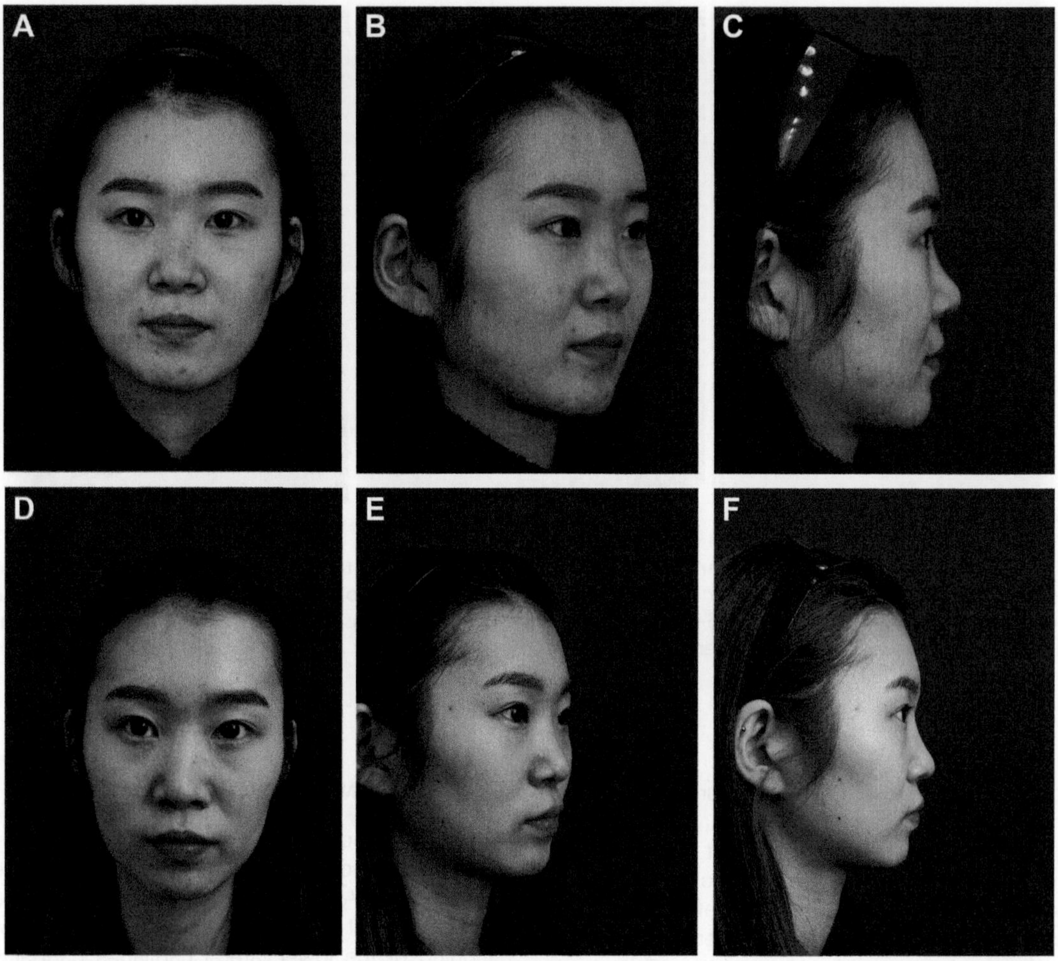

Fig. 12. Patient with a vertically oriented folded dermal graft for dorsal augmentation. (*A–C*) Preoperative views. (*D–F*) One year after dorsal augmentation surgery using a vertically oriented folded dermal graft and tip plasty with a derotation suture and conchal cartilage shield graft.

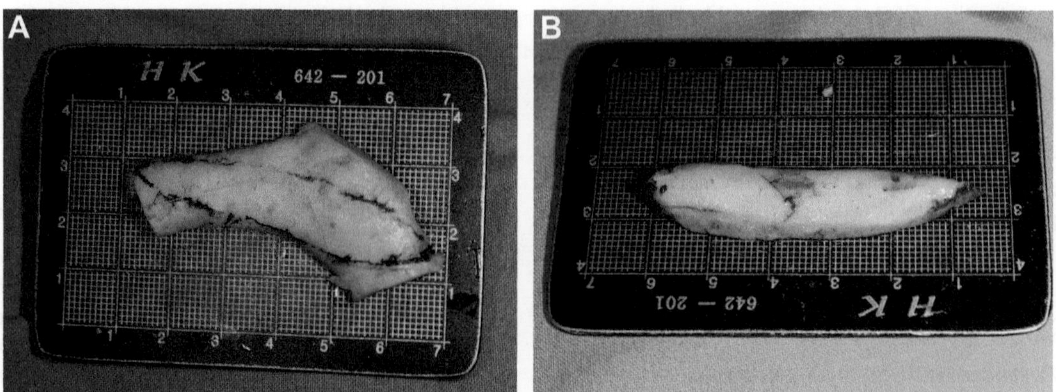

Fig. 13. Concentric carving of the costal cartilage to minimize the graft warping (*A, B*).

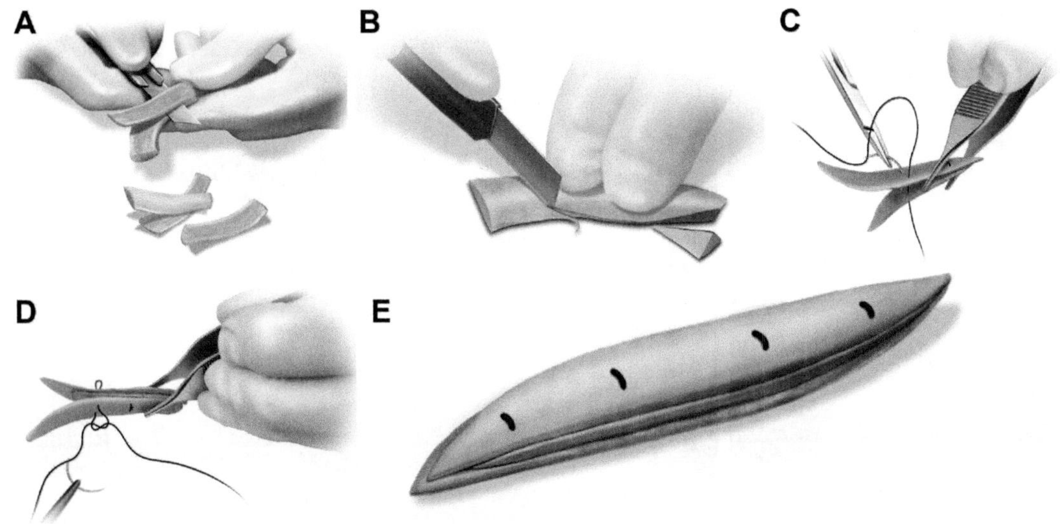

Fig. 14. Multilayered costal cartilage graft technique. (*A*) Harvested costal cartilage is sliced into thin pieces. (*B*) Top layer piece is being carved. (*C*) Two pieces of thinly sliced cartilage are gathered by absorbable sutures. (*D*) Several pieces of thinly sliced cartilage are stacked according to the desired height. (*E*) Final shape without warping.

should be beyond the pyriform aperture, reaching the medial maxilla.

Fixation of Caudally Repositioned Lower Lateral Cartilages to the Graft

The batten type of septal extension graft is technically less demanding for novice operators, with more stable outcomes. The most common donor site for septal extension graft is the septum. After firm fixation of the graft to the septal angle and caudal septum, released lower lateral cartilages are pulled caudally and fixed to the graft. Medial crura of lower lateral cartilages are fixed to the caudal portion of the graft, whereas dome is fixed to the anterior caudal end of the graft. To avoid extrusion of the graft end between domes, the lower lateral cartilages are fixed such that the domes are wrapped around the anterior caudal end of the graft using an interdomal suture (**Fig. 22**).

Pros and Cons of Septal Extension Graft

Septal extension graft enables robust projection and caudal rotation of the nasal tip. Also, this technique allows caudal projection of columella in patients with retruded columella (**Fig. 23**).

However, rigid nasal tip is a major disadvantage of this technique, and can induce the appearance of so-called witch tip when smiling. Unilateral batten-type septal extension graft can be the cause of gradual deviation of remnant septal L-strut, resulting in deviation of tip/columella and nostril asymmetry (**Fig. 24**). To avoid this common problem in Asian noses with weak and thin septal cartilage, the operator must perform an additional batten graft to the opposite side of the septal extension (**Fig. 25**).

DEROTATION GRAFT

Derotation graft[13,14] using auricular cartilage is placed between the fixed structure (dorsal septum) and caudally repositioned lower lateral cartilages (**Fig. 26**).

The procedures for the release of lower lateral cartilages and skin envelope are same as in septal extension graft, as described earlier.

Cymba concha is preferred for this graft because it is longer than cavum concha. Harvested cymba concha is divided into 2 pieces (**Fig. 27**). The pieces are used as a columellar strut graft and a derotation graft.

Preparation of the Harvested Cartilage

The upper piece of divided cymba conchal cartilage is folded along the midline and made into a straight strut through several sutures. The lower piece of harvested cartilage is used as the derotation graft.

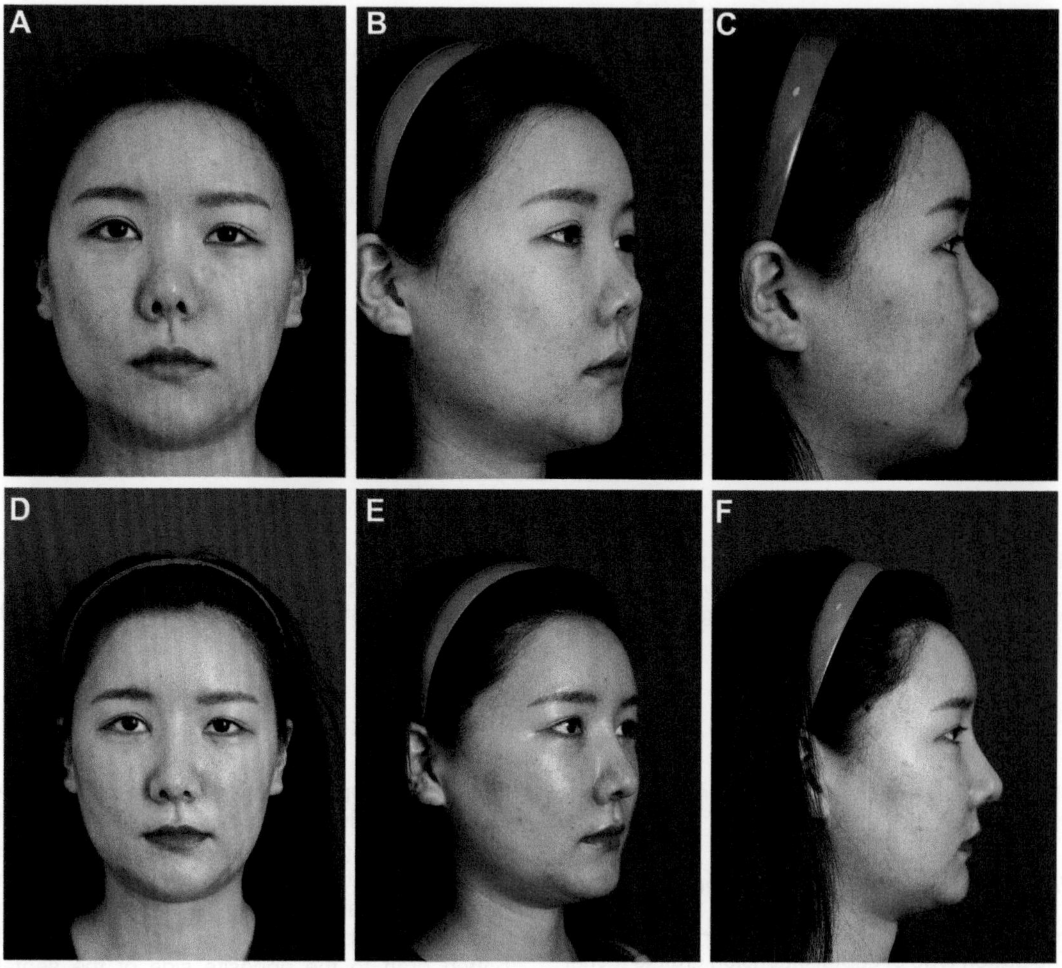

Fig. 15. Dorsal augmentation with a solid block costal cartilage. (*A–C*) Preoperative views. (*D–F*) Five months after lateral osteotomy, dorsal augmentation using block costal cartilage graft, and tip revision and columella projection with septal extension graft using costal cartilage, and rib cartilage extended shield graft.

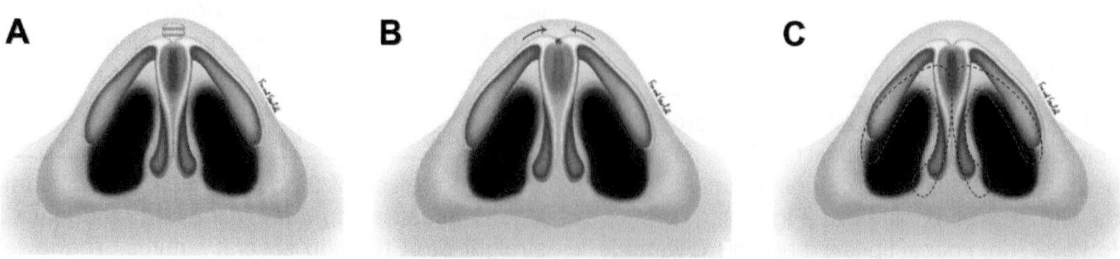

Fig. 16. Surgical techniques for the tip projection. (*A*) Cartilage onlay/shield graft. (*B*) Lengthening of medial crura by medialization of lateral crura (*arrows*). (*C*) Anterior suspension of lower lateral cartilages (*dotted lines*).

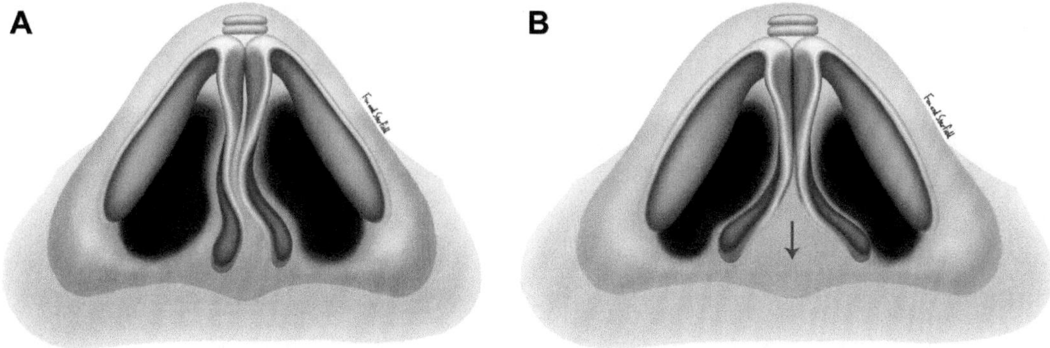

Fig. 17. Weak medial crura is often a cause for tip projection failure following cartilage onlay graft as the medial crura is twisted (A) or compressed (arrow of B).

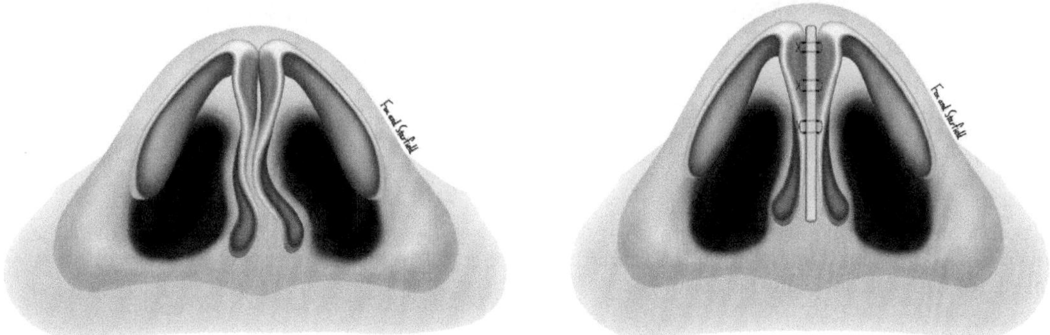

Fig. 18. Straightening twisted medial crura with columellar strut graft.

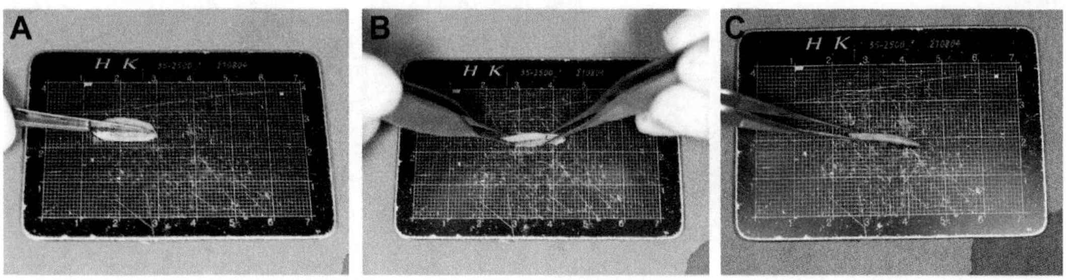

Fig. 19. Cymba conchal cartilage for columella strut graft. (*A*) The cartilage is cut half-thickness along the midline of concave side to allow for folding. (*B, C*) The cartilage is folded lengthwise and straightened with several sutures.

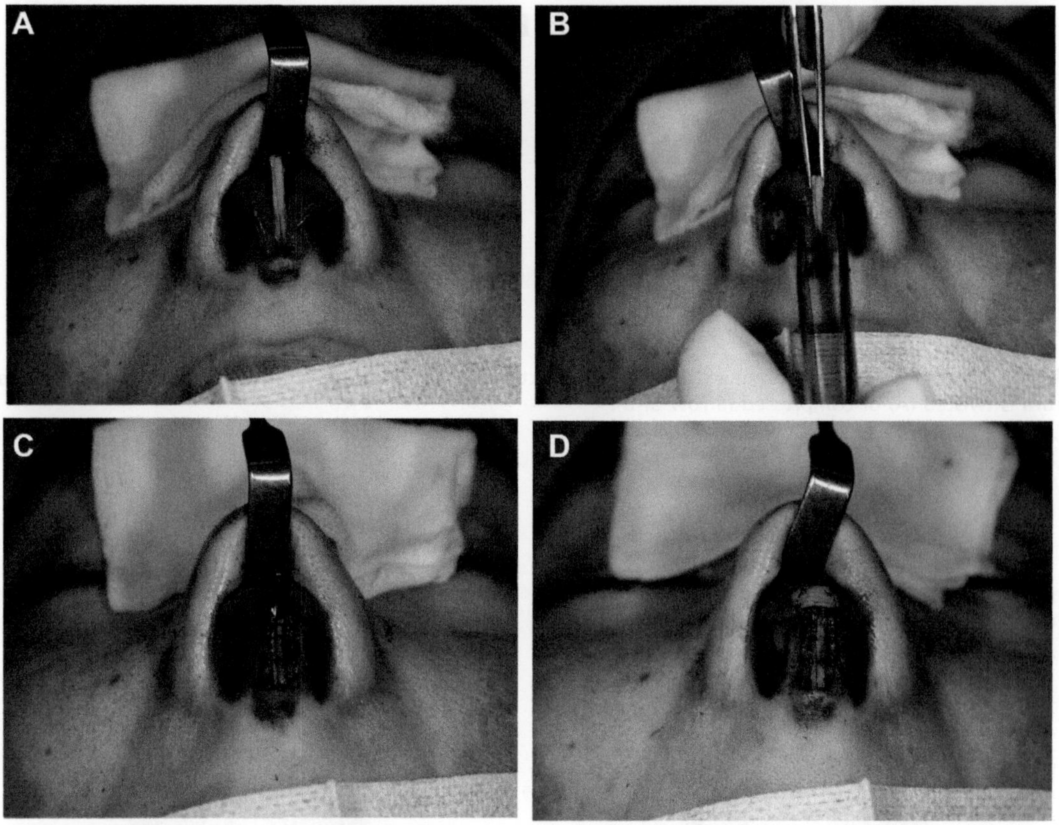

Fig. 20. Floating-type columellar strut graft. (*A*) Graft is placed between medial crura. (*B*) Graft being gently pushed posteriorly; the domes are pulled upward. (*C*) Intercrural fixation sutures and interdomal suture are applied. (*D*) Cartilage onlay graft is performed.

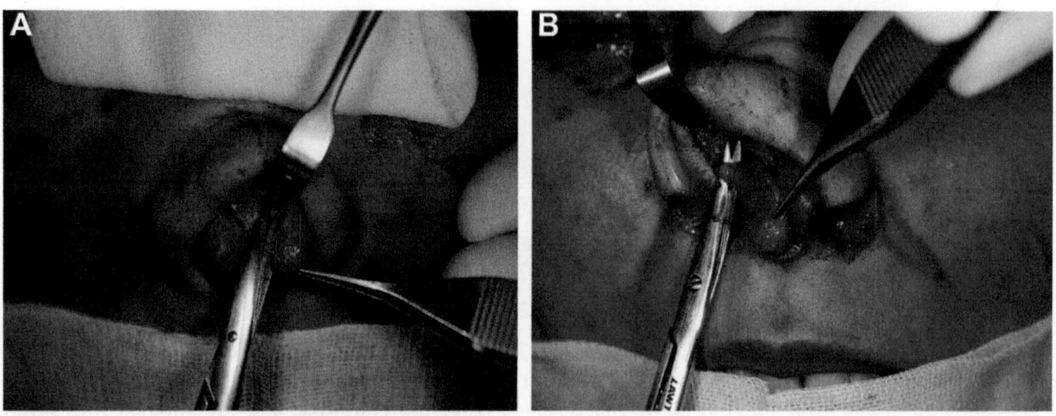

Fig. 21. Release of scroll area (*A*) and hinge complex (*B*).

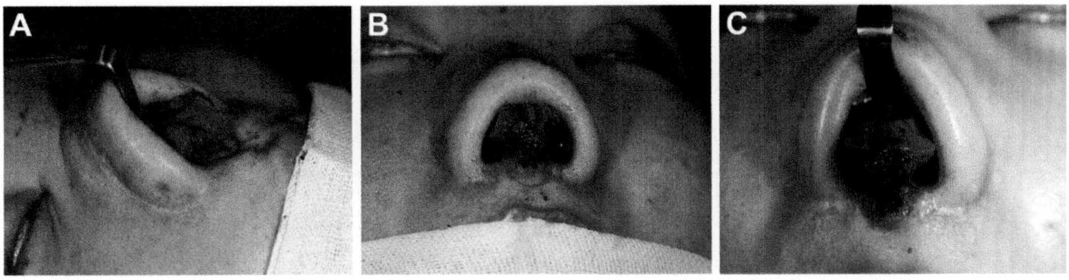

Fig. 22. Wrap-around fixation technique. The medial crura and domes wrap around the graft (*A, B*) end and are fixated using intercrural suture and interdomal suture (*C*).

Columellar Strut Graft and Derotation Graft

As shown in **Fig. 28**, after performing columellar strut graft, the lower lateral cartilages are pulled caudally with traction suture. The cephalic portion of the derotation graft is placed on the dorsal septum and upper lateral cartilages, and fixated with 5-0 PDS suture. The first suture is passed through the paramedian portion of the most cephalic portion of the graft, through the dorsal septum, passed back through the opposite paramedian portion of the graft, and tied in the midline. The subsequent 2 to 3 sutures are placed serially in the caudal direction. After the cephalic portion of the graft is sutured, the caudal portion of the graft is sutured to the underlying cephalic portion of lateral crura of the lower lateral cartilages.

The most important advantage of the derotation graft is that it allows supple and movable nasal tip while enabling enough tip lengthening (**Fig. 29**).

SUMMARY

Because of the thick skin envelope of Asian noses, implants can be safely used for nasal dorsal augmentation.

Implants for dorsal augmentation should be placed under the periosteum and the caudal end of the implant should be placed at the supratip area.

three-dimensional printed nasal implants can exactly fit the patients' nasal dorsal contours, decreasing the chance of deviation and malpositioning.

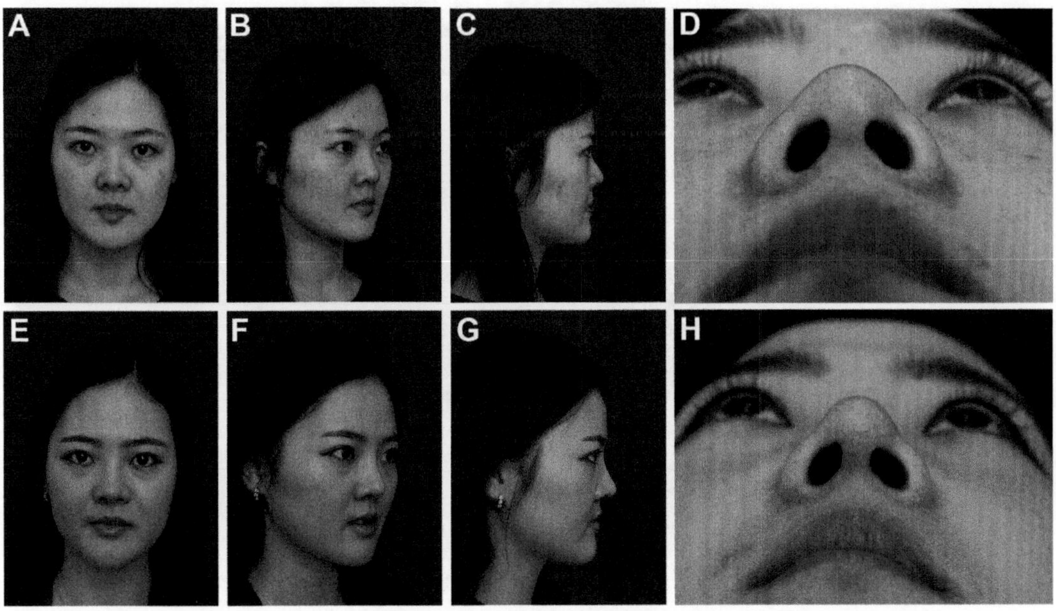

Fig. 23. Short nose correction with septal extension graft. (*A–D*) Before operation. (*E–H*) Six months after dorsal augmentation with silicone implant and tip plasty with septal extension graft using septal cartilage and septal cartilage onlay graft on tip.

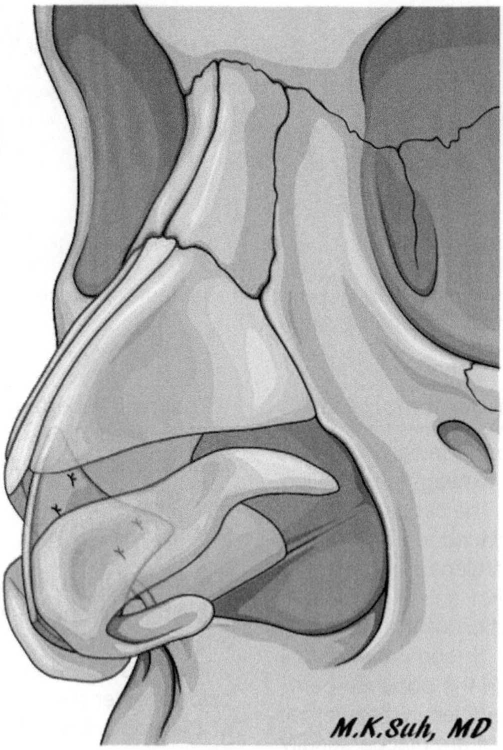

Fig. 24. Deviation of remnant septal L-strut and septal extension graft.

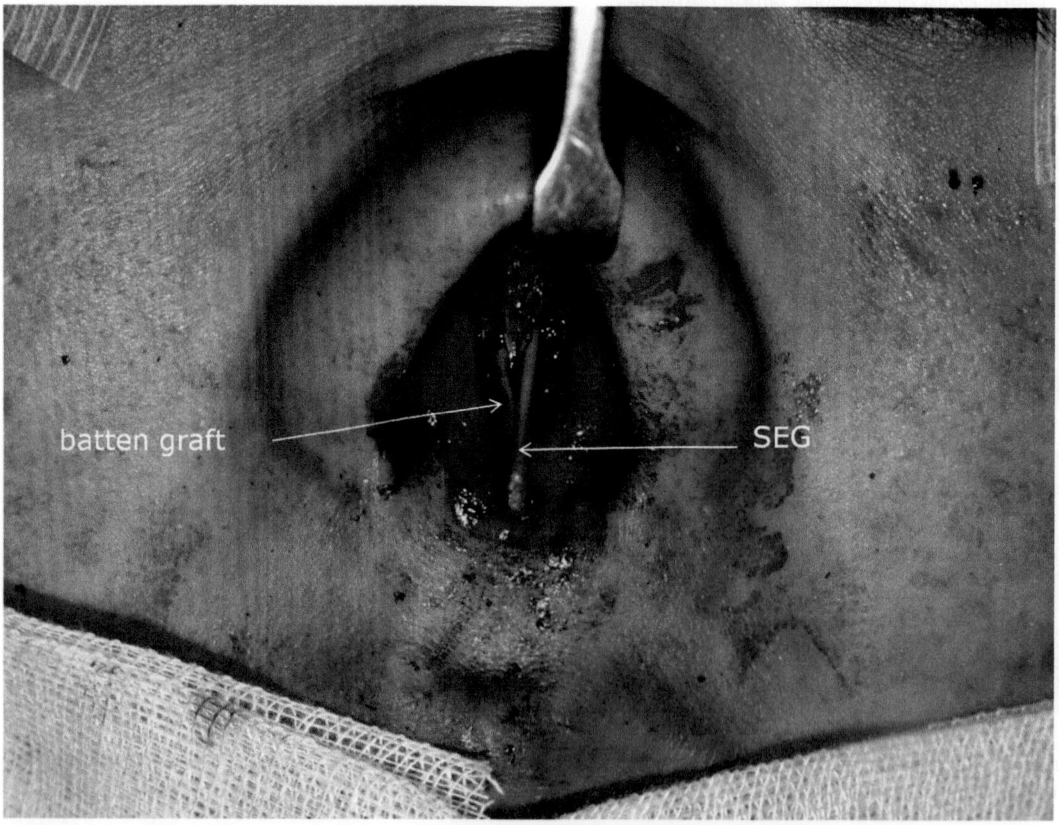

Fig. 25. Small batten graft is applied to opposite side of septal extension graft (SEG).

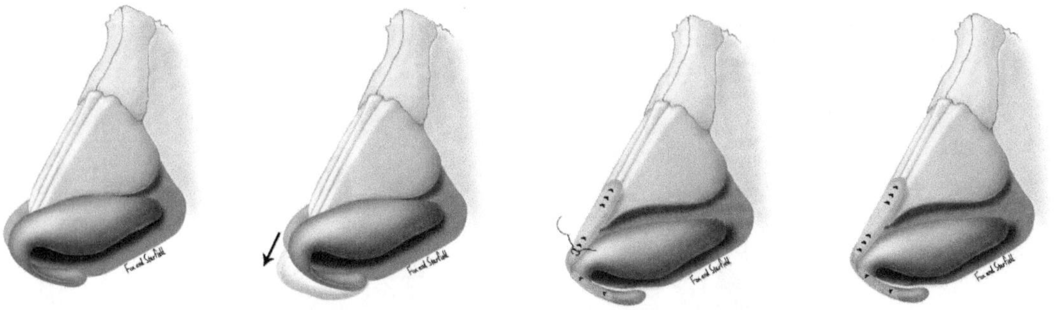

Fig. 26. Derotation graft and columellar strut graft using the conchal cartilage. Lower lateral cartilages are pulled caudally (arrow) and fixated with derotation graft.

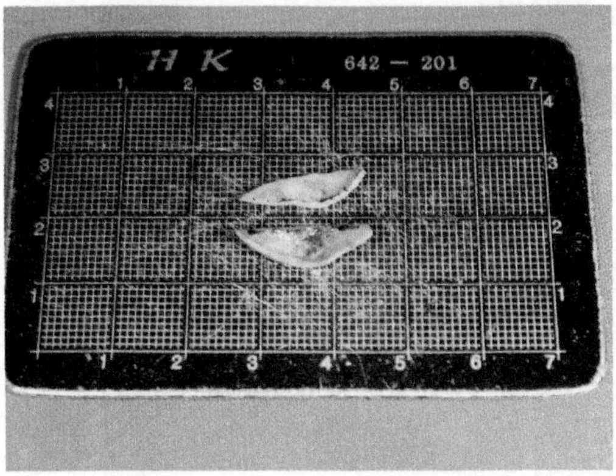

Fig. 27. Harvested cymba concha is divided into 2 pieces for derotation graft and columellar strut graft.

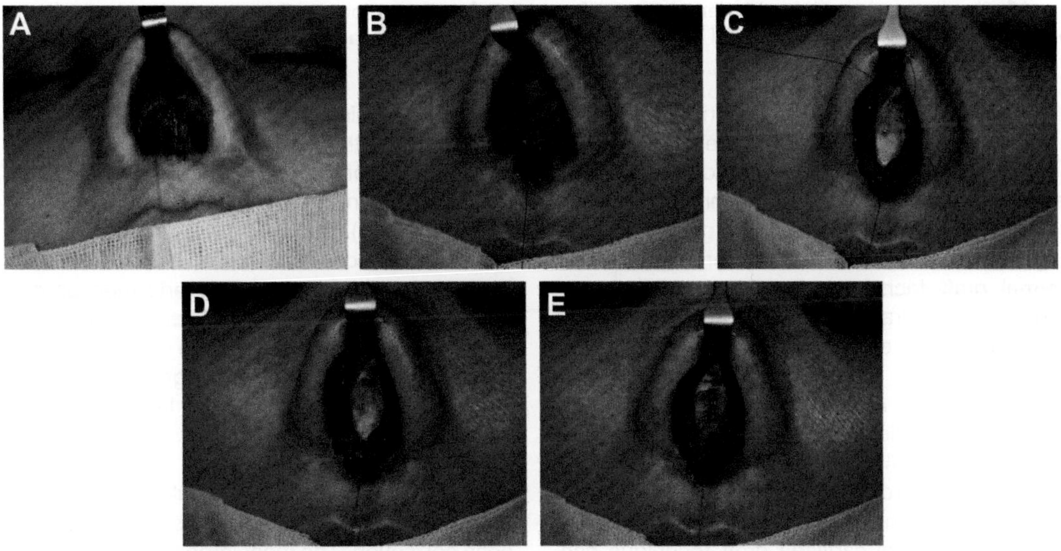

Fig. 28. Operative sequence for derotation graft. (*A*) The columellar strut graft is performed with folded conchal cartilage. (*B*) Lower lateral cartilages are pulled caudally with traction suture. (*C*) Derotation graft is placed on the dorsal septum and upper lateral cartilage. The first fixation suture to the underlying cartilage is started at the most cephalic part of the graft. (*D*) Subsequent sutures are placed serially. (*E*) The caudal portion of graft is now sutured to underlying lateral crura of lower lateral cartilages.

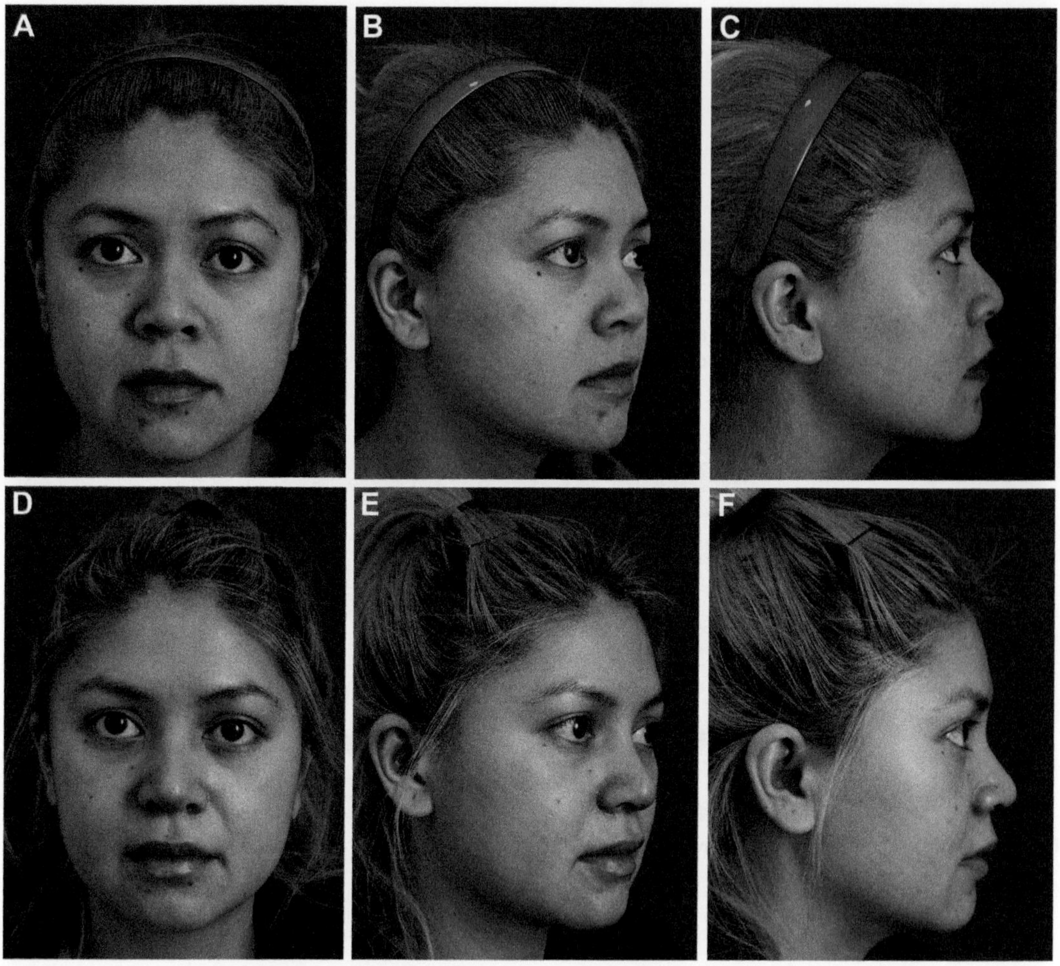

Fig. 29. Short nose correction with derotation graft. (*A–C*) Before operation. (*D–F*) Postoperative views after tip plasty with columellar strut graft and derotation graft with conchal cartilage and alar base reduction.

Autogenous tissues are appropriate for dorsal augmentation in patients with extremely thin dorsal skin, and in secondary operation for implant-related complications. A new technique to overcome high resorption of dermofat graft for dorsal augmentation is the vertically oriented folded dermal graft technique. The vertically oriented folded dermal graft augments the dorsal height not by the thickness but by the folded height of the graft.

The choice of autogenous material for major dorsal augmentation is costal cartilage. The typical solid block costal cartilage carving technique is performed according to the balanced intrinsic stress by using the core portion of the cartilage. Multilayered costal cartilage graft technique can be an effective alternative technique to solid costal cartilage graft for dorsal augmentation.

Projection of the nasal tip in Asian noses is accomplished through 1 or a combination of the following surgical techniques: cartilage onlay/shield graft on the dome of lower lateral cartilages, medialization of lateral crura (lateral crural steal), and suspension of lower lateral cartilages (septal extension graft).

For short nose correction, septal extension graft is the most commonly performed procedure in Asian countries. The first and the most important step of this technique is the repositioning of the lower lateral cartilages caudally. For caudal repositioning, lower lateral cartilage should be released from the scroll area and hinge complex.

Derotation graft using auricular cartilage is a useful alternative to septal extension graft for short nose correction. The most important advantage of derotation graft is that it allows supple and movable nasal tip while enabling enough tip lengthening.

CLINICS CARE POINTS

- Long L-shaped implants should be avoided. Implants for dorsal augmentation should be placed under the periosteum and the caudal end of the implant should be placed at the supratip area.
- To minimize high resorption of dermofat graft, the vertically oriented folded dermal graft is the choice of graft technique for dorsal augmentation in patients with thin skin.
- For dorsal augmentation using costal cartilage, the concentric carving technique or multilayered graft technique should be performed to avoid graft warping.
- It is common for the tip and columella to be deviated after unilateral septal extension graft in Asian noses from the deviation of remnant septal L-strut. To avoid this problem in Asian noses with weak and thin septal cartilage, the operator must perform an additional batten graft to the opposite side of the septal extension graft.
- Derotation graft can be a good solution to overcome the major disadvantages of septal extension graft, such as rigid nasal tip and witched tip appearance when smiling.

REFERENCES

1. Ahn JM. The current trend in augmentation rhinoplasty. Facial Plast Surg 2006;22:61–9.
2. Peled ZM, Warren AG, Johnston P, et al. The use of alloplastic materials in rhinoplasty surgery: a meta-analysis. Plast Reconstr Surg 2008;121:85e–92e.
3. Tham C, Lai YL, Weng CJ, et al. Silicone augmentation rhinoplasty in an oriental population. Ann Plast Surg 2005;54(1):1–5.
4. Suh MK. Deviated nose correction and functional rhinoplasty. In: Suh MK, editor. Atlas of Asian rhinoplasty. Singapore: Springer Publishing Company; 2018. p. 735–9.
5. Anna A, Augusto P, Bernardo I. The role of 3D printing in medical applications: a state of the art. J Healthc Eng 2019;2019:5340616.
6. Cho IC. Correction of contracted noses with unilateral cymbal cartilage and dermofat. November 8, 2015; 73rd congress of the Korean society of plastic and reconstructive surgeons, Seoul, Korea
7. Kim HK, Rhee SC. Augmentation rhinoplasty using a folded "pure" dermal graft. J Craniofac Surg 2013; 24(5):1758–62.
8. Toriumi DM. Dorsal augmentation using autologous costal cartilage or microfat-infused soft tissue augmentation. Facial Plast Surg 2017;33(2):162–78.
9. Namgoong S, Kim S, Suh MK. Multilayered costal cartilage graft for nasal dorsal augmentation. Aesthet Plast Surg 2020;44(6):2185–96.
10. Kridel RW, Konior RJ, Shumrick KA, et al. Advances in nasal tip surgery: the lateral crural steal. Arch Otolaryngol Head Neck Surg 1989;115(10):1206–12.
11. Suh MK. Optimal tip projection in Asian noses. In: Suh MK, editor. Atlas of Asian rhinoplasty. Singapore: Springer Publishing Company; 2018. p. 449–90.
12. Kim JH, Song JW, Park SW, et al. Tip extension suture: a new tool tailored for Asian rhinoplasty. Plast Reconstr Surg 2014;134(5):907–16.
13. Paik MH. Correction of short nose. J Korean Soc Aesth Plast Surg 2005;11(1):22–6.
14. Paik MH, Chu LS. Correction of the short nose using derotation graft. Arch Aesthet Plast Surg 2012;18(1): 35–44.
15. Byrd HS, Andochick S, Copit S, et al. Septal extension grafts: a method of controlling tip projection shape. Plast Reconstr Surg 1997;100(4):999–1010.

Special Consideration in Rhinoplasty for Deformed Nose of East Asians

Yong Ju Jang, MD, PhD*, Hyun Moon, MD

KEYWORDS

• Asian rhinoplasty • Deviated nose • Convex dorsum • Dorsal augmentation • Short nose

KEY POINTS

- Asian noses tend to have a weak and small cartilage framework and flat and thick nasal bone, thus resulting in a low radix and dorsal height. Hence, in most of rhinoplasty surgeries among Asians, augmentation is important.
- Augmentation of the nose should be achieved by framework augmentation and tip augmentation and dorsal augmentation.
- Typical Asian deformed nose has many different types: mildly concave nasal dorsum, severely concave or low nasal dorsum, wide nasal dorsum, deviated nose, convex nasal dorsum, saddle nose, short-nose deformity, and deformities involving irreversible damage of skin/soft tissue envelope and nasal skeleton are the most representative ones.
- Various kinds of techniques are needed to correct different types of deformities where a dorsal augmentation is a critically important concept to accomplish aesthetically pleasing surgical outcome.

INTRODUCTION

Despite the lack of general and scientific consensus on its definition, a deformed nose is characterized as one that has an obvious deviant shape. From a frontal view, a wide nasal dorsum and deviated nose can be considered as deformity. From a profile view, a hump or low-profile nose, saddle nose, upturned nose, long nose with ptotic tip, or a nose with columellar retraction can be problematic.[1] This article aims to address the important points for successful correction of deformed noses of East Asian individuals. Although there is huge variation, the tip of the East Asian is usually low and the lower lateral cartilages are small and weak.[2] The nasal bones are flat and thick, resulting in a low radix and dorsal height. Because the septal cartilage of some Asians is thin and small,[3] the size and quantity of harvestable septal cartilage may be inadequate for complex rhinoplasty procedures, increasing the need to harvest grafts from other sites. Hence, in most of rhinoplasty surgeries among Asians, augmentation is important.[4] Aesthetic perfection of the nose is determined by the height and shape of the nasal dorsum seen from the profile and frontal views, with its harmonious alignment with the nasal tip. The augmentation should be achieved by framework augmentation and tip augmentation and dorsal augmentation. In framework augmentation, spreader and septal extension grafts are added to the native septal cartilage, by which the surgeon can secure strong nasal bases that can withstand subsequent tip augmentation and dorsal augmentation.[5] Tip augmentation is usually performed with grafting procedures such as onlay grafting, shield grafting, and multilayer tip grafting using autologous cartilages. Once the desired height and shape of the tip is acquired by aforementioned procedures, subsequent dorsal augmentation should be done using various

Department of Otolaryngology, Asan Medical Center, University of Ulsan College of Medicine, Seoul, Korea
* Corresponding author.
E-mail address: 3712yjang@gmail.com

Facial Plast Surg Clin N Am 29 (2021) 611–624
https://doi.org/10.1016/j.fsc.2021.06.009

materials. Dorsal augmentation is the most frequently performed procedure in Asian rhinoplasty; it is critically important not only in simple cosmetic rhinoplasty but also in all types of rhinoplasties to achieve aesthetic perfection.[1] In this article, rhinoplasty procedures for different types of nasal deformities will be introduced.

TREATMENT STRATEGIES FOR VARIOUS FORMS OF DEFORMED NOSES

Mildly Concave Nasal Dorsum

Although the female population generally favors this type of nasal profile, men with mildly concave nasal dorsum prefer a straighter dorsal line, thus seeking rhinoplasty. Various types of dorsal implants can be used to augment this type of nose. For example, alloplastic implants such as thin silicone and expanded polytetrafluoroethylene (ePTFE) may be suitable. In addition, autologous materials such as fascia-wrapped diced cartilage, free diced cartilage, and glued diced cartilage are also adequate material.[1] The degree of augmentation desired by the patient must be determined by a thorough consultation. For example, patients desiring a slight augmentation may not require tip work, whereas patients desiring substantial augmentation should undergo tip augmentation before dorsal augmentation to create a harmonious tip–dorsum relationship (**Fig. 1**).

Severely Concave or Low Nasal Dorsum Without an Upturned Tip

This deformity is relatively common in the East Asian population (**Fig. 2**). The pathology underlying this deformity is a usually poorly developed cartilaginous dorsum and nasal bone. To beautify the profile line, this type of nose usually requires major septal reconstruction and tip augmentation before dorsum management. Augmentation of the nasal dorsum without reconstructing the poorly developed septal cartilage often causes the dorsum to sink under the weight of the dorsal implant.[1] Because the correction of deformity highly demands a significant quantity of graft materials, costal cartilage is considered the most ideal graft source. Among the methods used to enhance septal support, the authors prefer to sandwich a caudal septal extension graft, placed end-to-end with the caudal septum, between 2 extended spreader grafts, slightly extended dorsally and caudally.[5] If the increase in the tip height augmentation is insufficient, additional tip grafting is required.[6] Subsequent dorsal augmentation should be done thereafter. This article recommends costal cartilage for dorsal augmentation material, as it is already harvested for framework augmentation. For dorsal augmentation, an autologous costal cartilage can be used in a solid mono-block form or in diced cartilage. Although augmentation using a mono-block carved implant may seem simple, carving is actually difficult and the graft can be bent or warped during the postoperative period. Furthermore, it is difficult to create a natural-looking smooth dorsal contour. To avoid problems inherent to the solid carved cartilage, augmentation with finely diced cartilage is becoming increasingly popular. Diced costal cartilage is used for dorsal augmentation as fascia-wrapped implant, glued graft, and free diced cartilage.[7,8] The authors prefer the technique of glued diced cartilage. In this technique, bonding diced cartilage with fibrin glue is performed instead of placing it in a fascia sleeve. Thus, this technique requires a mold to create the desired shape. Manually molded glued diced cartilage graft using a half-cut syringe has been reported to be useful.[9] However, the false volume caused by fluid and glue around the diced cartilage is difficult to control with this method, and using a half-cut syringe makes this method cumbersome. Thus, the senior author developed a mold for the glued diced cartilage graft technique to get more refined control of the shape, thickness, and length of the diced cartilage implant for dorsal augmentation. The mold comprises the base template, guarding frame, and compressor (**Fig. 3**). In this technique, harvested autologous fascia/perichondrium or homologous fascia lata can be used as a covering material at the convex side of the implant to prevent dorsal irregularities. Making the dorsal implant starts with applying 1 or 2 drops of the fibrin glue onto the covering material placed on the base template, and the guarding frame of the mold is assembled. Then, a thin layer of diced cartilage is placed on top of the fascia or perichondrium, a second layer of glue is painted, an additional layer of diced cartilage is laid on top, and glue is painted over the second layer of diced cartilage. Finally, the compressor of the mold is applied and manually pressed. Through the small holes of the sidewall, excessive glue and fluid around the diced cartilage are drained and suctioned out. After carefully disassembling the molds, the graft for dorsal augmentation is obtained. The implant has a convex outer surface with or without a soft-tissue cap, whereas the undersurface has a concave shape conforming to the convexity of the nasal dorsum (**Fig. 4**). The graft is then placed onto the nasal dorsum usually in one piece but sometimes in a segmental fashion at the radix and supratip dorsum. Because molded diced cartilage graft with glue is in a semisolid state, it is important to

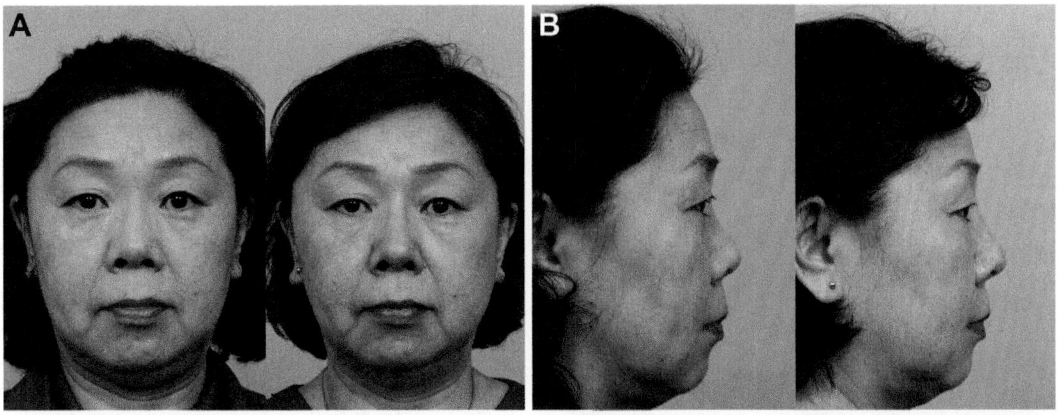

Fig. 1. A patient with a mildly concave nasal dorsum who was treated with a combination of septal extension graft, tip grafting, and dorsal augmentation with one layer ePTFE. Preoperative (*left*) and postoperative (*right*) views of frontal (*A*) and lateral photograph (*B*).

handle it cautiously so as not to break the molded cartilage implant. The final shaping of the implant can be achieved by gentle manual molding over the skin-soft tissue envelope.

Wide Nasal Dorsum

In a Caucasian nose, a wide nasal dorsum is often attributed to the broad nasal bone and cartilaginous dorsum, which requires the dorsal-width narrowing by osteotomy. However, in Asians, this deformity is usually associated with a flat low-profile nose with a poorly developed nasal skeleton, which cannot create a distinct brow-tip aesthetic line, thus giving an impression of a wide nasal dorsum (**Fig. 5**). In this case, osteotomy is not suitable to narrow the dorsum. Instead, dorsal augmentation is the mainstay for creating an aesthetically pleasing brow-tip aesthetic line.[10] Furthermore, subjects with broad nasal dorsum usually have thick skin and poorly developed alar cartilages causing an underprojected and amorphously defined nasal tip. For the correction of the broad nasal dorsum, a significant tip projection using septal extension graft with or without tip grafting should be done, and subsequent dorsal augmentation is needed to create a well-balanced brow-tip aesthetic line.

Deviated Nose

Correction of a deviated nose is a complex issue that cannot be simplified, where dorsal augmentation is often the neglected procedure.[11] Dorsal augmentation is one of the last steps in correcting deviated noses. To correct the deviation, procedures such as osteotomy or spreader graft are frequently used, but these maneuvers can cause dorsum irregularities in patients with thin skin. Moreover, surgical maneuvers to straighten

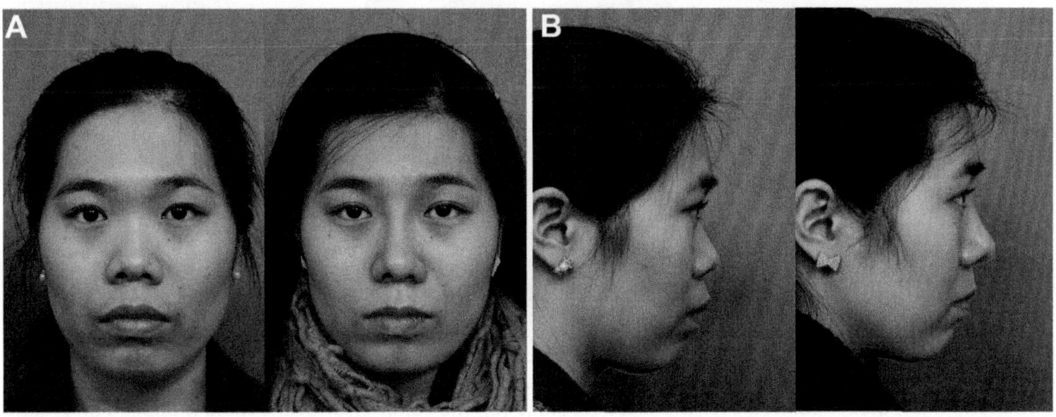

Fig. 2. A patient with severely low nasal dorsum: dorsal augmentation was done using 3 layers of ePTFE after tip augmentation. Preoperative (*left*) and postoperative (*right*) views of frontal (*A*) and lateral photograph (*B*).

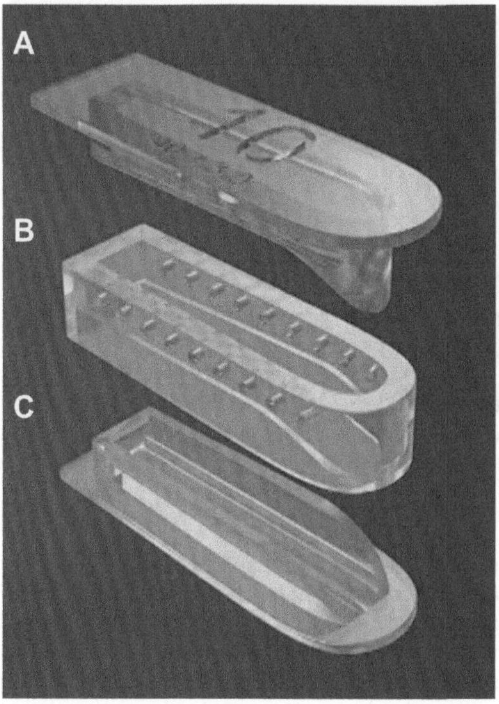

Fig. 3. A mold to fashion glued diced cartilage implant. It is composed of a compressor (*A*), a guarding frame (*B*), and a base template (*C*).

cartilaginous dorsum and bony dorsum cannot perfectly correct the deviated appearance of the nose. As such, when the underlying nasal skeleton is not straight in the midline, rather tiled, dorsal augmentation can neutralize and mitigate the deviated nasal skeleton, so that the final shape of the nose looks straight. Subjects with deviated nose also show contraction of the tissue and the soft tissue where their deviation was originally located; appropriate dorsal augmentation and camouflage can correct the soft tissue deformities that cause deviation. Implant materials for augmentation should be small in volume and soft. Because the correction of deviation requires extensive dissection and may weaken the underlying structure due to osteotomy and septal correction, dorsal augmentation with solid materials such as silicone or costal cartilage can easily be displaced or deform the underlying nasal skeleton by its weight. It is therefore recommended to use soft implant materials such as ePTFE, fascia, conchal cartilage, crushed septal cartilage, diced cartilage, and fascia-wrapped diced cartilage for dorsal augmentation (**Fig. 6**).

Convex Nasal Dorsum

The prevalence of a hump nose among Asian is lower than Caucasian, and dorsal convexity is generally small and less prominent. However, certainly, hump noses are also a significant issue in Asian rhinoplasty. On examination of the Asian noses, a typical hump or a humplike deformity can be identified. Therefore, it is desirable to define the deformities as a convex nasal dorsum, which can be classified into 3 types: a generalized hump, an isolated hump, and a relative hump with a low tip[12] (**Fig. 7**). A generalized hump represents the typical hump deformity commonly seen in Caucasian populations in which the curvature of

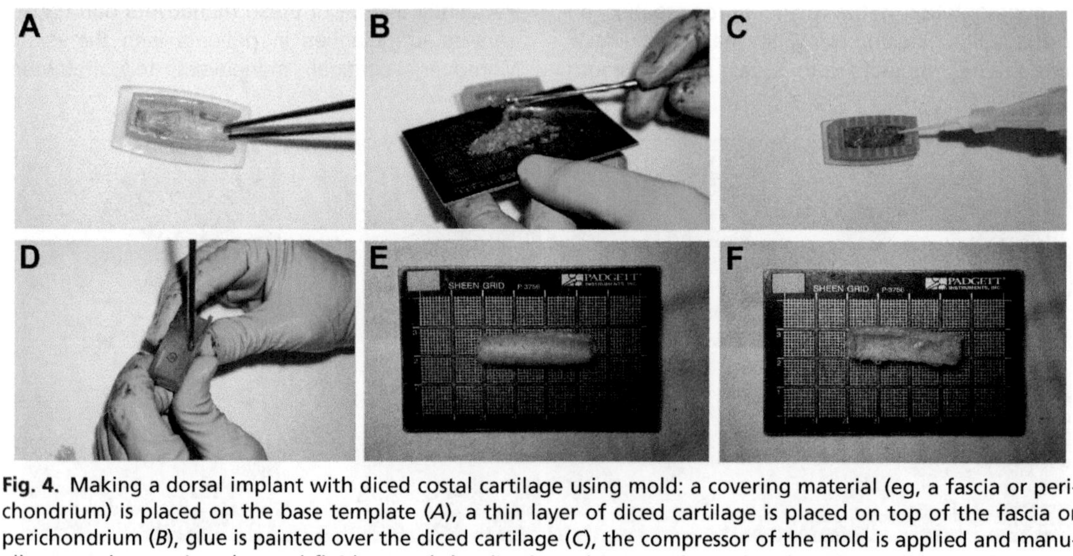

Fig. 4. Making a dorsal implant with diced costal cartilage using mold: a covering material (eg, a fascia or perichondrium) is placed on the base template (*A*), a thin layer of diced cartilage is placed on top of the fascia or perichondrium (*B*), glue is painted over the diced cartilage (*C*), the compressor of the mold is applied and manually pressed, excessive glue and fluid around the diced cartilage are drained and suctioned out (*D*), finally an implant with convex outer surface with fascia and concave undersurface is created (*E*, *F*).

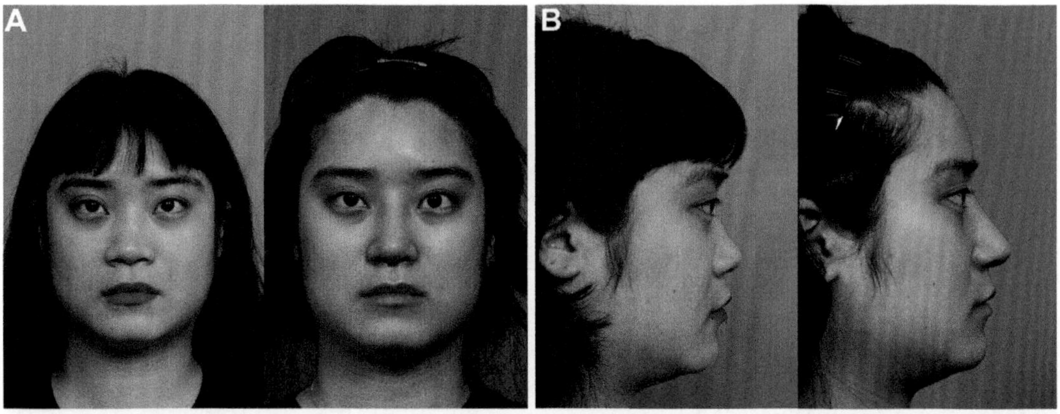

Fig. 5. A patient showing wide nasal dorsum was treated with a combination of a caudal septal extension graft and dorsal augmentation with glued diced costal cartilage covered with fascia. Preoperative (*left*) and postoperative (*right*) views of frontal (*A*) and lateral photograph (*B*).

the hump begins from the bony vault and extends to the cartilaginous dorsum in a gentle curve. An isolated hump represents an abrupt protrusion of a small hump in a triangular or round shape on the dorsal line. The hump is short, with most of it located around the rhinion. A relative hump with a low tip is seen in patients whose nasal dorsum is not very high but the nasal tip is severely underprojected, giving a false impression of a nasal dorsal hump. Because many Asians lack appropriate tip projection, the desired height of the tip should be set first during the correction of the convex dorsum, followed by the determination of the degree of hump reduction and augmentation of the radix and supratip according to the new tip height. The ordinary hump nose correction starts with conservative hump reduction. During the hump reduction, bony cap covering the cartilaginous hump is gradually removed, and subsequently exposed cartilage prominence should be reduced very carefully in an incremental fashion. Hump reduction is followed by elevation of tip height using septal extension grafts, with or without tip grafting (**Fig. 8**). This elevation, in turn, is followed by dorsal augmentation. A one-piece implant covering the area from the radix to the tip, such as silicone or mono-block costal cartilage dorsal augmentation, may not be suitable, as it tends to result in a convex nasal dorsum. Rather, the radix and the supratip nasal dorsum should be augmented as separate units as segmental augmentation[13] (**Fig. 9**). Materials considered adequate for augmentation include diced conchal cartilage with perichondrium, ePTFE, crushed septal cartilage, diced ear cartilage, and diced costal cartilage.

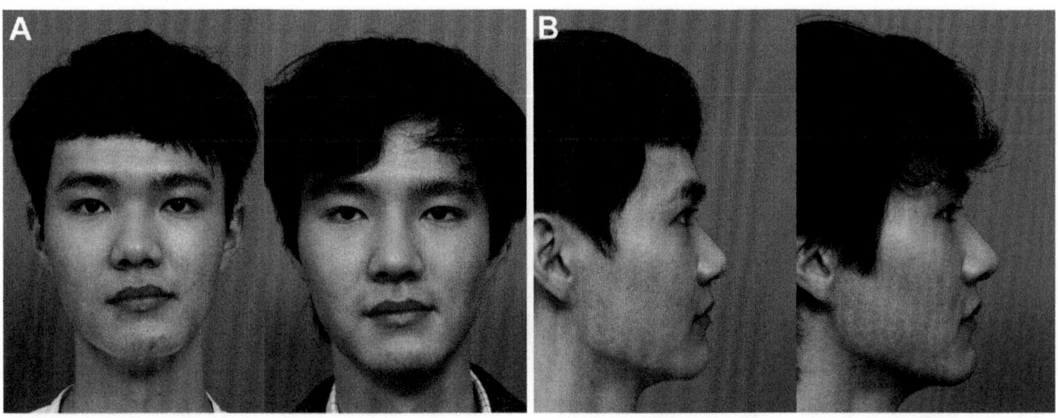

Fig. 6. A patient showing improved deviated nose corrected by the placement of left-sided caudal septal extension graft and left-sided extended spreader graft and subsequent dorsal augmentation with glued diced costal cartilage covered with fascia. Preoperative (*left*) and postoperative (*right*) views of frontal (*A*) and lateral photograph (*B*).

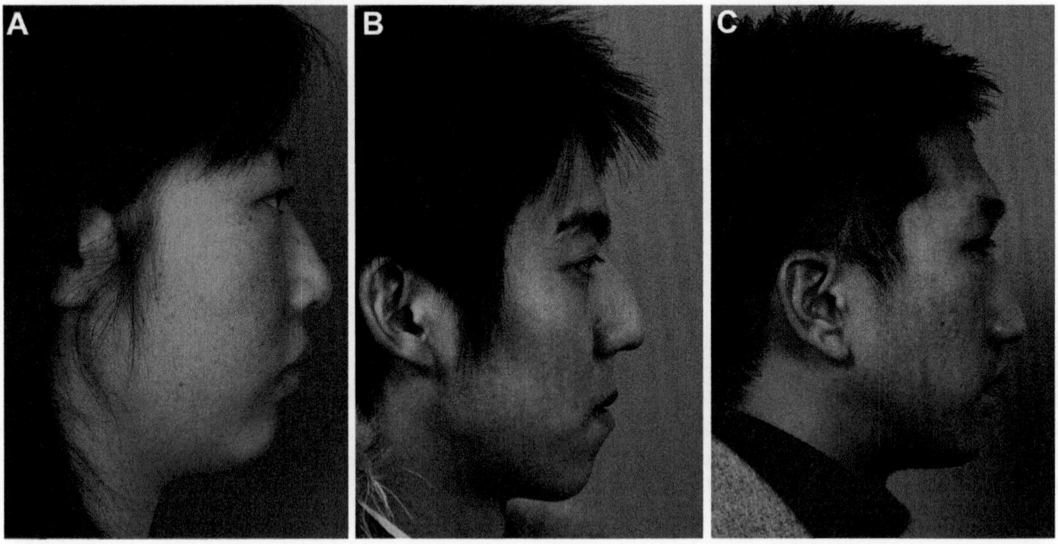

Fig. 7. Classification of Asian hump nose; a generalized hump (*A*), an isolated hump (*B*), and a relative hump with a low tip (*C*).

Saddle Nose

A saddle nose is usually a consequence of derangements of the supporting structure of the quadrangular cartilage, resulting in decreased dorsal and caudal height. It involves not only middle vault and dorsal depression but also loss of tip support and definition, columellar retraction, overrotation of the tip, and deprojection. Most saddle noses are associated with disorders of the septal cartilage.[14] Proper reconstruction of the septal supporting framework and additional dorsal augmentation is the mainstay of the treatment of both deformities. Saddle nose can be classified as a minor or major saddle nose. Managing a minor saddle nose with a relatively strong septal framework requires strengthening of the caudal septum with a bony batten graft[15] and augmentation of the nasal dorsum using crushed septal cartilage or diced conchal cartilage with perichondrium via an endonasal approach. Septal cartilage can be obtained with the fewest additional scars. Despite its ease of accessibility, the quality and quantity of this cartilage is often less ideal in a patient with saddle nose. Conchal cartilage is another material that can be easily accessed but its elasticity and intrinsic curvature make it less suitable for weight bearing. Hence, conchal cartilage is usually used for tip grafting or minor dorsal augmentation (either in stacked form, fascia-

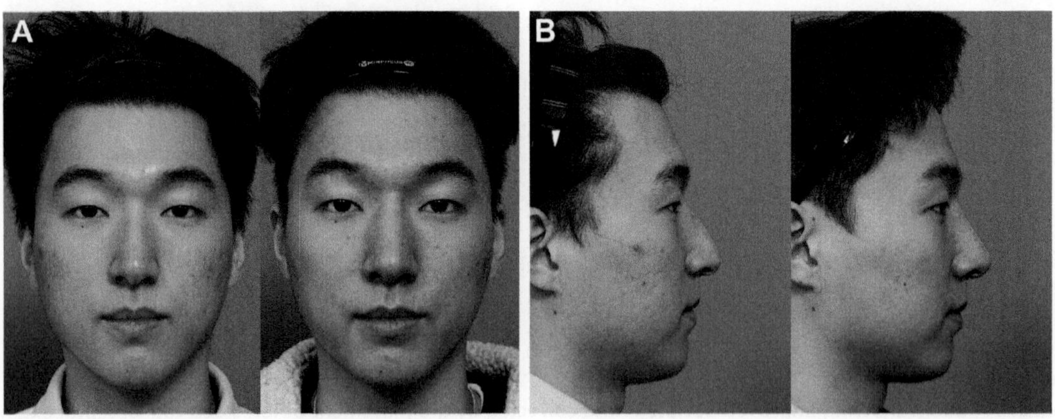

Fig. 8. A patient showing an improved hump nose after hump reduction, tip augmentation with caudal septal extension graft, and dorsal camouflage with crushed septal cartilage and fascia. Preoperative (*left*) and postoperative (*right*) views of frontal (*A*) and lateral photograph (*B*).

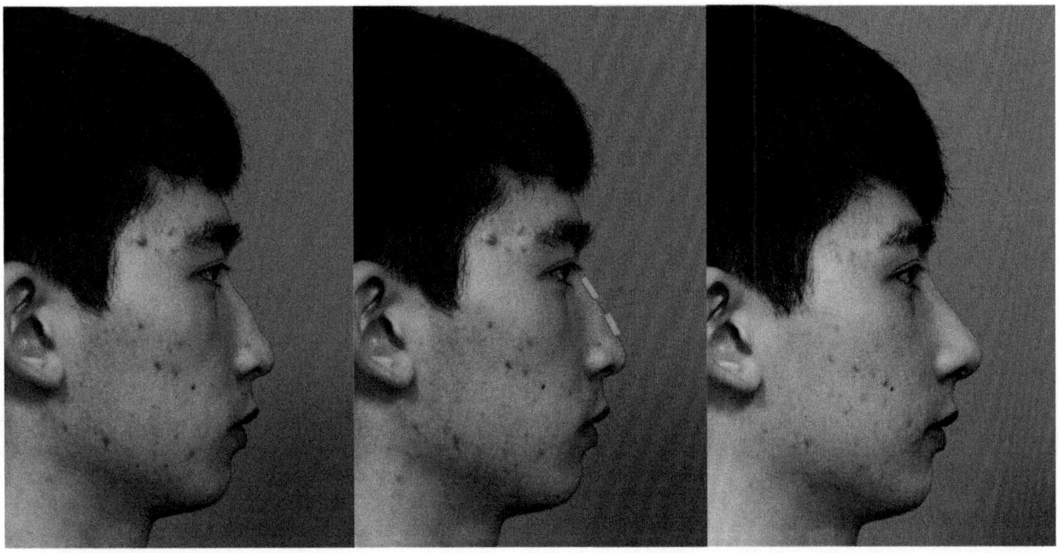

Fig. 9. A patient with a favorable aesthetic change in the nasal dorsum after segmental dorsal augmentation with perichondrium-attached diced ear cartilage.

wrapped diced form, or glued diced cartilage). Kim and Jang have described a dorsal-augmenting method involving diced conchal cartilage with perichondrium attachment, which is suitable for patients having moderate-to-thick skin[16] (**Fig. 10**). In patients who have a severe saddle nose, where the septal framework is deemed not strong enough, the first step in the rhinoplasty surgery is to go for a major septal reconstruction, in which a solid foundation is established. Major septal reconstruction can be done in several different ways depending on the condition of a remaining L-strut and the availability of cartilage.[5,17] First is the placement of one extended spreader graft combined with one caudal septal extension graft, where they are sutured on different sides of the existing L strut (**Fig. 11**). The extended spreader graft (the spreader graft extending beyond the caudal border of the anterior septal angle) is sutured beside the nasal septum. A caudal septal extension graft is placed on the contralateral caudal septum and meets the extended spreader graft. The caudal septal extension graft is then suture fixated with the extended spreader graft, septum, and soft tissues around the anterior nasal spine. This method has been used when the remaining dorsal L strut is curved and relatively thick grafting cartilage is available, mainly, autologous costal cartilage. This technique is also useful when there is nostril asymmetry caused by off-centered or dislocated caudal septum, where the caudal septal extension graft is placed at the side of the wider nostril. Second is the combination of the bilateral extended spreader grafts and one caudal extension graft, where the bilateral extended spreader grafts are sutured on both sides of the dorsal strut with one caudal extension graft sandwiched between them; caudal septal extension graft is positioned end-to-end with the native caudal septum. Further anchoring of the caudal extension graft can be done by simply suturing the basal part of the graft with the nearby soft tissue or passing the suture through the hole on the anterior nasal spine (created by a sharp-ended towel clip). Sometimes, lateral buttress grafts (a short batten-type graft) are placed below the extended spreader graft and suture-fixated at the junction of the caudal

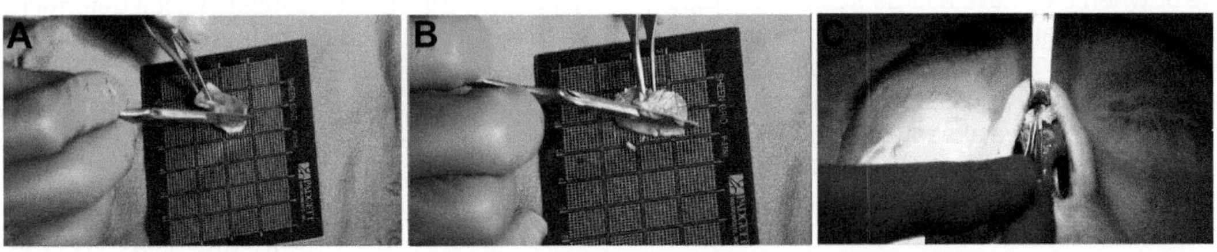

Fig. 10. Intraoperative views of diced conchal cartilage with perichondrium attachment.

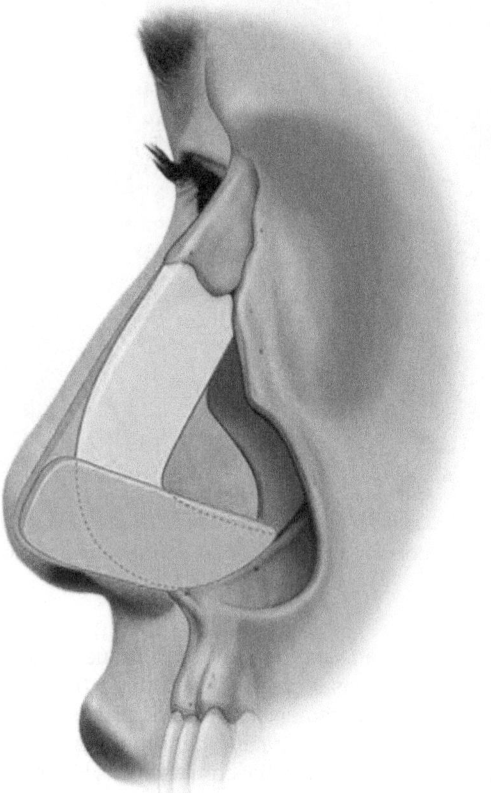

Fig. 11. A caudal septal extension graft placed side-to-side with the caudal septum. Placement of one extended spreader graft combined with one caudal septal extension graft, where they are sutured on different sides of the existing L strut.

septum and basal part of the caudal extension graft on one side or bilaterally (**Fig. 12**); this can prevent lateral displacement of the caudal extension graft and provide further stabilization. The most commonly used material for major septal reconstruction is autologous costal cartilage harvested from the sixth or seventh rib, which is by far the most versatile autologous material for major reconstruction. Third is the use of an integrated dorsal implant and columella strut technique (**Fig. 13**), which is indicated when the patients with saddle nose have no remaining septal cartilage or when they have a large septal perforation, where the septal mucosal dissection for grafting extended graft and septal extension becomes extremely difficult and carries an increased risk of further injury to the already damaged septal mucosa. Using the integrated dorsal implant and columellar strut allows surgeons to bypass the problematic cartilaginous septum and enables them to reconstruct the lower two-thirds of the nose. To make an integrated dorsal implant and columellar strut made of costal cartilage, one mono-block dorsal implant is suture fixated with a columella strut to form the new cartilaginous L strut. The dorsal implant part can be inserted directly into the subperiosteal pocket above the nasal bone spanning the entire nasal dorsum. With regard to the columella strut part, this could be suture fixated in front of the anterior nasal spine or simply be inserted into the space between the divided medial crura. Placement of the integrated implant usually creates a gap between the new straight dorsal strut and the native depressed nasal dorsum, which should be filled with spare cartilage in crushed or diced form to secure stable positioning and prevent potential hematoma formation in this dead space (**Figs. 14 and 15**). Even after major septal reconstruction using aforementioned methods, the dorsal shape might still be concave to some degree. In this case, additional onlay grafts for dorsal augmentation could help achieve the ideal dorsal height. Different materials could be chosen for this purpose, such as autologous, homologous, or alloplastic materials, based on the surgeon's preference and accessibility. The most commonly used autologous material is the same material we use for septal reconstruction, that is, autologous costal cartilage. An underprojected tip and a columella retraction are very common in severe saddle nose patients. Simple tip-suturing techniques can sometimes be helpful in refining a tip definition but are not so reliable in projecting the tip. Usually, tip grafting techniques are necessary if further tip projection is desired after septal reconstruction and elongation. Multilayer cartilaginous tip grafting techniques can be useful for further tip augmentation and derotation[18] (**Fig. 16**). Other methods that can also be useful in modifying the infratip contour by changing the nasolabial angle include a premaxillary graft. Precise recognition of the different underlying pathologies in a particular saddle nose and choosing the reconstruction material and method accordingly are the most important tasks for rhinoplasty surgeons when treating this condition.

Short-Nose Deformity

A short nose is one of the most difficult deformities to correct, and it requires the use of a multitude of challenging surgical techniques for adequate correction (**Fig. 17**). A short nose most commonly develops as a sequela of nasal surgery, especially after dorsal augmentation with silicone.[19] In addition, overly aggressive rhinoplasty maneuvers that include extensive septal cartilage work are more likely to result in a short nose. Corrective

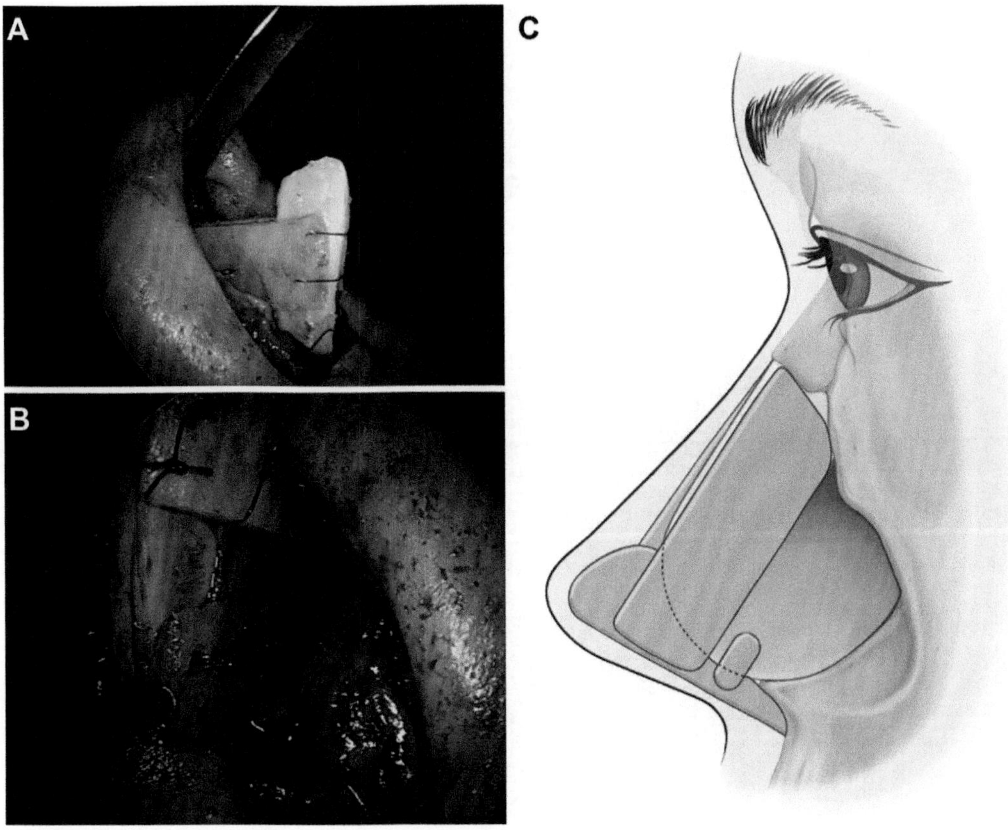

Fig. 12. A lateral buttress graft. Intraoperative views (*A, B*) and an illustration (*C*). Combination of the bilateral extended spreader grafts and one caudal extension graft, where the bilateral extended spreader grafts are sutured on both sides of the dorsal strut with one caudal extension graft sandwiched between them. A lateral buttress graft is suture fixated at the junction of the caudal septum and basal part of the caudal extension graft on one side.

surgery aims for the actual extension of the nose length, while simultaneously creating an illusion of a longer nose. Short noses should be corrected by adhering to the surgical principles of lengthening the central and lateral segments, tip grafting to lengthen the nose, and dorsal augmentation.[20] For the correction of a short nose, the authors usually place extended spreader grafts on both sides of the dorsal strut and the caudal septal extension graft between the extended spreader grafts. The caudal septal extension graft, which is sandwiched between the dorsal grafts, is placed in an end-to-end manner with the caudal septum. The septal extension graft should be appropriately designed so that it does not project the tip too much and widen the nasolabial angle, instead lengthening the tip lobule portion. If lengthening of the central compartment is not combined with adequate lengthening of the lateral compartment, the nose may look pinched and unnatural. It is therefore important to address the lateral compartment of the nose accordingly to attain an aesthetically harmonious surgical outcome. Lateral compartment elongation is performed by caudally mobilizing the lateral crus from the scroll area after careful dissection of scar tissue, followed by suture stabilization with the elongated central compartment. However, in a severely scarred nose, the mobility of the lower lateral cartilage cannot be gained even after dissection between the lower and upper lateral cartilage. In this perplexing situation, covering both sides of the already-lengthened central compartment may become difficult. To overcome this problem, the midline structure can be covered by performing cartilage flap technique modified from the dome division technique in which both sides of a medially based cartilage flap are developed by incising and dissecting off the lateral crust of the lower lateral cartilage from the underlying vestibular skin and rotated medially to cover the extended spreader graft[20] (**Fig. 18**). Because a short nose is usually accompanied by a concave nasal dorsum, dorsal augmentation is a crucial surgical

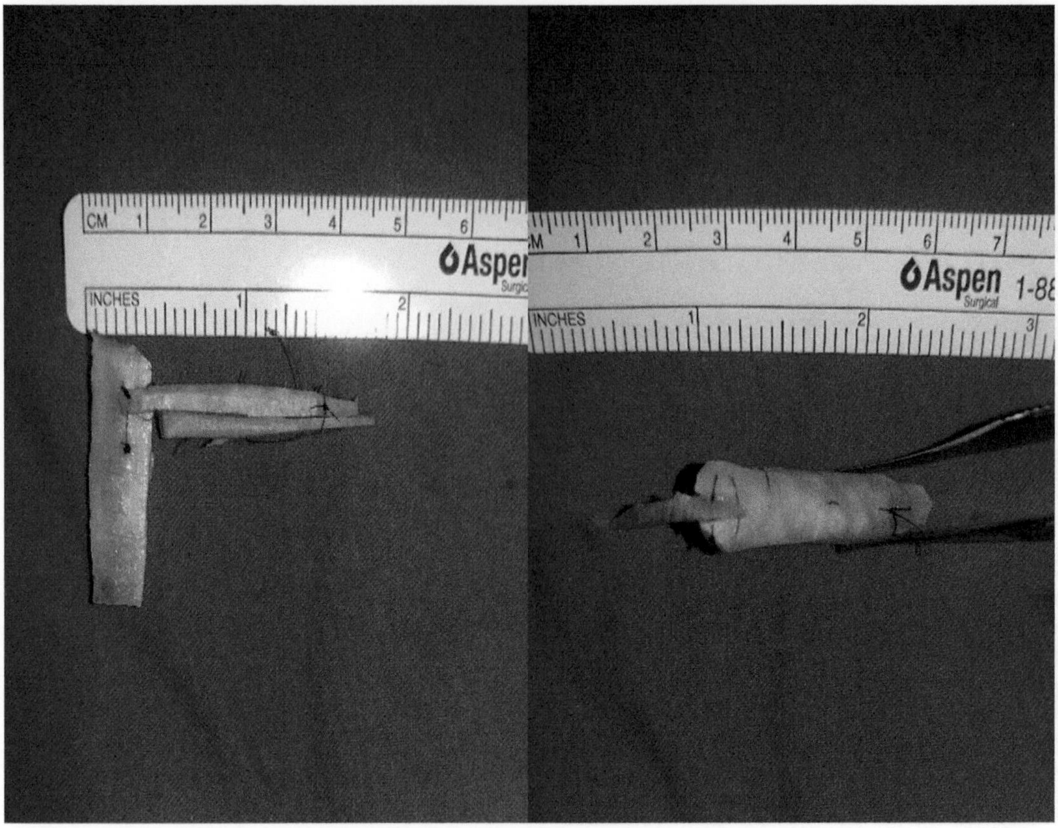

Fig. 13. Intraoperative views of an integrated dorsal implant and columella strut graft.

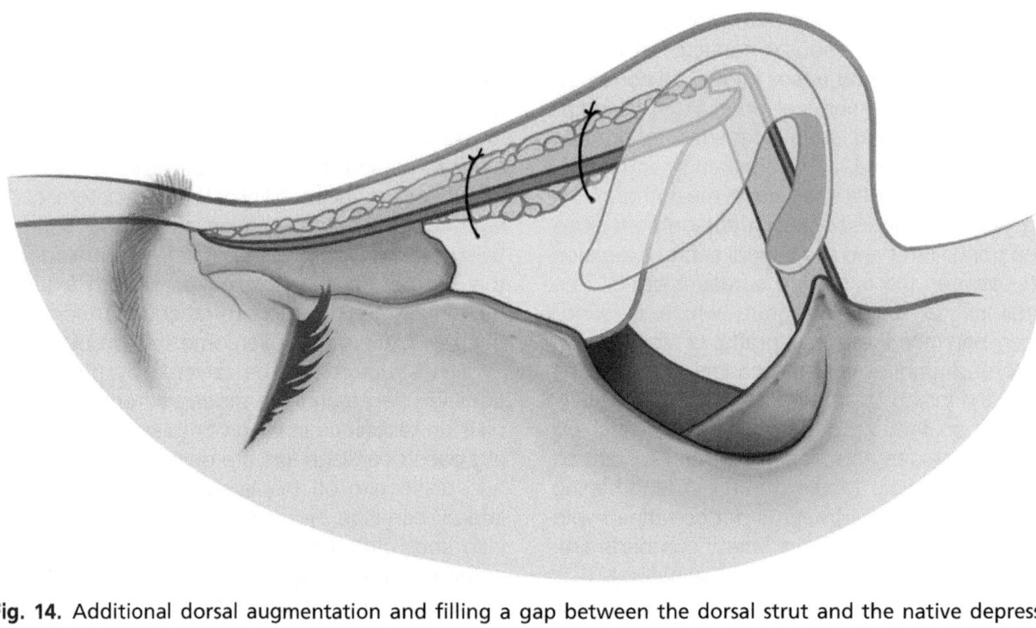

Fig. 14. Additional dorsal augmentation and filling a gap between the dorsal strut and the native depressed nasal dorsum with spare cartilages.

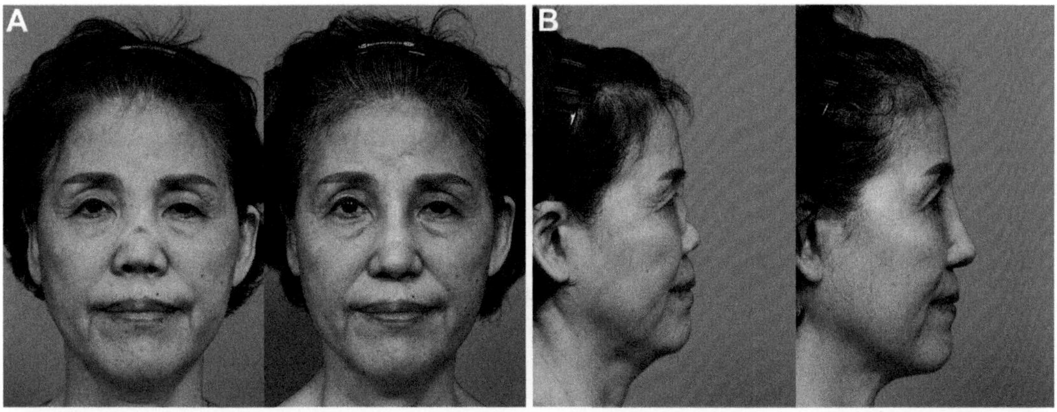

Fig. 15. A patient with an improved saddle nose deformity after reconstruction with an integrated dorsal implant and columella strut and dorsal augmentation with glued diced costal cartilage covered with fascia. Preoperative (*left*) and postoperative (*right*) views of frontal (*A*) and lateral photograph (*B*).

procedure because the nose seems longer after the correction of the dorsal concavity. The nasal dorsum should be augmented using an implant the surgeon feels most comfortable with. When additional derotation is needed, shield graft or the multilayer tip grafting technique is useful. In performing this maneuver, the first cartilaginous shield graft layer is placed at the caudal surface of the media or the middle columella and secured. Additional shield graft layers are then placed on the caudal aspect of the first layer. In correcting a short nose, the most important determining factor for the success of the operation is the condition of the skin/soft tissue envelope. The nasal skeleton can be elongated through extended spreader grafting, tip grafting, and dorsal augmentation. However, if the overlying skin is severely thickened and has lost its normal elasticity because of repeated inflammation and contraction, the lengthened nasal skeleton cannot be adequately redraped with skin, causing a problem in suture approximation of the transcolumellar incision. In this case, the surgeon should reduce the length of the central segment or remove tip grafts to ensure easier, tension-free closure. The soft tissue of the internal alar surface is often insufficient when short nose is associated with severe alar retraction. In such cases, a composite graft that includes cartilage and skin from the cymba concha or cavum concha can be placed to compensate for the inner lining deficiency.

Deformities Involving Irreversible Damage of Skin/Soft Tissue Envelope and Nasal Skeleton

This deformity is one of the most catastrophic complications of rhinoplasty with alloplastic implants and is usually caused by repeated infection and extrusion of the implant through the columellar skin, which results in the destruction of the medial crus and severe retraction of the columella.[19] When the columellar retraction is mild and the medial crus of the alar cartilage looks intact, severe columellar retraction can be treated with the placement of caudal septal extension grafting and additional shield grafting (**Fig. 19**). However, in severe columellar retraction with no skin, a major reconstruction with a forehead flap may be the best option for treatment. In this surgical procedure, the deformed and missing alar cartilage

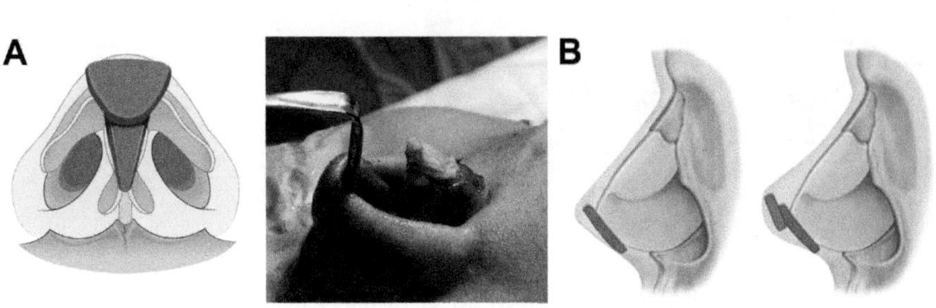

Fig. 16. Multilayer tip grafting technique. An illustration of basal view and intraoperative view (*A*) and profile views (*B*).

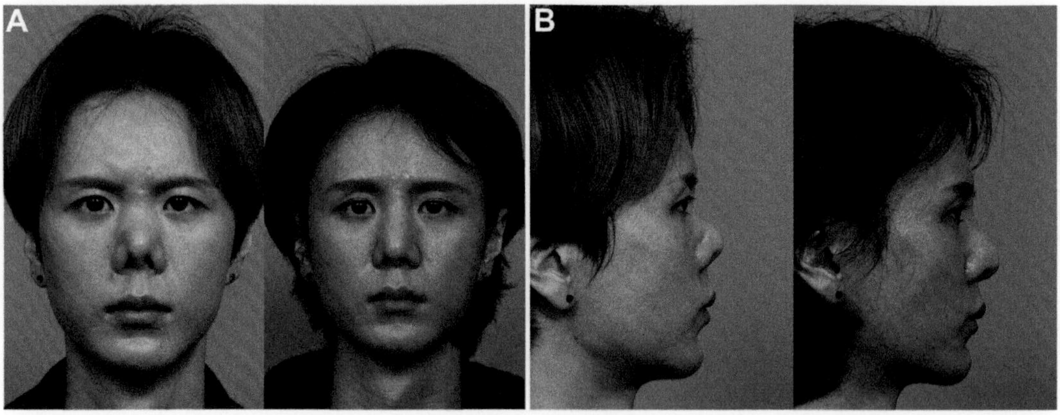

Fig. 17. A patient with a short nose deformity who was treated with a combination of extended spreader grafts and caudal septal extension graft, followed by dorsal augmentation using glued diced costal cartilage. Preoperative (*left*) and postoperative (*right*) views of frontal (*A*) and lateral photograph (*B*).

framework is reconstructed with costal cartilage after resecting the deformed skin and the adjacent normal skin of the lower third to perform the nasal subunit reconstruction. The resected skin can be used as a hinge flap for inner lining. If the use of skin flap is not sufficient for the inner lining, a septal mucosal flap or an ear cartilage composite graft can also be used. Then, a forehead flap designed to fill the skin defect is applied and rotated to the skin defect. The nasal skin of the deformed nose due to alloplastic implant-related complications usually has injured vasculature; thus, it is recommendable to perform a pedicle division of the forehead flap after waiting a little longer (4–6 weeks) than in the case of cancer reconstruction.

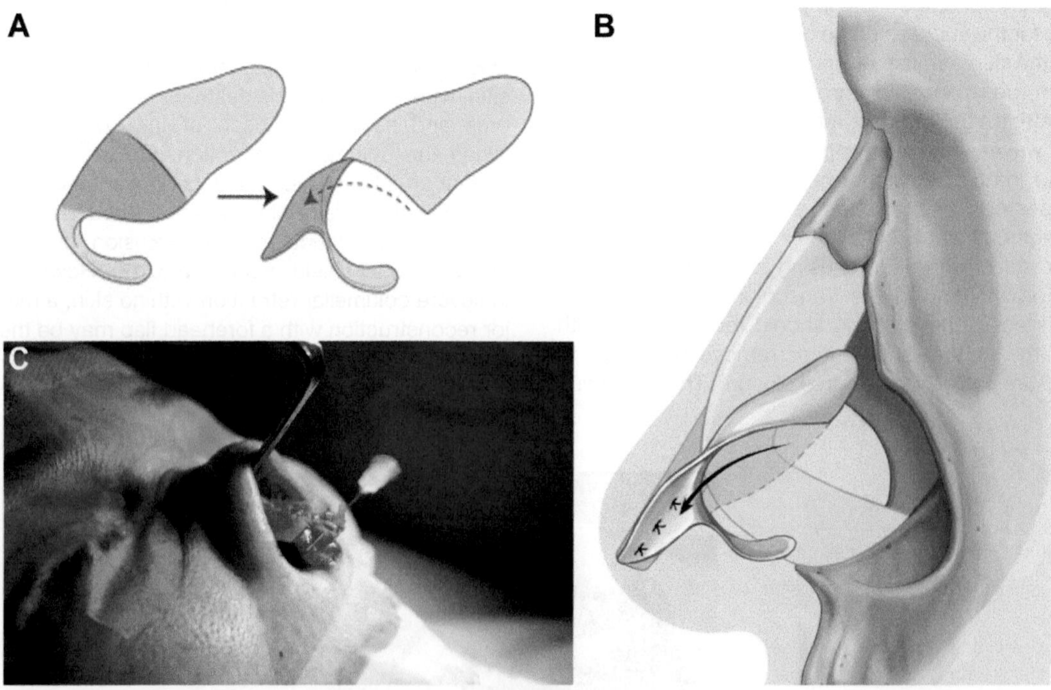

Fig. 18. Illustrations (*A, B*) and an intraoperative view (*C*) of cartilage flap technique in which both sides of a medially based cartilage flap are developed by incising and dissecting off the lateral crust of the lower lateral cartilage from the underlying vestibular skin and rotated medially to cover the extended spreader graft.

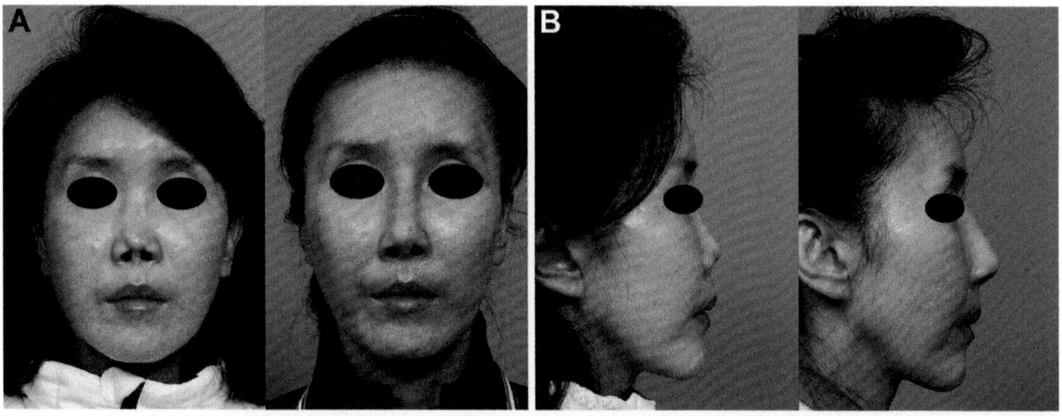

Fig. 19. A patient with a retracted columella treated with caudal septal extension grafting and shield grafting. Concave nasal dorsum was augmented with glued diced costal cartilage covered with fascia. Preoperative (*left*) and postoperative (*right*) views of frontal (*A*) and lateral photograph (*B*).

SUMMARY

The key concept in Asian rhinoplasty is augmentation in all different forms of nasal deformities. Augmentation of the nose consists of framework, tip, and dorsal augmentation. Septal extension grafting and tip grafting are 2 maneuvers with profound importance in augmentation of lower two-thirds of the Asian nose. Dorsal augmentation is a central concept in beautifying all different types of deformed noses, even the hump nose. Among various implant and graft materials, costal cartilage is most preferred due to its versatility and adequate amount.

CLINICS CARE POINTS

- To avoid problems in dorsal augmentation inherent to the solid carved costal cartilage, augmentation with finely diced cartilage in the forms of fascia-wrapped implant, glued graft, and free diced cartilage is becoming increasingly popular. For the correction of the broad nasal dorsum, a significant tip projection using septal extension graft with or without tip grafting should be done, and subsequent dorsal augmentation is needed to create a well-balanced brow-tip aesthetic line.
- Because many Asians lack appropriate tip projection, in order to create a well-balanced profile line, the desired height of the tip should be set first during the correction of the convex dorsum, followed by the determination of the degree of hump reduction and augmentation of the radix and supratip.
- The combination of the bilateral extended spreader grafts and one caudal extension graft sandwiched between them, positioned end-to-end with the native caudal septum, is the most reliable and versatile technique for straightening and reinforcing the deformed septal cartilage framework.

REFERENCES

1. Jang YJ, Yoo SH. Dorsal augmentation in facial profiloplasty. Facial Plast Surg 2019;35(5):492–8.
2. Jang YJ, Alfanta EM. Rhinoplasty in the Asian nose. Facial Plast Surg Clin North Am 2014;22(3):357–77.
3. Kim JS, Khan NA, Song HM, et al. Intraoperative measurements of harvestable septal cartilage in rhinoplasty. Ann Plast Surg 2010 Dec;65(6):519–23.
4. Na HG, Jang YJ. Use of nasal implants and dorsal modification when treating the East Asian Nose. Otolaryngol Clin North Am 2020 Apr;53(2):255–66.
5. Chen YY, Jang YJ. Refinements in saddle nose reconstruction. Facial Plast Surg 2018;34(4):363–72.
6. Jang YJ, Kim SH. Tip grafting for the Asian Nose. Facial Plast Surg Clin North Am 2018;26(3):343–56.
7. Jang YJ. Dorsal augmentation using costal cartilage: what is the best way? Clin Exp Otorhinolaryngol 2019;12(4):327–8.
8. Yoo SH, Jang YJ. Rib cartilage in Asian rhinoplasty: new trends. Curr Opin Otolaryngol Head Neck Surg 2019;27(4):261–6.
9. Tasman AJ, Diener PA, Litschel R. The diced cartilage glue graft for nasal augmentation. Morphometric evidence of longevity. JAMA Facial Plast Surg 2013;15(2):86–94.

10. Na HG, Jang YJ. Dorsal augmentation using alloplastic implants. Facial Plast Surg 2017;33(2):189–94.
11. Cho GS, Jang YJ. Deviated nose correction: different outcomes according to the deviation type. Laryngoscope 2013;123(5):1136–42.
12. Jang YJ, Kim JH. Classification of convex nasal dorsum deformities in Asian patients and treatment outcomes. J Plast Reconstr Aesthet Surg 2011;64(3):301–6.
13. Jang YJ, Moon H. Special consideration in the management of hump noses in Asians. Facial Plast Surg 2020;36(5):554–62.
14. Hyun SM, Jang YJ. Treatment outcomes of saddle nose correction. JAMA Facial Plast Surg 2013;15(4):280–6.
15. Kim DY, Nam SH, Alharethy SE, et al. Surgical outcomes of bony batten grafting to correct caudal septal deviation in septoplasty. JAMA Facial Plast Surg 2017;19(6):470–5.
16. Kim JH, Jang YJ. Use of diced conchal cartilage with perichondrial attachment in rhinoplasty. Plast Reconstr Surg 2015;135(6):1545–53.
17. Lee HJ, Jang YJ. Correction of saddle and short noses. Curr Opin Otolaryngol Head Neck Surg 2016;24(4):294–9.
18. Jang YJ, Min JY, Lau BC. A Multilayer cartilaginous tip-grafting technique for improved nasal tip refinement in Asian Rhinoplasty. Otolaryngol Head Neck Surg 2011;145(2):217–22.
19. Jang YJ, Kim SA, Alharethy S. Failure of synthetic implants: strategies and management. Facial Plast Surg 2018;34(3):245–54.
20. Lan MY, Jang YJ. Revision rhinoplasty for short noses in the Asian population. JAMA Facial Plast Surg 2015;17(5):325–32.

UNITED STATES POSTAL SERVICE®

Statement of Ownership, Management, and Circulation (All Periodicals Publications Except Requester Publications)

1. Publication Title	2. Publication Number	3. Filing Date
FACIAL PLASTIC SUREGERY CLINICS OF NORTH AMERICA	013 – 122	9/18/2021
4. Issue Frequency	5. Number of Issues Published Annually	6. Annual Subscription Price
FEB, MAY, AUG, NOV	4	$412.00

7. Complete Mailing Address of Known Office of Publication (*Not printer*) (*Street, city, county, state, and ZIP+4®*)
ELSEVIER INC.
230 Park Avenue, Suite 800
New York, NY 10169

Contact Person
Malathi Samayan
Telephone (*Include area code*)
91-44-4299-4507

8. Complete Mailing Address of Headquarters or General Business Office of Publisher (*Not printer*)
ELSEVIER INC.
230 Park Avenue, Suite 800
New York, NY 10169

9. Full Names and Complete Mailing Addresses of Publisher, Editor, and Managing Editor (*Do not leave blank*)

Publisher (*Name and complete mailing address*)
DOLORES MELONI, ELSEVIER INC.
1600 JOHN F KENNEDY BLVD. SUITE 1800
PHILADELPHIA, PA 19103-2899

Editor (*Name and complete mailing address*)
Stacy Eastman ELSEVIER INC.
1600 JOHN F KENNEDY BLVD. SUITE 1800
PHILADELPHIA, PA 19103-2899

Managing Editor (*Name and complete mailing address*)
PATRICK MANLEY, ELSEVIER INC.
1600 JOHN F KENNEDY BLVD. SUITE 1800
PHILADELPHIA, PA 19103-2899

10. Owner (*Do not leave blank. If the publication is owned by a corporation, give the name and address of the corporation immediately followed by the names and addresses of all stockholders owning or holding 1 percent or more of the total amount of stock. If not owned by a corporation, give the names and addresses of the individual owners. If owned by a partnership or other unincorporated firm, give its name and address as well as those of each individual owner. If the publication is published by a nonprofit organization, give its name and address.*)

Full Name	Complete Mailing Address
WHOLLY OWNED SUBSIDIARY OF REED/ELSEVIER, US HOLDINGS	1600 JOHN F KENNEDY BLVD. SUITE 1800 PHILADELPHIA, PA 19103-2899

11. Known Bondholders, Mortgagees, and Other Security Holders Owning or Holding 1 Percent or More of Total Amount of Bonds, Mortgages, or Other Securities. If none, check box → ☐ None

Full Name	Complete Mailing Address
N/A	

12. Tax Status (*For completion by nonprofit organizations authorized to mail at nonprofit rates*) (*Check one*)
The purpose, function, and nonprofit status of this organization and the exempt status for federal income tax purposes:
☒ Has Not Changed During Preceding 12 Months
☐ Has Changed During Preceding 12 Months (*Publisher must submit explanation of change with this statement*)

13. Publication Title: FACIAL PLASTIC SUREGERY CLINICS OF NORTH AMERICA

14. Issue Date for Circulation Data Below: AUGUST 2021

15. Extent and Nature of Circulation		Average No. Copies Each Issue During Preceding 12 Months	No. Copies of Single Issue Published Nearest to Filing Date
a. Total Number of Copies (*Net press run*)		195	180
b. Paid Circulation (*By Mail and Outside the Mail*)	(1) Mailed Outside-County Paid Subscriptions Stated on PS Form 3541 (Include paid distribution above nominal rate, advertiser's proof copies, and exchange copies)	126	116
	(2) Mailed In-County Paid Subscriptions Stated on PS Form 3541 (*Include paid distribution above nominal rate, advertiser's proof copies, and exchange copies*)	0	0
	(3) Paid Distribution Outside the Mails Including Sales Through Dealers and Carriers, Street Vendors, Counter Sales, and Other Paid Distribution Outside USPS®	20	16
	(4) Paid Distribution by Other Classes of Mail Through the USPS (e.g., First-Class Mail®)	0	0
c. Total Paid Distribution [*Sum of 15b (1), (2), (3), and (4)*]	▶	146	132
d. Free or Nominal Rate Distribution (*By Mail and Outside the Mail*)	(1) Free or Nominal Rate Outside-County Copies included on PS Form 3541	33	31
	(2) Free or Nominal Rate In-County Copies Included on PS Form 3541	0	0
	(3) Free or Nominal Rate Copies Mailed at Other Classes Through the USPS (e.g., First-Class Mail)	0	0
	(4) Free or Nominal Rate Distribution Outside the Mail (*Carriers or other means*)	0	0
e. Total Free or Nominal Rate Distribution (*Sum of 15d (1), (2), (3) and (4)*)		33	31
f. Total Distribution (*Sum of 15c and 15e*)	▶	179	163
g. Copies not Distributed (*See Instructions to Publishers #4 (page #3)*)	▶	16	17
h. Total (*Sum of 15f and g*)		195	180
i. Percent Paid (*15c divided by 15f times 100*)	▶	81.56%	80.98%

* If you are claiming electronic copies, go to line 16 on page 3. If you are not claiming electronic copies, skip to line 17 on page 3.

16. Electronic Copy Circulation		Average No. Copies Each Issue During Preceding 12 Months	No. Copies of Single Issue Published Nearest to Filing Date
a. Paid Electronic Copies	▶		
b. Total Paid Print Copies (Line 15c) + Paid Electronic Copies (Line 16a)	▶		
c. Total Print Distribution (Line 15f) + Paid Electronic Copies (Line 16a)	▶		
d. Percent Paid (Both Print & Electronic Copies) (16b divided by 16c × 100)	▶		

☒ **I certify that 50% of all my distributed copies (electronic and print) are paid above a nominal price.**

17. Publication of Statement of Ownership
☒ If the publication is a general publication, publication of this statement is required. Will be printed in the NOVEMBER 2021 issue of this publication. ☐ Publication not required.

18. Signature and Title of Editor, Publisher, Business Manager, or Owner
Malathi Samayan - Distribution Controller *Malathi Samayan* Date 9/18/2021

I certify that all information furnished on this form is true and complete. I understand that anyone who furnishes false or misleading information on this form or who omits material or information requested on the form may be subject to criminal sanctions (including fines and imprisonment) and/or civil sanctions (including civil penalties).

Printed and bound by CPI Group (UK) Ltd, Croydon, CR0 4YY
08/05/2025
01864697-0017